Trouble in Mind

# Trouble in Mind

*An Unorthodox Introduction to Psychiatry*

## Dean F. MacKinnon, M.D.

Associate Professor
Department of Psychiatry and Behavioral Sciences
Johns Hopkins University School of Medicine
Baltimore, Maryland

The Johns Hopkins University Press

*Baltimore*

© 2011 The Johns Hopkins University Press

All rights reserved. Published 2011

Printed in the United States of America on acid-free paper

9  8  7  6  5  4  3  2  1

The Johns Hopkins University Press

2715 North Charles Street

Baltimore, Maryland 21218-4363

www.press.jhu.edu

Library of Congress Cataloging-in-Publication Data

MacKinnon, Dean F.

Trouble in mind : an unorthodox introduction to psychiatry / Dean F.
MacKinnon.

    p. ; cm.

Other title: Unorthodox introduction to psychiatry

Includes bibliographical references and index.

ISBN-13: 978-0-8018-9806-8 (hardcover : alk. paper)

ISBN-10: 0-8018-9806-4 (hardcover : alk. paper)

ISBN-13: 978-0-8018-9807-5 (pbk. : alk. paper)

ISBN-10: 0-8018-9807-2 (pbk. : alk. paper)

1. Psychiatry. 2. Mental illness. I. Title. II. Title: Unorthodox introduction to
psychiatry.

[DNLM: 1. Mental Disorders. 2. Brain—physiopathology. 3. Mental
Processes—physiology. 4. Psychiatry—methods. WM 140 M158t 2011]

RC454.M24 2011

616.89—dc22        2010013272

A catalog record for this book is available from the British Library.

*Special discounts are available for bulk purchases of this book.*
*For more information, please contact Special Sales at 410-516-6936 or*
*specialsales@press.jhu.edu.*

The Johns Hopkins University Press uses environmentally friendly book
materials, including recycled text paper that is composed of at least 30
percent post-consumer waste, whenever possible. All of our book papers are
acid-free, and our jackets and covers are printed on paper with recycled
content.

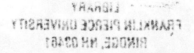

*To Linda Ryan, assistant extraordinaire*

Mind, n. A mysterious form of matter secreted by the brain. Its chief activity consists in the endeavor to ascertain its own nature, the futility of the attempt being due to the fact that it has nothing but itself to know itself with.

—AMBROSE BIERCE, *The Devil's Dictionary* (1911)

The human brain is the most public organ on the face of the earth, open to everything, sending out messages to everything. To be sure, it is hidden away in bone and conducts internal affairs in secrecy, but virtually all the business is the direct result of thinking that has already occurred in other minds.

—LEWIS THOMAS, *The Lives of a Cell* (1974)

# Contents

# Preface

Pundits periodically pitch spitballs at my profession. Psychiatry, they say, rates somewhere between hocus pocus and a threat to Western civilization. Mental illness is a social construct, psychotherapy is a scam, pharmaceuticals only dull the pain, involuntary hospitalization and electroconvulsive therapy —barbaric! If these critics could spend a month on the wards with me and see how treatment restores life to suffering patients and brings relief to their families, perhaps they would shed their ignorance. Or, perhaps not: over-valued ideas can be extremely stubborn.

One theme of psychiatric criticism I find harder to dismiss. When critics expose the logical foundation of modern psychiatry and find it to be a rickety edifice, constructed by committees with conflicting agendas, ungrounded in the firmament of psychology and neurobiology, I think they have a point. Psychiatrists are, literally, physicians for the mind, but psychiatry has no coherent concept of the mind. Although we help people regardless, we are often called on to explain the nature of mental illness to a patient or family or a student or a non-psychiatric colleague or the general public. We have little to offer but a lot of hand-waving about the biopsychosocial model, allusions to notoriously unreliable scientific findings, and vague metaphors about computers and "chemical imbalances."

Other fields of medicine have not only a firmer logical foundation, but also better metaphors that truly and simply capture the function of the organ: the heart acts as a pump, the kidney as a filter, the lungs as a sort of bellows, nerves as an electrical system, and so on. Beyond those simple images, one can readily explain that the pump distributes oxygenated blood to tissue, the filter maintains fluid balance, the bellows brings fresh oxygen to the blood, the nervous system activates muscles and transduces environmental stimuli. The popular idea that our heads house a computer processor—the brain is the hardware, the mind is the software—conveys accurately that brains and computers process information, but explains nothing about why it is necessary to process information. A computer is absolutely indifferent to the information it processes, or whether it processes information at all. What is the adaptive function of information for a person? What are the consequences of a failure to grasp, construct, retain, use, refine, revise, weigh, or interpret information? These consequences, and the symptoms, deficits, behaviors, and harms they produce, are the domain of psychiatry.

Psychiatry has no deficit in factual knowledge. One can find a thick textbook to suit every need and budget. The gap on the psychiatric bookshelf can be found between these encyclopedic monoliths and textbooks on neuroscience and psychology that provide access to the basic sciences behind psychiatry, without addressing the conceptual weakness at the heart of psychiatric knowledge. This book will help you to think more critically about a patient's problem, to offer reasoned judgment and more effective help, and perhaps to find the gems amidst the jetsam in the psychiatric literature.

I offer in this book an unorthodox view of mental life and mental illness. I portray mind as a function of the brain and place psychiatric problems into a working system. Although unorthodox with respect to the field of modern psychiatry, the general approach resembles that of a traditional introductory psychology text that begins with elementary processes that orient and move us in the world, and works up to the synthetic processes that define who we are as human beings.

Psychiatry is a practical art, and it owes its therapeutic power not to a sound basis in biology or psychological theory, but to serendipitous discovery, the creative application of empathy, a working knowledge of the forces that motivate behavior, and a rigorously empirical approach to clinical research. Most textbooks of psychiatry usefully compile knowledge across the biopsychosocial spectrum, about recent discoveries, modes of empathic healing, behavioral science, and clinical research. To define mental illness, they use the official manual of psychiatric diagnosis, the *Diagnostic and Statistical Manual of Mental Disorders* (DSM) (American Psychiatric Association 1994). They provide handy tables that list the rules, or DSM diagnostic criteria, that define each disorder. They present data from research that employ these definitions of psychiatric disorder. In this way, they teach about psychiatric disorders and their treatment. They do not, however, integrate knowledge into a systematic model of mind.

The orthodox approach to psychiatry neglects the nature of mind and mental illness. This is unusual in medicine; most fields place a strong emphasis on the natural function of bodily organs in health and disease. Other fields of medicine define a disease by its pathological cause or by the biological process it disrupts. Not psychiatry. Psychiatry explicitly avoids theoretical definitions of disorder. The definitions of disorders in the DSM include mainly the surface phenomena of mental illness—symptoms, behaviors, and measures of performance—that by consensus agreement characterize a diagnostic entity (Jensen and Hoagwood 1997).

The DSM has been and remains a useful resource for clinicians, scientists, and administrators, but nature did not define the DSM's official diagnostic criteria; committees negotiated them (Widiger and Clark 2000). The DSM definitions of mental illness capture the typical patterns but falter when a case is atypical or complicated. Intellectual dependence on DSM diagnostic definitions leaves psychiatrists flummoxed by uncertainty. Complex cases are said to have "comorbidities," which begs the question whether the presence of more than one diagnosis in the same person at the same time implies they are part of the same disorder (Wittchen 1996). Atypical cases typically receive a "not otherwise specified" (NOS) diagnosis. Although the NOS designation may be the diagnosis most faithful to the information one has, one sacrifices the power of empirical clinical research when one uses it. There are no data at all to inform us about the cause, prognosis, and effective treatment for a NOS diagnosis. What should one do for a patient who has an amorphous diagnosis? How does one develop an organized approach to the treatment of two or three or five comorbid psychiatric disorders?

In most fields of medicine, uncertainty about a patient's illness presents a puzzle to be solved. Puzzles generally require a logical approach and work best if the parts fit together precisely. To solve medical puzzles, clinicians typically apply the logic of biochemistry, genetics, physiology, pathogenesis; also microbiology, if an infection is involved. Thus an acute failure of kidney function might be traced to an excess of myoglobin in the bloodstream, which is evidence of damage to muscle tissue, which in turn might be the first clue that the patient has a rare genetic deficiency in a mitochondrial enzyme that causes breakdown of muscle cells under conditions of metabolic stress. Connecting the dots in this way does not resolve the renal failure, nor does it permit us to remove the genetic cause of the problem, but it does provide an explanation to counter fearful uncertainty, and a basis to give the patient sound advice on how to avoid such problems in the future. Clinical reasoning of this sort shows the beginner where to start to understand an individual patient, and the expert how to think through a challenging case. When a clinician can form a hypothesis about a disease by logical deduction and prove it by a definitive test, the model of disease as puzzle is most apt.

A person who has a mental illness presents the clinician not so much with a puzzle to be solved as with a text to be read and understood. Many texts, like many people, do not yield their meaning to a direct, logical approach, of the sort that allowed us to trace diminished, micturition to muscle breakdown to mitochondria. Text almost always hosts ambiguities to be untangled by the reader, and similarly a person's actions and statements about his or her thoughts, feelings, and intentions require interpretation. When the clinician does achieve sufficient understanding to diagnose and treat a patient, the ambiguity often remains. Diagnostic hypotheses in psychiatry are rarely subject to proof or disproof. Treatment manages, but rarely provides a definitive cure for a mental illness.

The lack of a sound theoretical basis for psychiatry becomes embarrassingly obvious when a clinician tries to explain mental illness to a patient or a patient's family. To invoke an empty idea, like the widespread notion that some mental illness is the result of a "chemical imbalance," is to apply the sort of circular explanation used since ancient times ("your melancholia is the result of an excess of black bile") and properly abandoned by modern medicine. Thus, the atheoretical approach to psychiatry that has become the de facto foundation of all orthodox psychiatric knowledge, has had unintended, corrosive consequences for psychiatric education (Andreasen 2007), for clinical research (van Praag 1997), and indeed for psychiatry's integrity as a medical discipline (Galatzer-Levy and Galatzer-Levy 2007).

Why has theory been left out of modern psychiatry? Theories at one time defined psychiatry. During the era of psychoanalytic dominance in about the middle third of the twentieth century, the unique features of a patient's inner life formed the heart of professional interest and were not an excuse merely to apply a noncommittal, "not otherwise specified" diagnosis. Psychoanalytic theories explain mental suffering in terms of the interplay between unseen and immeasurable entities like the ego, id, and superego (Freud 1949; Rieff 1979). They possess an appealing logic, can be rich in imagery and metaphor, and can lead troubled people out of deep distress. However, psychoanalytic theory is of limited benefit to patients who have serious mental illnesses involving psychosis, mood swings, or addictions or who otherwise lack the ability to engage in a cooperative endeavor like a therapeutic relationship (Malmberg and Fenton, 2001). For better or worse, the psychoanalytic approach has largely been supplanted by the pragmatism of biological psychiatry (Shorter 1996), with its arsenal of effective psychopharmaceuticals, and behavioral psychology, which aims to recondition patients toward healthy living.

As an approach to severe mental illness, purely psychodynamic theories have a fundamental flaw. Such theories tend to exist outside of natural law, in a model of mind not closely related to any recognizable activity of the brain (Kandel 1998). Casting aside abstract theories, psychiatry for nearly the past half-century has held to the faith that the methods of biological science will ultimately reveal the workings of the brain as they have revealed the workings of the heart, lungs, liver, kidneys, and immune system. When one hears that research has associated a disorder with a particular genotype, or an atypical anatomic pattern of metabolic activity, or high or low levels of a neurotransmitter—without having any idea how to link these findings to the clinical expressions of mental illness—one learns potentially significant facts, but not how to apply them to understand the nature of mental illness. Although the technology of discovery has produced an immense body of knowledge, biomedical sciences have not yet achieved for psychiatry what has been achieved in other fields: a mechanism to explain illness (Insel and Quirion 2005).

It is conceivable that the theoretical gap between brain processes and mental illness might forever exceed the reach of technological advances. When concepts of mental illness lag behind the technology employed to study them, progress hinges not on data acquisition, but on the development of a better idea of how to make sense of existing data (Kendler 2005).

In this book, I have approached mental illness with a model of mental life that employs a broad view of biology. At the level of the individual cell or organ, or organisms in general, biological explanations tend to be mechanistic. At the level of the individual, in his or her environment, as a member of a social group and species, mechanistic explanations prove less useful than narrative explanations. A plausible narrative explanation respects the known laws of nature while providing some freedom to speculate. Its truth is measured by the useful ideas it generates, rather than by its resilience against efforts to disprove it in detail.

Stories have value, even for scientifically reverent clinicians, when they help one to see meaningful connections between phenomena and to communicate to others the significance of the phenomena one can measure and observe (Richards 1992). How might one blend mechanistic and narrative modes of knowledge into a plausible explanation that sheds light on the nature of mental phenomena? A plausible description of how the brain organizes light sensation into visual perception, for example, will sketch the basic, well-established principles of connectivity between retina, thalamus, and cortex, while bypassing cutting-edge, finely detailed ideas about the functional organization of sensory neurons that distract from the narrative aim of understanding mental, not neuronal phenomena. The end result is a potentially useful concept about the nature of information—an abstract concept, irreducible to mechanistic explanation, but vital if one is to see the brain as an organ with a functional role.

A narrative can be valued by the degree to which it captures the salient facts and organizes them to reveal meaningful connections between them. Narratives risk veering into fantasy and dogma, but if the focus remains on its ultimate purpose—to understand mental illness within the context of the organic functions of the brain—a plausible narrative may be not only a useful way, but also the only way at present to make sense of this fascinating and confusing discipline. Darwin's theory of evolution is a powerful narrative by this definition, in that it reveals in general how all organisms may be related. At the time Darwin developed his theory (Darwin 1859), science was still a century short of uncovering its molecular mechanisms (Watson and Crick 1953). It may be a century or more before we can develop elegant scientific concepts adequate to explain mental phenomena the way molecular genetics explains evolution. But we cannot wait that long. Patients need a coherent psychiatry now.

For the student or trainee, this book should serve as a supplement to and not a substitute for a standard textbook of psychiatry to consult as a practical clinical reference and study guide for exams. To learn to see the mind as an organic function, and the phenomena of mental illness in their functional contexts, should enhance the reader's comprehension of the knowledge to be found in a standard psychiatric textbook. Whether or not the reader takes care of patients who have mental illness, this book will demystify the field and thus give any future clinician, in whatever specialty, more confidence when dealing with a mentally ill patient.

Any biologically savvy reader who is curious about how the mind goes about its business, how it goes wrong, and what can be done about it may gain a clearer sense of the power and limits of our knowledge. Clinical trainees who have moved beyond the introductory phases may find this book to be a link between clinical experience and the published knowledge base. Colleagues may appreciate the effort here to weave a coherent but simplified explanatory model.

In brief, the model I present in this book integrates the elements of perception and recognition of objects, appetite and arousal, motion and its regulation, into the substrate of mental phenomena. Mental phenomena such as attention, memory, learning, and the emotional/motivational forces of reward and defense all have biological functions salient to survival and propagation. These same mental phenomena, tasked with coping with both the world and the internal reflections of past and anticipated experience, construct mental models of reality to accomplish functions more abstract and complicated, involving choice, belief, planning, and relationships with other people.

To link the theoretical ideas about mental illness in the main text to the standard psychiatric references, they are cross-referenced to appendix A, which describes the major psychiatric diagnoses as defined in the DSM. But the study of mental illness is incomplete unless the knowledge is tested with real patients. To that end, I have added appendix B as a brief guide to psychiatric assessment, so the student-clinician may approach a patient prepared to ask the right questions at the right times and glean greater understanding from the patient's responses.

Finally, I have added a glossary as a handy reference to some of the technical terminology in general use in psychiatry, psychology, and neuroscience, as well as for other familiar terms used with a specific technical connotation in this book, and a few unfamiliar terms I have used in hopes of emphasizing the estrangement of my model from the DSM. Thus, to refer to symptoms (as opposed to DSM syndromes) I have replaced terms like *depression* and *anxiety* that have such broad meanings that they essentially have no meaning, with terms that I believe more precisely refer to a symptom, such as *dejection* and *dread*. I have also used some rare, or coined words like *hyperfluency* to refer to pressured speech, and *avulsion* to refer to thought withdrawal, again because I believe they have connotations more consistent with my model of psychopathology, and also because I want to inject some freshness into a sometimes stale psychiatric vocabulary.

# Acknowledgments

So many fellow faculty members will recognize their ideas in these pages that a collective thank you is in order, especially to those who have taught the Johns Hopkins medical students with me, and me with the medical students. Any authority I can bring to these ideas I owe to my patients, and to the teammates, students, residents, colleagues, and mentors who have worked with me to help them.

A book like this is in some ways the culmination of a lifelong journey. Among my earliest guides to the life of the mind were Judy Kreiling and Bob Markwood, who taught me that science and creative writing go together very well. Alan Kors and Philip Rieff at Penn taught me to think critically about the mind and what it can do; Larry Squire at UCSD taught me how to go from just thinking about the mind to exploring it. Here in Baltimore, George Gallahorn and Phillip Slavney in their distinctive ways steered me to a safe harbor from which I could take such excursions. Peter Rabins and Ray DePaulo at Hopkins both provided essential moral support for this project. For their constructive criticism of the manuscript in its various drafts, I thank Eric and Roberta Anderson, Jay Baraban, Tony Carlino, Ray DePaulo, David Edwin, Paul McHugh, Barbara Schweizer, Beth Winter, and the editors and reviewers at the Johns Hopkins University Press. Although the writing is entirely my own, Drs. McHugh and Slavney, through their dogmatically anti-dogmatic approach to psychiatry, must be acknowledged as silent co-authors, anywhere my discussion of the four types of mental problem—disease, vulnerability, behavior, and adversity—echoes their four perspectives of psychiatry.

Finally, words cannot begin to express my gratitude to my wife, Catherine Washburn, and our sons, Ian, Jared, and Peter (and quasi-sons Jack and Masayuki as well), for their patience with me while I spent many an evening and weekend tinkering with the text.

Trouble in Mind

# CHAPTER ONE

# Organic Mind

Many people confuse psychology and psychiatry. The two have surprisingly little to do with each other. Psychology refers to the study of the mind, a field of inquiry encompassing a set of theories that inform research and clinical work. Psychiatry refers to a field of medicine. Psychiatrists care for people who have mental illness. Psychiatric research leans on other scientific disciplines, such as epidemiology, genetics, and neurobiology. Psychiatrists do, of course, employ principles of behavioral psychology, but no more than many other kinds of physicians. Psychological theories about the nature of perception, knowledge, attention, memory, motivation, attachment, and a variety of other mental phenomena tend to have limited, if any, place in the standard, modern psychiatric approach to mental illness.

For a variety of reasons, psychiatry can be and tends to be practiced without reliance on psychological concepts. Rule-based diagnostic practices make it possible to discern a patient's mental illness via a symptom checklist, and this in turn points to effective treatment options, vetted by randomized, double-blind, placebo-controlled clinical trials. Psychiatrists rarely have the time to delve into a patient's personal trials, in part because insurance tends to cover only brief visits to assess symptoms and renew prescriptions. Medical students who go into psychiatry often have relatively little education in psychology, compared to their education in biochemistry, anatomy, genetics, and physiology. The growing scientific power to probe the genome, and to observe the brain in action, seems to support the promise that neurobiology, not psychology, represents the future foundation of psychiatry. All of these factors render psychology seemingly inessential in the treatment of mental disorder.

But this professional neglect of psychology perpetuates a fundamental error. To neglect the study of the mind is to neglect the theoretical foundation of psychiatry's core mission: the treatment of mental illness.

One might object: perhaps the problem for modern psychiatry is not the neglect of psychology, but the relative immaturity of neurobiology. In time, psychiatry will have a thoroughly neurobiological basis. Research has begun to reveal the neurobiology of the major mental illnesses like schizophrenia, bipolar disorder, obsessive-compulsive disorder, and dementia, and also has begun to gain traction in knowing the anatomical components of temperament, the cellular mechanisms of learning and behavior, and the molecular biology of the brain's response to stress and trauma. Naturally, the biological science behind psychiatry lags behind the development of biological science across the rest of medicine. The brain is difficult to study. It is less accessible to measurement by researchers, compared to other organs. It has no moving parts and emits little measurable substance to collect and analyze. Isn't it just a matter of time before we overcome these technical obstacles and develop a bioassay for the phenomena of mental life?

No more than it was just a matter of time before the early alchemists discovered a philosopher's stone to transmute lead into gold. Many philosophers have argued eloquently that mind cannot be reduced simply to a mere activity of the brain (Jackson 1986); albeit not everyone shares this belief in the irreducibility of mind (Churchland 1994).

A modern account of mind must respect neurobiology, but mind has qualities that cannot be reduced to neurobiology (Nagel 1974). Consider free will: the nearly universal sense that we think and act as independent agents, as opposed to being mere slaves of material or supernatural forces. Free will makes no sense neurobiologically. One may accept that the laws of nature govern the brain, along with everything that arises from it. If so, then the sum total of our physical being, hence our experience, must have been determined by the collected physical interactions of the atoms that comprise us. When a neurotransmitter activates a neuron that moves a muscle, this follows from a long chain of molecular and cellular events determined by physical and chemical forces. At what point do one's thoughts, feelings, or intentions acquire the power to impose a new force on the neurotransmitter molecules that will ultimately move our bodies to act? Or is our sense of control over our bodies merely an illusion, and mental life a side effect of physical forces over which we have no real control? Such arguments notwithstanding, even the most ardent believers in the physical basis of all reality think, act, and feel as if they were free to choose their attitudes and actions, including psychiatrists, who should know better (Miresco and Kirmayer 2006).

Our thoughts do not seem to obey the laws of physics, nor can logical algorithms represent our feelings and desires. An idea can seem to come from nowhere, a random event may seem ripe with meaning, and an inscrutable motive can override all biological imperatives to eat, to propagate, and even to survive. Most people assume that their thoughts, feelings, and intentions represent their own free will, as if these phenomena of mental life were somehow immune from the causal laws of nature. Those who feel less confident in the universality of the laws of nature think about mind as something more than brain, when they regard the mind as an aspect of an immaterial soul or spirit.

Whatever one thinks about free will, mind over matter, or spirit over flesh, one may still see mind as fundamentally irreducible to brain, for practical reasons. Mind lives within each of us, privately. Our brains are uniquely wired, and our experiences are unique as well. Yet, the individual mind has no meaning apart from other minds. The unique and personal, yet communal aspects of mental life imply that the methods of physical science can, at best, explain observations about mental life in general, not the meaning of an experience for an individual. The apt analogy, perhaps, is to a book. One could decompose this book into pulp, centrifuge and electrophorese the pulp into its molecular components (or, if this is an e-text, analyze it down to patterns of semicolon use and pixel density), compare these data to the results of the analysis of other books, and draw some conclusions about the makeup of books, but one would probably learn a lot more by just reading it.

So, while neurobiologists strive to reveal the molecular secrets of the mind, and the rest of us await their discoveries, we all behave as if the mind is more than mere brain activity. We prove this every time we search our souls, weigh our options, or follow our bliss. Our own psychological experiences should lead us to doubt that we can ever adequately understand the mind through purely mechanism-focused inquiry. How can one hope to understand *mental illness* without a firm grounding in the study of the *mind?*

Psychiatry without psychology is like medicine without physiology. Can one practice medicine without a physiologic theory about how organs function? Of course. In the vast majority of cases, a computer could render a diagnosis using only a symptom checklist, some physical measurements, a panel of laboratory studies, and an algorithm (Shortliffe et al. 1979). The art of medicine, and the need for physiologic reasoning, begins when the cases get harder to solve, when information is insufficient, or ambiguity leads to conflicting courses of action, or the patient fails to respond as predicted.

The art of *psychiatry*, and the need for *psychological* reasoning, begins when the cases get harder to solve, when information is insufficient, or ambiguity suggests conflicting courses of action, or the patient fails to respond as predicted. A psychiatrist applies psychological reasoning to predict whether a paranoid patient believes in her delusions strongly enough to act on them, or to know what to say to retain the trust of a manic patient whose exuberance has just soured into hostility, or to help a patient's spouse understand why someone who has crippling obsessions habitually drinks to oblivion, or to teach a patient why people like him find good news stressful. An overview of psychiatry filtered through psychological concepts should help sharpen the clinical wit of anyone who encounters people with mental illness.

Does this entail forcing a non-biological perspective into medicine? It depends how you define *biology*. Although psychology is not and may never be completely grounded in mechanistic neurobiology, psychological phenomena have real implications for survival. Mental phenomena are truly biological in the sense that they represent essential functions of the organism.

An expansive view of biology, ranging from cells to selves to human habitats, is needed in order to capture all of the phenomena relevant in psychiatric practice. Mental illness is not always a disease of the brain. It is true that brain pathology, known or inferred, accounts for much severe mental illness. But a person whose brain operates within normal parameters might be considered mentally ill if the person tends to have inappropriately exaggerated or muted responses to stress. A person who has a normal brain might in effect choose to behave in a mentally ill manner, by surrendering to urges to perform self-destructive acts. Or a person who has a normally functioning brain and responds appropriately and behaves adaptively in general may nonetheless experience painful mental illness under the burden of overwhelming adversity. All too often patients have complex mental illness: a malfunctioning brain, superimposed on a vulnerable disposition, leading to adverse experience that motivates self-destructive acts.

What does the mind do? What are the mental tasks a brain must perform in its capacity as a vital organ? Is mental experience merely an entertaining side effect of brain activity, or does it improve our chances to adapt, survive, and procreate?

This book aims to make the case that the mind is a vital organic function with its own properties that contribute in tangible ways to human adaptation. The major mental functions depend on known structures and mechanisms of the brain. Mind has a shape and structure. The domain of mental life begins with the sensory points of entry from the outer world and with molecular and cellular communication from the body that give rise to arousal and appetite. It ends at the point where it coordinates purposeful motion. These *elements* of mental life are interrelated and develop over time. The *integration* of these elements gives rise to the functions that define the systems of mental life: memory, executive function, and emotion. These functions, along with the simpler elements of mental life, comprise working memory, and thus are the substrates of our subjective experiences of thought, intention, and feeling.

The first two levels of the model of mind describe functions common to many higher mammals. The remaining functions are almost exclusively human. These *synthetic* extensions of mind construct an internal model of reality that permits us to act intelligently in the face of uncertainty. Because we rarely have all the facts, or have time to use the facts we have, we guide our behavior using beliefs and assumptions along with factual knowledge. Because we cannot always predict what other people might do, we employ behavior that elicits cooperation and thus narrows the range of likely possibilities. Synthetic phenomena are computationally the most complex within the mind, as they engage aspects of elementary and integral functions all at once in the construction of a subjective model of reality that helps us predict how a course of action now may bring satisfaction in the future.

Each component of mental life described throughout the book is illustrated by a description of some of its disruptions. The reader may note that these disruptions fall into the class of one or a combination of four general types, as laid out in Table 1.

*Table 1.*  Typology of Mental Disorders

| | Disease | Vulnerability (Dimensions) | Behavior | Adversity (Life Story) |
|---|---|---|---|---|
| What a patient . . . | HAS | IS | DOES | ENCOUNTERS |
| Core function | Cerebral faculties | Traits | Adaptive actions | Personal development |
| Logic | Categorical: rules | Quantitative: excess or deficit | Teleological: ends | Narrative: meaning |
| Model | Biomedical | Probability | Conditioning | Interpretative |
| Process | Etiology → Pathology → Syndrome | Potential → Provocation → Response | Antecedent → Behavior → Consequence | Setting → Sequence → Outcome |
| Treatment aim | Remedy | Guidance | Interruption | Rescripting |
| DSM diagnoses | Schizophrenia, bipolar disorder, Alzheimer disease | Personality disorders, intellectual disability | Alcohol abuse, anorexia nervosa, paraphilia | Grief, Adjustment disorders |

*Source:* Adapted from McHugh and Slavney, *The Perspectives of Psychiatry* (1998).

Disrupted biological processes cause much of mental illness. One may consider them *diseases* in the sense that they are imposed on people, and that the resulting symptoms tend to have a common form regardless of the attitude or culture of the patient. Hallucinations, obsessions and compulsions, memory loss, and derangements of arousal exemplify disease in this sense.

Innate *vulnerabilities*, or traits, set up some individuals for recurrent mental problems. For several critical aspects of mental life, a pattern of biologically normal but maladaptive responses to life and social challenges signifies a propensity to have problems rather than an active disease state. An innate overabundance of emotional volatility or paucity of intellectual capacity places one at long-term risk for distress and maladaptive behavior. Thus, low intelligence, biases toward inertia, avoidance, and impulsiveness are examples of attributes of mental life that contribute to psychiatric problems; anankastic and histrionic personalities are examples of the long-term entrenchment of temperamental traits.

Many disruptions can best be understood as expressions of *behavior*. The person who has a behavioral problem, in contrast to the person who has a disease or vulnerability, perpetuates the disruption through voluntary activity. In many cases, the impetus for the behavioral disruption may be a disease process or it may have its source in a person's vulnerabilities or life experiences; indeed, the pain that motivates maladaptive behavior in some people might drive almost anyone to want to drink, or visit a doctor with psychosomatic ailments, or contemplate putting an end to life. Nonetheless, the harmful consequences of behavior result from the behavior. If one could prevent or discourage the person from carrying out the behavior, the troublesome drive might remain, but the harmful effects would go away. Addictions, anorexia and bulimia, suicidality, psychosomatic complaints, and parasuicidal behavior all have complex causes, but the harms that result are a direct result of what the person does.

In combination with the other three causes of psychiatric problems, and sometimes in the absence of other biological disturbance, vulnerability, or maladaptive behavior, psychiatric problems may arise as a result of *adversity* a person encounters in life. Adversity that shakes up one's sense of meaningful purpose in life can lead to suffering and maladaptive behavior. Examples of mental problems attributable to adversity, or ineffective ways to cope with adversity, include demoralization, shame, dissolution, guilt, and denial.

In practice, of course, it is rare for a psychiatric patient to have only one kind of problem. Biological disruptions that produce one symptom often contribute to a host of symptoms. Personality vulnerabilities that ignite one maladaptive behavior often inflame several. The pursuit of psychiatric treatment for any and all problems often requires a major adjustment in a person's sense of purpose in the world, as the identity must shift to encompass the new role of psychiatric patient. To try to help the reader make sense of mental illness, this book starts with the biggest question of all: what is the purpose of mind?

## 1.1. Why Mind Matters

The brain produces mental function as somatic organs produce digestive, cardiac, renal, immunological, reproductive, and other bodily functions.

An organic function helps an individual survive and a species carry on. Digestive, cardiac, renal, immune, and reproductive functions have obvious utility. Even the simplest organisms have to take in and distribute metabolic necessities, excrete selected waste products, avoid or cope with adverse environments, and pass on their genes. The development of sophisticated organs to serve these functions permits the growth of more complex and better-adapted creatures that thus gain a reproductive advantage. What does the mind do? To begin to see the mind as the function of a vital bodily organ, consider the struggle for life in its elements.

In terms of Newtonian physics (to get down to basics), life is a struggle for order against entropy. Every organic function serves to create, maintain, defend, and propagate order against a universe that moves inexorably toward disorder. In life, raw carbon, oxygen, hydrogen, and other chemical elements form orderly proteins, carbohydrates, lipids, and nucleic acid chains. These complex chemicals organize into working cells, and cells into a working body.

Entropy destroys order; it represents death for the intricate workings of a living organism. Organs, tissues, cells, molecules dissolve into simple, digestible chemicals. Order comes at a price: to maintain order in a closed system the system must increase disorder elsewhere. An organism that consumes plants, animals, or microbes maintains order for itself because the organic sources of fuel, once consumed, digested, and metabolized, become far less organized. An organism may delay the ultimate victory of entropy by acquiring and using energy from the environment.

Order thus requires energy. Well-adapted organisms optimize the intake of energy relative to its expenditure. Organisms without brains do this by trial and error. For the simplest plants and microbes, being caught without resources in a hostile environment generally means death for the individual. These species compensate when they reproduce prodigiously and allow the environment to select their better-equipped variants.

However, even plants and microbes derive information from the environment, whether a plant that turns its leaves in the direction of solar photons, or a hungry paramecium that moves along a chemical gradient, propelled by the presence of nutrients. Complex organisms use photo- and chemoreceptors too, but they rely more on the ability to detect order—hence stored energy—among the objects in the environment. An orderly object in nature is potentially a source of energy for an organism. Thus to be able to sort the orderly potential sources of energy from the random, spent residua of entropy reduces error for an individual organism and hence aids survival. The brain helps the organism to detect orderly objects, to initiate and modulate efforts to acquire their stored energy, and to retain information about how to obtain resources in the future. Fewer trials and less error mean a better return on effort and longer, richer individual survival.

To take full advantage of a brain, an individual organism must defend itself from harm. A brain requires a huge investment of energy. The investment pays off only if the organism survives long enough to make use of the information and skills the brain has acquired. Thus, the brain also stays attuned to signs of disorder in the environment that speak of possible danger—an unexpected howl, lumbering shapes amid the underbrush, a rancid odor from a water source. Without the ability to mobilize the body to defend itself, a brain might not be worth the energy it costs to maintain it.

Brainy species that communicate and cooperate have additional advantages. Information about the successful experiences of one individual reduces wasted effort by other members of the group. Ants secrete pheromones and bees dance to inform colony members and hive mates where to find food sources. Information about threat preserves the species: termites generate vibrations to alert their nest mates to danger. Higher up the evolutionary ladder, cooperative arrangements and communication methods become more complex and individualized, and more flexible across different environments.

Humans use symbols as signals to others and also to know one another. We can condense our own internal experiences—perceptions, thoughts, feelings, intentions, memories, beliefs—into time- and energy-efficient signs and symbols. We can pass along to others not only information about sources of energy and danger, but also precise information about the qualities of the objects we have encountered.

The ability to communicate about internal states and the qualities of objects has contributed to the development of social cooperation. We can tell others what we need and learn what they need. Information about thoughts, feelings, and intentions also adds depth to information about the world. When we communicate our subjective reflections on the objective world we provide richer and more nuanced information, and reduce trial and error for others. Symbolic communication—language—has made it possible to transmit information over time and space, so that people we never even meet help us survive and prosper from the experiences they had long ago and far away.

A brain allows an organism to adapt its actions to its environment; it optimizes the search for energy and defends its adaptations. A brain that is equipped to communicate and cooperate with others optimizes resources and defense for others, and gains in return. A brain that can detect, retain, recall, and communicate efficiently about remote and internal events uses a special set of functions that occur abundantly only in humans, and partially in only a few other mammals: these are called mental functions, or mind. When we describe someone as "mentally ill" or "out of her or his mind" or behaving "mindlessly," we mean that the person's problem is abnormal or inappropriate or inadequate or painful or erroneous thoughts, feelings, and intentional actions.

As a philosophical aside, awareness of internal states—self-consciousness—appears to play an important role in human adaptation, but a self-conscious mind poses problems for evidence-based science. Self-consciousness defies clean measurement. One can never be certain that two people share the same thought, feeling, intention, or belief, even when they say the same thing, and score the same on a psychometric scale. But the lack of good measurement does not mean subjective states are inessential. One could, perhaps, try to engage with other people without reliance on qualitative, language-bound, messy subjective data, but it would involve a lot more trial and error.

In the account that follows, the emphasis will be on mind as an organic function—how, based on the basic rules of neurobiology, psychology, and the constraints of brain anatomy, can we account for reflection, learning, and decision making? How can the mind determine from its own internal activity whether to take action, and what actions to take, and assess whether the actions aid or hinder the ends of survival and propagation? What are the processes by which raw information is converted to purposeful motion? What motivates a person to disobey the commands of immediate bodily needs and desires? And how does dysfunction in these processes produce psychiatric problems?

## 1.2. A Brain Primer

### *The Five-Cent Tour*

The goal of this quick trip through the brain is to point out where and with what processes the brain produces the mind. Some details about deep structures and molecular machinations have been left out, as are many anatomic landmarks, in favor of a streamlined sketch. Thus, much of the following has been abstracted from other texts, listed in the Additional Reading section at the end of this book. Readers without interest in neurobiology may find this helpful but not essential to grasp the rest of the book; readers with in-depth knowledge of neurobiology may find it useful just to skim this section.

The brain is the center of the nervous systems of the body. *Sensory* nerves convey information about the environment to the brain and *motor* nerves translate signals from the brain into instructions for individual units of muscle to contract. The sensory and motor systems are thus organized centrally, in the brain.

In contrast, the *autonomic* nervous systems have an organizational structure distributed throughout the body. They are networks of nerves to and from vital organs, including blood vessels and endocrine glands. They carry general information from the periphery about physiologic states, and convey general impulses to stimulate or inhibit the actions of vital organs. Autonomic activity contributes to *interoception* (Saper 2002), that is, the perception of the body's internal status and *allostatic regulation* of the internal environment to match physiologic performance to present circumstances (McEwen 1998).

There are two functionally opposed autonomic nervous systems. States of alarm and excitement activate the *sympathetic* system. Using as its key signaling molecule *norepinephrine* (noradrenalin), sympathetic stimulation shunts blood and other metabolic resources to the muscles and inhibits energy-conserving (vegetative) functions like digestion, to prepare an endangered organism to fight or flee from immediate danger.

The *parasympathetic* system also connects to visceral organs, but has the opposite effect from its counterpart. It promotes blood flow to and smooth muscle activity in the visceral organs to enhance the extraction, storage, and conservation of metabolic energy. Sympathetic activation, for example, raises the heart rate and blood pressure, while parasympathetic activation slows the heart and lowers blood pressure. In the sexual response, the reflexive opposition of parasympathetic activity, which is associated with sexual arousal, to sympathetic activity, which produces orgasm, vividly demonstrates their dynamic integration. The vasovagal response, another illustration of sympathetic/parasympathetic opposition, occurs when a sudden loss of sympathetic tone results in unopposed parasympathetically mediated (via the vagus nerve) slowing of the heart and shunting of blood to visceral organs. Less blood flows to the brain, producing lightheadedness and fainting—the melodramatic swoon.

Parasympathetic neurotransmission is largely cholinergic, mediated by the neurotransmitter *acetylcholine*. Nicotine, incidentally, mimics the action of acetylcholine in some parts of the parasympathetic system, which may account in part for its putative calming effects, as well as for the ease with which one can become physically dependent on it.

As the focus turns to the brain, three main topographical domains emerge. The *brainstem* links the brain to the rest of the nervous system and body. The *midbrain* contains centers of coordination and communication among brain structures. The *cortex* covers the surface and is the virtual interface between the inside and outside worlds: information flows in, action flows out of the cortex. The Byzantine matrix of arcanely named nerve centers in the midbrain and brainstem may be referred to collectively as *subcortical structures*. Both autonomic systems interact with subcortical structures, and thus carry information to the brain about the status and activities of the visceral organs.

One can observe also a split down the middle of the brain, from front to back, into hemispheres that are linked together by a central highway of cross connections, the *corpus callosum*. The hemispheres have rough mirror symmetry anatomically and are asymmetric in some functions such as language, which is centered in the left hemisphere in most people. To fully understand the brain's interactions with the environment, it is necessary to know all about these asymmetries. However, this quick tour bypasses the asymmetry and laterality of functions, as they are not essential details to the model described here.

Hiking is a fine way to explore a terrain. If one were an insect, encountering a brain on display, one could land on the surface of the cortex and explore on foot. Figure 1 traces the path it might take. The insect explorer alights first

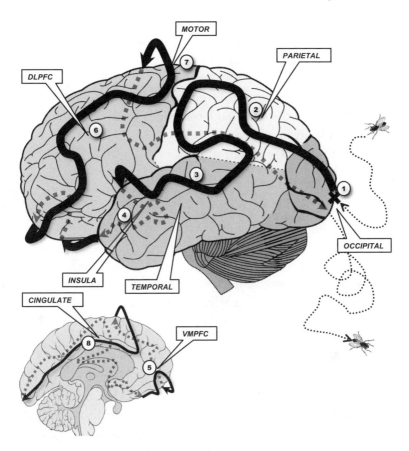

*Figure 1*. Path across the cortex, as described in the text. The arrows trace the wanderings of our insect explorer from the initial landing point on the (1) occipital cortex up to the (2) parietal, down and around to the (3) temporal, behind to the (4) insula, down and forward and in between the hemispheres to the (5) VMPFC, and then out, around, and up across the (6) DLPFC. Traversing the (7) motor cortex, our explorer slips again between the hemispheres to navigate the (8) cingulate cortex, emerging finally at the occipital lobe. *Lower image*: Patrick J. Lynch, medical illustrator; C. Carl Jaffe, M.D.

at the place where a visual image would first arrive at the cortex, in the aft, or *occipital* region. It ascends from there, across the wide expanse of the *parietal* cortex, where much of the processing of sensory input takes place. At the peak, it has reached the *central sulcus*, a fissure that divides the parietal lobe from the *frontal* lobe. If the skull were transparent, the central sulcus would appear to run roughly from ear to ear across the scalp. Turning back, heading downhill, around another bend, it encounters the shelf of cortex of the *temporal* lobe, which projects on the lower half of each side of the brain and coordinates auditory sensation, language, logic, multimodal perception, and memory. Advancing along the upper surface of the temporal cortex, the intrepid insect finds a gap, and crawls through it to find the *insula*, an island of cortex tucked behind the temporal lobes, which receives information about the state of bodily organs (Critchley et al. 2004).

One leaves the insula by advancing forward and down behind the temporal lobe, toward the bottom surface of the brain, and thus arrives at the *prefrontal cortex*, a vast region that stretches to the foremost tip of the brain, and continues around and up to cover almost the entire front half of the brain. The path traverses the *ventromedial prefrontal cortex* (VMPFC), where information about states of bodily arousal interacts with other highly processed sensory and motor functions (Groenewegen and Uylings 2000). The VMPFC is thus associated with motivation and emotional life (Price 1999). Note that the VMPFC encompasses another region one might read about, known as the *orbitofrontal* cortex because of its proximity to the eyes ("orbits," to the anatomists).

If the traveler scurries forward, out around the tip and back up the side, it crosses the *dorsolateral prefrontal cortex* (DLPFC). Embedded in this region of cortex are the encoded instructions one uses to scan the environment, plan, and undertake actions. The two regions of the prefrontal cortex together are commonly associated with *executive* functioning, which encompasses both the elements of motivation embedded in the VMPFC and the sequencing of perceptions and plans in the DLPFC (Davidson and Irwin 1999).

As the path continues along the outer edge of the DLPFC, heading back in the direction of the parietal lobe, it crosses *premotor* areas where simple actions are encoded, and arrives ultimately at the *motor strip*, from which the individual outputs that stimulate muscle fibers originate. This strip of cortex has an organization that corresponds roughly to the anatomic layout of the body: outputs that activate muscles within one limb are clustered together, as are those for the face, torso, and so on. Across the central sulcus that divides the frontal lobe from the parietal lobe, one would observe a similar map in the parietal lobe that reflects the individual components of sensation from the periphery of the body.

The circuit of the cortex is completed by venturing between the two halves of the frontal lobe, to explore the *cingulate* cortex. This strip runs along the midline on each hemisphere, parallel to the corpus callosum, and integrates sensory, motor, and internally generated signals (Paus 2001).

This circuitous trip across the surface of the brain, like a quick jaunt through the woods, has provided some landmarks but little understanding of the life beyond the surface. To learn more, one can pick a spot anywhere on the cortex and obtain a core sample, to find out about the connections to that cortical location. In reality, describing the connections within and beneath cortical regions would be an impossibly complex task unless one were to narrow the focus. The following discussion leaves out a great many connections essential to integrated mental activity, but less salient to a basic grasp of the logic of functional neuroanatomy.

Beneath the surface anywhere on the cortex one encounters cells that connect to and communicate with other cells, both near and far, to form a vast network. Most have either local connections within the cortex or project to distant areas of cortex; others project to and receive input from subcortical structures. One can infer from the connections within the cortex that the organization of cells with respect to one another within and across regions of the cortex is likely to be essential to its function, but this does not (yet) help one to understand the logic behind the functional organization of cortex (Fingelkurts et al. 2005). Although the effort to try to understand the relationship of structure and function in the brain occupies many great minds, one may perhaps gain a rough, workable idea from a few general observations about the routes of these connections within the cortex, and between cortex and subcortical structures. The first thing to notice, as one traces connections beneath a variety of areas of cortex, is that specific areas of cortex engage reciprocally with specific subcortical structures. The occipital, parietal, and parts of the temporal cortex all communicate extensively with the *thalamus*, a large cluster of clusters of nerve cells in the center of the brain. More precisely, different parts of the cortex connect with specific clusters, or *nuclei*, that comprise the thalamus (Jones 2001).

The peripheral inputs to these thalamic nuclei derive from the various sensory modalities. So, for example, visual stimuli from the eye connect to cells within the lateral geniculate nucleus of the thalamus, which, in turn, connect to the occipital cortex. Sonic stimuli from the ear travel to the medial geniculate nucleus and then to a region of temporal cortex. Stimuli from the skin project to other areas of thalamus, which then communicate with the foremost region of the parietal cortex mentioned above, on the side of the central sulcus opposite the motor strip. We revisit these connections in a later section on perception.

In contrast, if one takes a sample of the cortex just across the central sulcus, from the motor strip, one traces many of these connections to the *basal ganglia*. These nuclei are situated around the thalamus (in a region commonly called the *striatum*, for its striped appearance in anatomic section) and, like the thalamus, have extensive reciprocal connections with specific areas of cortex. Basal ganglia structures also connect in complex ways with one another, and with other subcortical structures like the *cerebellum* (from the Latin: "mini-brain"), a separate structure with its own cortex that sits beneath the occipital lobe and is a center for sequencing, conditioning, and coordination. As one might infer from their connections, and learn from the study of patients who have damage in these areas, the basal ganglia are essential for the organization and regulation of motion and action-related learning (Packard and Knowlton 2002).

If one now continues down the motor strip into the insula, tucked behind the temporal lobe, one finds its cortical neurons tethered by subcortical connections to nuclei in the brainstem and *hypothalamus* (a set of clustered brain cells that sit below the thalamus), which thus involve this region of cortex in the processing of information about the physiologic state of the body. We will learn more about the hypothalamus in sections on arousal and appetitive functions.

Elsewhere on the cortex, it becomes more difficult to define the function of a cortical region simply based on the ultimate sources for its subcortical connections. The subcortical structures that communicate primarily with cingulate and frontal cortical regions are nuclei in the *limbic system*, an old (some say archaic) term for several important nuclei deep in the brain. In contrast to structures like the thalamus and hypothalamus that receive raw data from the environment and bodily organs, limbic structures receive information already processed by other regions of cortex, and mediate interactions between these and the frontal region, cingulate region, and parts of temporal cortex. These structures are thus essential to the integration of elementary mental functions into memory, drive, and emotion (Critchley 2005).

The two limbic structures of greatest interest to us in mental life and illness are the hippocampus and amygdala (Phelps 2004). The *hippocampus* consists of a pair of seahorse-shaped structures deep in each temporal lobe. It integrates signals from all senses, as well as internal signals, and is a necessary element in the formation of conscious memory (Holscher 2003). The *amygdala* is an almond-shaped pair of clustered nerve centers just in front of each hippocampus. Its chief function appears to be to translate information about autonomic and physiologic states into an adaptive state of arousal for action (Cardinal et al. 2002). We will look at these structures in later sections, when discussing mental functions having to do with emotion, drive, and memory.

## Meatware

One could regard the brain thus far as a computational device, designed mainly for information processing. Like a computer, the brain has units that take in and compile data, operate on the data, and generate output, and it even performs self-monitoring to incorporate into its calculations information about the state of the device itself. But brains are far more than fancy calculators. Their circuits are made of biological stuff, not metallic conductors. Their information content is defined not only by the binary logic of a circuit diagram, but also by the dynamic physiologic state of the conductors and the context in which the system operates.

Computers typically perform the same operation repeatedly, exactly the same way, ad infinitum. In contrast, the repeated use of a brain circuit alters the performance of the circuit, so the same input on two separate occasions will likely yield a different outcome. This quality is inherent in the biological makeup of the components of the circuit. Thus to understand the biological basis of mental life it is necessary to know something of the biology of its smallest units.

What biological circuitry transmits information throughout the brain? The brain, along with the rest of the nervous system, is comprised of individual cells—*neurons*—and other cells that support the neurons. Neurons often resemble microscopic trees, with rootlike *dendrites*, a long, trunklike *axon*, and branching projections. At the tip of each twig of each branch the neuron forms a link, or *synapse*, with another neuron. The heart of the neuron, called the *soma*, houses the cell *nucleus*, maintains the cell, and resides somewhere between dendrites and axon.

Individual neurons in the brain comprise the elements of a vast network. With a few exceptions (initial sensory input from transducer cells and final motor output to muscle cells), a neuron carries a signal from one set of neurons to another set of neurons. A *network* can be thought of as the unique pattern of neurons that would result if you could trace the connections between a given neuron and all the neurons it signals, and the neurons they signal, and so on. The brain is more than a network—it is a network of networks.

If one looks at a brain cut open, one notices darker regions on the surface and in clusters centrally, and lighter regions in between. The darker part, or "gray matter" of the brain refers to the cortex and subcortical structures. Neuronal nuclei and synaptic connections between neurons are located in the cortical and subcortical gray matter. As described earlier, some neurons synapse locally with other neurons in the same region; others send out long axon projections to other parts of the cortex, or to subcortical structures, or out to the spinal cord and beyond. The lighter part of the brain, or "white matter" refers to the synapse-free region beneath the cortex through which these long axons run—white because the axons are wrapped in layers of pale-colored, *myelin*-enriched *oligodendrocytes* that insulate the axons.

The wiring in a simple electrical circuit tends to have fixed conductive properties, under standard environmental conditions. The conductive properties of neurons change markedly with use. At low levels of signal from incoming (presynaptic) neurons a receiving (postsynaptic) neuron may conduct no impulse at all. But when the intensity and rapidity of an incoming signal passes a given threshold, a rapid inflow of charged particles (sodium ions) occurs in the postsynaptic neuron, and this neuron becomes an active conductor. Because the neuron tends to hold a different charge inside than exists on the outside, as soon as it opens molecular portals on its surface, sodium ions are drawn in by the opposite electrical charge within the neuron. The neuron goes from being in a different charge state than its surroundings (the polar opposite electrically), to being more in tune with its surroundings; so it is said to *depolarize*.

Once it has depolarized at the synapse, the neuron opens channels all down its axon to its terminal branches, producing a chain reaction of depolarization, or *action potential*. When the action potential reaches the terminal branches, it stimulates the neuron to release specialized chemicals called *neurotransmitters*. Neurotransmitters travel from the synapse to the next neuron, via a space called the *synaptic cleft*. They then interact with specialized neurotransmitter receptors on the receiving neuron.

If there is a sufficient quantity of the neurotransmitter in the synaptic cleft to cause a chemical change in the receptors, the receiving neuron reacts. Some neurotransmitters stimulate a new action potential in the postsynaptic neuron, and some inhibit an action potential. After depolarization, the neuron resets by pumping out the sodium ions and restoring the resting charge. The synapse resets by either removing or breaking down neurotransmitter molecules remaining in the synaptic cleft.

Having reviewed the gross structure of the brain and the mechanisms of neuronal function, we can now add an additional dimension to the model of brain functioning, vital to the understanding of how the brain generates mental functioning: neurotransmitter systems.

There are several neurotransmitter systems, each with a unique distribution through the brain and nervous system, and each serves a unique set of functions. The focus here is on the systems best known to be salient to mental functioning.

Some neurons primarily encode information. These include neurons within the cortex and others that connect the cortex to subcortical structures. Information-encoding neurons tend to employ neurotransmitters like *glutamate* that promote depolarization in the receiving neuron and *gamma-amino-butyric acid* (GABA) that inhibit depolarization. The integration of activating and inhibiting influences on neurons and networks enriches the potential for finely tuned responses. As we will learn later, networks that include glutamate-mediated neurotransmission can alter their qualities through repeated use and thus constitute the major components of information retention in the brain (Chklovskii et al. 2004).

Drugs that affect these neurotransmitters might have an enhancing or suppressive effect on the acquisition or use of information in general. However, there are actually few clinical applications for drugs that promote depolarization by enhancing glutamate or inhibiting GABA. Overexcitement of neurons tends to have bad consequences, including globally unmodulated neural activity that leads to seizures or neuronal damage (excitatory neurotoxicity). On the other hand, inhibition of activity in these systems can be useful clinically. Drugs that enhance GABA—the benzodiazepines mainly—and a few drugs that inhibit glutamate have wide clinical application as sedatives and neuromodulators, or seizure-suppressive agents. GABA-enhancing drugs, when given during an event like a medical procedure, can also induce a limited state of amnesia, by blocking the retention of information.

Not all neuronal networks encode information. Other sets of neurons emanate primarily from subcortical structures and have generally activating or inhibiting effects on populations of neurons (Hurley et al. 2004). The *monoaminergic* neurotransmitters *serotonin*, *dopamine*, and *norepinephrine* have long been a central focus in biological theories of mental illness, and they form the basis for much of our psychopharmacology. Monoaminergic neurons originate in many subcortical structures, including the raphe nucleus (serotonin), locus coeruleus (norepinephrine), and ventral tegmental and substantia nigra (dopamine). Neurons in these nuclei all are activated by communication between them and other subcortical structures, and ultimately with cortex. Thus sensory, motor, and interoceptive (internal sensation) states normally engage the monoaminergic nuclei whenever heightened cortical arousal would have an adaptive purpose.

The three monoaminergic systems differ by the anatomic connections to and radiations from their principal nuclei, and by differences in their engagement with their end receptors in the cortex. Their general functional effects, however, are probably similar. When an element of one of these systems has been activated, the result is an additional stimulus to some cortical locus that serves to facilitate activity of neurons at that point or over that region. Behaviorally, the end result of heightened monoaminergic arousal tends to be heightened mobilization for action (dopamine), heightened cognitive acuity (norepinephrine), and/or heightened capacity to modulate action (serotonin) (Robbins 1997).

Altered function in these monoaminergic neurotransmitters and pathology in their subcortical points of origin are associated with symptoms that reflect their influential role in the regulation of cognition, emotions, and behavior. Suicide and aggression, specifically, have been associated with perturbations in serotonin (Mann 2003; Davidson et al. 2000), psychosis and addiction with dopamine (Sawa and Snyder 2002; Wise 2008), and anxiety and mood disorders with norepinephrine (Schildkraut 1965; Sullivan et al. 1999).

*Acetylcholine*-releasing (*cholinergic*) neurons also contribute to cortical arousal but in contrast to the monoaminergic systems, the cholinergic system acts primarily to arouse activity in subcortical structures and secondarily to arouse cortical regions (Sarter and Bruno 2000). Long cholinergic projections within the brain effect communication between certain subcortical structures and cortex, and others are limited to local and mediating influences, for example, on dopamine-secreting neurons. Anti-cholinergic drugs are useful for correcting the inhibitory effects on motor activation that can occur via dopamine blockade. Pro-cholinergic agents appear to have beneficial effects in slowing the progress of Alzheimer disease, perhaps by enhancing the acetylcholine-mediated arousal of subcortical structures involved in memory, such as the hippocampus.

A host of other molecules serves to translate the physiologic state of the body into adaptively useful information (Rossi 1996). The hypothalamus sits at the center of this chemical network. Its neurons radiate to emit a variety of polypeptide neurotransmitters (comprised of short amino acid chains) to points throughout the brain, and specifically, to the pituitary (by way of direct neuronal input and by release into a local vascular pathway) to control the release of hormones in organs throughout the body. The specific activities of these molecules, with a few exceptions, work at a level removed from direct influence by or on mental life. From the perspective of mental life, the important thing to know is that the body communicates its status to the brain, and the brain translates this into hormonal signals that convey information useful in the conduct of mental life, by influencing the brain's level of activity, locally and generally. Because we will learn more about the nature of this information in the section on arousal, only a few of the relevant molecules will be mentioned here.

It is well known that perturbations in hormone functions, such as excess or deficiency of *thyroid-* and *cortisol-*related hormones, can produce significant psychiatric symptoms. These effects occur in several common disease states, in which low quantities of the hormone (Hashimoto thyroiditis—thyroid, Addison disease—cortisol) or excess quantities (Grave disease—thyroid, Cushing syndrome—cortisol) cause systemic and mental illness. We return to the cortisol system in the following section, in the discussion of stress. Perturbations in the hormones that govern sexual functioning can also profoundly affect the state of mental arousal, whether normal and cyclical as in the menstrual cycle, or the product of the ingestion of androgenic steroids—male sex hormones—by athletes. Although these hormones derive from organs outside the brain, they are regulated by polypeptide hormones secreted from the brain by the hypothalamus and pituitary.

Another polypeptide neurotransmitter system significant in mental function is the *endorphin* system. Aside from its great influence in the nervous system, this system is accessible by pharmacologic agents. Plant-derived and synthetic endorphin analogs—opium and its family of drugs—are among the most widely used and abused pharmaceuticals. The endorphin system (named to reflect the significance of its ENDogenous mORPHINe-like chemicals) has widespread influences, including a critical role in the pleasure response and in the relief from pain-associated states of arousal.

## The Plastic Brain

Most bodily organs tend to wear down with age, even under the best of circumstances. A well-kept brain tends to function better with age (up to a point). The brain has the capacity to retain within its permanent structure a useful map of the optimal path to survival in the world, and to revise it over time to make it even more useful (Pascual-Leone et al. 2005).

The newborn emerges from the sensory deprivation chamber of the womb with little if any information established in the brain, not because of a paucity of neuronal connections, but because of too many indiscriminant connections. Although the brain continues to grow for a time after birth, it adds mainly structural and supporting cells. For example, oligodendrocytes, which wrap axons in a protective myelin sheath, take years to reach full maturation.

Maturity thus emerges not from expansion of the neural substrate of networks, but from the protection of useful networks and the atrophy of unused connections (Johnson 2001). It begins when the infant brain begins to record patterns of association between sensations, actions, and changes in body states. Over a lifetime, one acquires a set of permanently entrenched patterns—the anatomic basis of the last memories to go when one has a degenerative dementia such as Alzheimer disease. Similarly, one acquires a set of permanently entrenched emotional and behavioral responses through a combination of frequent use and disuse of alternative responses. Thus one develops the stubborn stability of character and worldview that characterize middle age. But is that all there is to life? Can't adults still learn and grow?

Neurobiologists used to think that an adult brain could produce no new neurons. They now know that new neurons and connections can be formed well into advanced adulthood, so in a healthy brain there may always be new cellular material with which to learn new things. The persistence of *plasticity* —the functional restructuring of synapses, hence networks—suggests the capacity for new learning is integral to adaptive living. As long as the capacity for plasticity exists, new links can be established, and thus add new twists to old memories.

Unused connections wither, heavily used connections grow stronger. Thus, experience alters the structure of the brain (Kandel 2001). The logic of this process is illustrated in Figure 2. Each time a neuron depolarizes it has the potential to change the way its network will respond the next time it depolarizes. Rapid and repeated stimulus from incoming neurons *potentiates*, or enhances, the likelihood of future depolarization from that input. A potentiated neuron will fire more readily when its dendrites receive stimulus from heavily used inputs, but will continue to fire at the normal threshold when stimulated by other occasional incoming impulses that have not undergone this potentiation. A counterpart process in which the converging impulses inhibit, or depress the size of depolarization, has a similar net effect of recording in the neuronal connections information about past activity.

When two or more neurons converge on and affect the reactivity of another neuron, the process is called an *association*. Associations occur in cortex and certain subcortical structures. A potentiated (or depressed) neuron in an association has undergone a change in the kinds of glutamate receptors expressed at synapses. Association varies across neuron types and locations (Castro-Alamancos and Connors 1997). Plasticity in hippocampus neurons is essential for memory consolidation, but not for long-term retention (Eichenbaum 2000). Plasticity in cortical neurons maintains the association permanently, without active hippocampal involvement (Buonomano and Merzenich 1998). We will investigate the relationship of plasticity to memory more thoroughly in a later section.

A moderate degree of monoaminergic arousal enhances performance and information retention, but overarousal harms the brain (Sapolsky 1996). Excessive intensity and duration of monoaminergic arousal brings on the *stress response*.

Humans often seem to swim in a sea of stress. The stress response arises from the inescapability of threat-triggered arousal. One might argue that its pervasiveness in humans is a natural consequence of the highly advanced human ability to anticipate future events. A person can become aware of and physiologically provoked by not only immediate threats, but also future threats, many of which may never materialize. Immediate threats can be managed in the short term by evasive or defensive action, but future threats cannot.

A classic laboratory experiment illustrates the point that the inescapable anticipation of threat produces stress (Weiss 1970). Two rats are kept isolated in identical, restrictive cages. They can do virtually nothing but spin a wheel with their forepaws. Each rat has an electrode on its tail that administers a shock. Each rat receives a series of simultaneous, identical shocks. However,

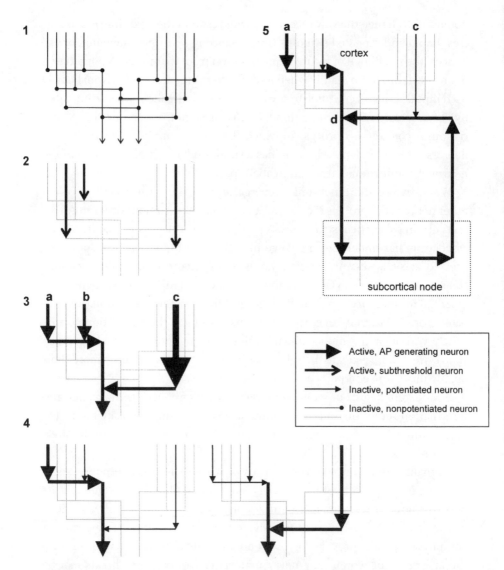

*Figure 2.* How potentiated associations are made and reinforced. (1) Tabula rasa: all neurons have potential for potentiation. (2) Subthreshold stimuli fail to ignite action potentials (AP) in network. (Note that inactive elements of the network are now portrayed as thin, arrowless lines for clarity.) Moderate stimuli at the threshold of activation ignite an AP but do not lower the threshold to pass along a stimulus in the future (not shown). (3) Strong stimuli paired (a + b), or a single very strong stimulus (c), ignites action potentials *and* lowers the threshold for future stimulation from these sources, creating a newly potentiated network. (4) A stimulus from any element of the potentiated network activates the same output. Stimuli (a) and

one rat sees a light before the shock, and then may delay or diminish the shock by working the wheel. The other rat sees no cues and thus has no way to anticipate the shock or to influence its delivery. Again, both rats receive the same shocks at the same times. The rat that has no influence and no warning cues develops the stress response.

How does one know the rat is stressed? High levels of cortisol accompany the stress response and produce widespread toxic effects (Jessop 1999). The stressed rat exhibits a known consequence of stress, such as a stomach ulcer. Why don't both rats become stressed? At the start of the experiment, both rats likely experienced an unpleasant state of pain and alarm upon receiving the shock. Over time, however, the rat given cues and control of the shock enters a state of anticipatory alarm when a cue is presented for an impending shock. The subsequent surge in monoaminergic tone induces the rat to spin the wheel frantically to defer the shock. Thus the rat has a finite period of time in which to be aroused to anticipate the shock, and has motivation to expend energy to control it. After the shock, the rat can relax until the next appearance of the cue.

Meanwhile, the other unfortunate, uncued rat has no way to anticipate the shock and no way to act on the anticipation of a shock, thus no cue to stand down from a state of arousal. There is no end point to the anticipation of a shock; hence the rat remains in a state of stress. In physiologic terms, this rat has maintained high levels of norepinephrine secretion over an extended period. In addition to its cortically arousing effects, norepinephrine stimulates activity in the *hypothalamic-pituitary-adrenal* (HPA) axis (Charney 2003).

The end result of the activation of the HPA axis is the release of cortisol (and related hormones) from the adrenal glands. Cortisol has widespread physiologic effects, including mobilization of glucose stores from the liver

(c) are not completely interchangeable because they would have many other connections not in common, but in this pathway, their net effects are the same. So if (a) was the visual stimulation from a hornet and (c) was the tactile/pain stimulation of its sting, any unexpected stinging sensation might induce one to look for hornets, and the sight of a hornet would be inseparable from the memory of the sting. (5) Output following stimulus (a) in cortex excites a neuron to a subcortical node, which projects back to cortex and ultimately re-excites the same output pathway at point (d). The net effect is the same as if the stimulus that enters the network at point (c) were active. By this re-entrant path, the painful arousal of a hornet's sting in the past ensures that any sign of a hornet in the present will persist in working memory, no matter what else is going on.

and diversion of amino acids from protein-building to energy consumption (Sprague and Power 1950). In a state of truly prolonged threat, such as a famine or siege, the ready availability of physiologic resources may prove life saving even if maintenance of this state impairs long-term survival and quality of life.

Prolonged exposure to high levels of cortisol has physiologically damaging effects, however. Because cortisol inhibits the creation of new protein, tissue comprised of cells in which there is high turnover tends to waste and weaken. The immune system falters and stomach ulcers develop. The damage is magnified in the brain. Certain populations of overexcited neurons are vulnerable to toxicity as a direct result of overstimulation, and cortisol inhibits the growth of new neurons to take their place (McEwen 2003).

Physiologic, as opposed to stress-induced cortisol is normally secreted on a circadian schedule, and controlled by feedback. When one is awakened in the morning by the normal surge in cortisol, the effect is transient because the hormone penetrates the brain and induces the HPA axis to switch itself off. Stress-induced cortisol elevation is maintained by the continued signals of threat and thus is not tightly controlled by feedback while the threat persists. Elevated cortisol in the brain is associated with a variety of dysfunctions of emotional arousal (Steckler et al. 1999; Charney et al. 1998).

This survey of the basic functions of the brain has highlighted important cortical and subcortical landmarks, and cellular processes that contribute to the processing of information, adjustment to environmental conditions, and retention of information. In the following chapters, we will look at the elements of mental life, at how the information-processing aspects of brain functioning are linked to the major inputs and output—sensory and bodily input, and motor output. In later sections on topics that relate to the systems of mind, we turn to how these informational elements combine, over time, to produce adaptive changes in the brain, and to guide behavior.

## 1.3. Summary: Organic Mind

*Mind* refers to the information-processing functions of the brain. Mind aids the survival of an individual and its species by collecting, processing, and checking the information an organism may use to find resources and avoid harm. In addition to sensory information about the effect of the environment on the individual here and now, the mind retains information about the effect of this and other environments in the past, and predicts the likely outcome of actions in the future, based on information the mind gathers from other minds. To put it another way, mind has the unique property of serving as the information-processing function of the brain, and as a source of information itself.

There are four major ways mental function goes wrong: from a disease, or malfunction of brain activity; from vulnerability conferred by one's traits; by the choice of maladaptive behaviors; or by encounters with adversity. In an individual patient, any or all of these kinds of dysfunction may occur at once, to form a complex clinical problem.

The brain receives input from the body (interoception) and from the environment (sensation). The autonomic nervous system conveys information about the state of the body, and governs the automatic, adaptive response to stress. The brain exerts influence in a number of ways, but voluntary motor activity is the final, elemental outcome of mental processing.

The functions of the various regions of the cortex, or outer layers of the brain, can be understood by their connections to deep brain, or subcortical, structures. Sections of the occipital, parietal, and temporal cortex process raw sensory information from eyes, skin, and ears, respectively, all relayed through specialized regions of the thalamus. The insula receives interoceptive input about the state of the body. Motor cortex connects reciprocally with basal ganglia structures. Many cortical regions receive information processed in other brain regions, and exert their influence primarily on other brain regions. The ventromedial prefrontal cortex, cingulate cortex, and medial temporal lobe receive much of their input from hippocampus, amygdala, and other deep subcortical structures, and thus integrate information from inside and outside worlds. Large swaths of dorsolateral prefrontal cortex, parietal, and temporal lobes receive critical input from other cortical areas, and are devoted to higher-order processing of perceptions and actions.

Plasticity refers to the brain's capacity to alter its function through structural self-modification, either by the growth of new neurons or from changes in the potential of an existing neuron to respond to a stimulus. Potentiation occurs when two or more inputs to a neuron change the threshold at which that neuron will fire in the future, generally by shifting the population of glutamate receptors in the receiving neuron. Potentiation can either occur over the short term or leave a permanent record of experience in cortical neural networks.

The stress response is induced by prolonged and unpredictable threat and/or privation. The body's response to stressful circumstances can adversely affect plasticity. Stress causes a physiological alteration in bodily functioning, mediated by glucocorticoid hormones such as cortisol. While adaptive in some circumstances, the net negative effect on plasticity may be to render the brain less adaptive, hence exacerbating mental illness.

# CHAPTER TWO

# Elementary Mind

The mind has two main sources of input: sensation, stimulated by the environment, and arousal, stimulated by signals from the body. The mind has one main conduit for output: orchestrated skeletal muscle contraction. To make sense of the world, to respond to bodily needs, and to move effectively in the environment, these elemental strands of mental life must come together. When they do, they generate *information*: an emergent phenomenon connecting the physical properties of the world we inhabit to the biochemistry of our bodies.

Emergent phenomena have properties that cannot be adequately explained in the same language and logic that explains their simpler mechanisms. All subatomic particles obey the laws of physics, but the laws of physics are overmatched by even simple phenomena contained in the periodic table, such as the fact that fluorine (atomic number 9) has properties more in common with chlorine (number 17) than with its immediate neighbor neon (number 10). Brains obey the laws of physics and biochemistry, but when our brains attach personal significance to the phenomena we observe, the urges that move us, and the things we do, we add something to the world that would not have existed without cerebral processing, and which cannot be reduced to the physics of light, sound, and pressure transduction and the biochemistry of sodium ions and serotonin.

How do we manufacture information from the raw materials of cerebral activity? How, for example, do we transform a fleeting retinal flicker into the image of a soaring bird? The short answer is, we can't, without the help of the other elementary aspects of mental life. Nor can we interpret hunger pangs as a yen for pistachio ice cream, based solely on the quality of the visceral sensations. Nor can we differentiate picking up a baby from lifting a sack of potatoes, using only the sequence of motions we undertake. Somehow we must learn how to identify what we perceive, pursue what we need, and act with purpose.

The mind is more or less a blank slate at birth, though the tabula is not quite rasa. Our brains do come equipped with sense-specific virtual maps, embedded in the cortex and subcortical structures. The first bit of information we can derive from sensation thus consists of the locations within the brain, down to specific sets of neurons, which immediately become active at an encounter with a specific stimulus. The final bit of information output consists of the specific arrays of cortical neurons in the motor strip that, at any given moment, send signals out to the muscles they control.

But none of this is useful to the naïve neonate. Sensations reach the newborn cortex with minimal organization and thus with little value as a source of information. Infantile movements appear uncoordinated, if not random. The capacity for organization and coordination depends on neuronal maturation, but also on rich encounters with the environment. Hubel and Wiesel, in their classic experiments (Hubel 1982), demonstrated that kittens, blinded temporarily for several weeks after birth, fail to develop full visual perception after the blinders are removed. Therefore, sensory stimulation must play a critical role in the organization of raw input into useful perception.

Learning to draw information from experience is not as simple as filling an empty vessel with knowledge—we not only lack knowledge at birth, we lack the vessel to hold it. Eventually, when we become sentient beings, we grow adept at dialectical learning. We start with some bit of information (thesis), note when it fails to be true (antithesis), and from that we acquire a more sophisticated body of knowledge (synthesis). But how can an infant imbue the world and body with information, when there is no information to begin with, no thesis as a point of reference? The answer, as will be described in the following sections, is that the information content of something we sense develops from the arousal state of the body at the time we sense it, and from the way our sensory experience and body state changes as a result of the things we do when we sense it.

A few words on terminology, before moving on. Sensation is not the same as perception, and motion is not interchangeable with action. *Sensation* refers to the raw cortical representation of the physical properties of the world. *Perception* refers to the process of pattern recognition that transforms these raw sensations into meaningful units of information, capable of engagement by the *cognitive* faculties that, as we will see, feed memory, motivation, and executive functions. The end result of a cognitive process is the recognition of a pattern of sensory data as a meaningful object. The word *object* here denotes any identifiable unit of mental life: anything in one's perception or memory or imagination, animal, mineral, vegetable, construct or concept, that has some qualities to differentiate it from other objects. In other words, an object is anything one can name. Sensation acquires raw data about the qualities of things in the environment; they become objects only after the mind has processed them into organized perceptions.

An object may also constitute an *objective*, the purpose for which one conducts any coordinated action. *Motion* refers to a sequence of muscle contractions, independent of the purpose that activated them. Motion, in other words, is directed toward no specific object; it implies no objective. *Action* refers to a particular sequence of goal-directed motions. Transitive verbs are, in general, actions ("I'm kicking the habit," "Gamblers, place your bets," "She solved the differential equation"), whereas intransitive verbs ("The pitcher balked," "The batter walked," "Weaver squawked") harbor ambiguity about the purpose of the motor activity, and might even refer to unintentional motions—mistakes or automatic or reflexive responses.

In contrast to sensory raw data, which the brain maps to some quality of the world, motor impulses map to the musculoskeletal structure of the body. Whereas the brain performs a kind of pattern analysis to ascribe significance to sensation, the purpose of action derives from the cortically embedded instructions to program the timing, accuracy, and precision of the muscle movements that must be coordinated to carry it out (Grafton and Hamilton 2007). The term *action program* denotes these encoded sequences of movements that produce the coordinated pursuit of an objective: whether to examine it, consume it, manipulate it, acquire it, destroy it, or avoid it.

The primal forces of physiology animate the system; without some internal signal to lend significance to objects, and to fuel objectives, nothing happens. Thus the fact that we assign any significance at all to an object has much to do with our present state of *arousal*. The body becomes aroused by a variety of circumstances—strong appetites, pain, fear, pharmacologic agents—but this general sort of arousal conveys very little information other than the fact that the body wants something badly. The specific objective we will pursue, or object we will invest with significance, derives from the state of appetite or a specific physiologic need. The map for appetitive information exists in part within the cortex (specifically, the insula), in part within the architecture of the hypothalamus, and in part within the chemical or neuronal signals of a specific need in the body system, as for food, water, warmth, companionship, stimulation, and so on.

So, once again, how do the powers of perception and action develop in the absence of an organized curriculum? How does the mind teach itself to perceive objects and perform purposeful actions? The mind must organize itself according to the world it encounters. Repeated exposure to patterns of sensation and interoceptive signals of bodily need, at a time when one is also performing a series of motions, establishes a linkage in the mind (stored in the brain's neuronal networks) between the things one senses, feels, and does frequently. A perception acquires meaning as an object because one tends to do certain things to or with it. Motions become linked into sequences of programmed actions when they tend to produce predictable changes in sensory patterns and arousal states, repeatedly, that is, when they attain their objectives. The qualities of these objects and actions stem directly from the form and degree of appetite and arousal that drove the action and found the object salient.

Later in this book, in encounters with the integral systems of mind—memory, executive function, and motivation—we will see that these objects and action programs become the basic building blocks that form the rest of mental life. Although the elements of perception, action, and drive may seem far removed from clinical psychiatry, there are mental dysfunctions that arise in these processes. Moreover, in the effort to describe an organic basis for all of psychiatry, it is essential to have some biologically plausible model, however speculative, to account for phenomena we typically take for granted.

Most disruptions of the elements of mind result from pathological processes. Global disruption of arousal due to metabolic, infectious, or toxic insult ren-

*Table 2.*    Elementary Mind: Basic Input and Output Functions

| Function | Description | Disruptions |
|---|---|---|
| Arousal | Constitutive and responsive enhancement of cortical activity and the likelihood of action | Anergia, agitation, delirium |
| Appetite | Need-driven selection of specific cortical pathways to motivate behavior | Disorders of sleep, eating, sex, visceral function |
| Perception | Pattern detection from raw sensory input | Hallucinations, illusions, pseudo-sensory symptoms, pseudohallucinations |
| Cognition | Higher-order pattern detection from perceptions | Low intelligence, agnosia, disorganization |
| Motion | Generation of coordinated muscle activity independent of purpose | Catatonia, pseudomotor symptoms, dyskinesias |
| Action | Control of initiation and cessation of goal-driven motion | Obsessions/compulsions, extra-volition, apraxia |

ders a person confused and delirious. Problems of both appetitive and general arousal are common in syndromes of depression and mania and suggest that the root cause of these syndromes may rest within the mechanisms of arousal and appetite. Problems with perception in the form of hallucinations, and with purposeful action in the form of catatonia, are common in the syndrome of schizophrenia. A few elemental disruptions can occur in a normally operating brain. These include pseudosymptoms of sensory and motor loss that may arise with acute emotional distress. Low intelligence implies a relatively impaired capacity to organize and accurately differentiate perceptions. Chronic psychosis may erode socially shared concepts of meaningful thoughts and actions. Table 2 summarizes the components of the elementary mind.

## 2.1. Not Shaken, Stirred: Inappropriate Arousal

What differentiates coherence from confusion? How do physiologic signals and environmental cues stir the brain to action? Disruption in the regulation of this process of arousal gives rise to common and often dangerous mental disturbances.

Arousal is comprised of distinct mechanisms that set the general, background tone of brain activity, and other mechanisms that alter the level of activity, according to shifting phases of need (Jones 2003).

In a waking brain, *tonic arousal* maintains the brain in readiness for all other functions. Tonic arousal arises largely from the activity of subcortical cholinergic projections (medial septal nucleus, nucleus basalis) to cortex and other subcortical structures. In the sleeping brain, a limited state of tonic arousal defines the rapid eye movement (REM) sleep stage, when dreaming occurs. One can observe this process at work in the *electroencephalogram* (EEG) of a conscious (or dreaming) person (Llinas and Ribary 1993).

An EEG measures the electrical activity in the brain, via electrodes placed around the scalp. Compared to the relatively indolent oscillations in the EEG of a person in deep sleep, a waking EEG reveals something perhaps counter-intuitive about the way the brain maintains consciousness. A waking EEG reveals rapid, synchronized activity across the entire brain, at a pace of about 40 cycles per second (40 Hz). This rapid, rhythmic signal corresponds to the constant cycle of activity between cortex and the major subcortical structures (like the thalamus). It takes about a 40th of a second for a thalamic neuron to signal cortex and for the cortex to send a return signal. The rhythm of these oscillations has been tied to the nature of conscious perception (Joliot et al. 1994).

Absent the tightly paced activity, there would likely be more randomness in the interactions between neurons: one neuron might be active while another is unreceptive (that is, refractory to stimulation for a brief time after depolarization). Such randomness would interrupt circuits and introduce chaos, as in fact occurs with patients who are delirious or intoxicated and is revealed in their disrupted EEG patterns. Picture an orchestra playing in perfect synchrony, each musician playing a series of designated notes at the same time to produce a powerful, complex tone—like the synchronous cycles in the waking EEG—versus the cacophony of an orchestra in the warm-up before a symphony, when the pitch rises and falls randomly and the notes from one musician become lost in the noise.

The fact that the activities of the conscious brain occur in a regular, staccato pattern may challenge one's personal experience that consciousness feels like a fluid stream of thought. Instead, it appears to be more like a movie or an animated cartoon. Filmed movies consist of long strips of still images projected at a pace of 24 frames per second, which produces the illusion of motion in the characters on screen. But one no more sees these figures on a screen actually move than one sees anything move. Just as we assemble the perception of motion from a series of still movie images, we construct the continuity of consciousness out of a series of 40 Hz cycles of synchronized cortical activity (Llinas and Ribary 2001). Our brains automatically impose the quality of movement on objects that shift position in our sensory fields during the brief interludes between thalamocortical cycles.

The other arousal process, *phasic arousal*, serves as a volume control on the brain, that is, it alters the intensity of arousal on demand. Intense hunger, thirst, heat, cold, pain, injury, alarm, or threat conveys urgent signals to the hypothalamus, amygdala, and autonomic systems that, in turn, signal the brain to arouse the body for action. These signals travel from subcortical structures to the cortex, by way of monoaminergic neurons, among other bio-active chemicals. This general mechanism of arousal stimulates heightened attention to sensory stimuli and readiness for motor activity (Aston-Jones and Cohen 2005).

Phasic arousal varies to a mild degree throughout any moderately stimulating day and tends to increase in short bursts on demand (for example, to sharpen one's alertness while preparing to cross a busy street). Phasic arousal disengages upon satisfaction of the drive that triggered its onset (Robbins 1997). When the hypothalamus no longer conveys signals of intense need, or the source of environmental threat is eliminated, the monoaminergic systems no longer receive these urgent signals, and arousal diminishes appropriately. Some kinds of prolonged phasic arousal may lead to the stress response, described in the section on brain plasticity.

### Anergia

Anergia—the absence of energy—can be differentiated from other, physiologic forms of fatigue. Pure muscle fatigue reflects a deficit in the energy stores available to the muscles. After muscular exertion, it may take time and nutritional energy to reset the biochemical mechanisms of contraction. Sympathetic activation throughout the body can overcome an energy deficit directly by increasing the blood flow—hence oxygen and nutrients—to muscle tissues. We describe fatigue defined as sleepiness in the section on appetite. Pathological fatigue is a symptom of some neurological disorders, such as myasthenia gravis, in which there is failure of nervous stimulation of muscles (Chaudhuri and Behan 2004).

Mental illness can contribute to fatigue indirectly, for example, via malnutrition. Some illnesses (for example, depressive disorders) diminish appetite, and others (such as schizophrenia) induce impoverishment. In either case, there may be interference with proper nutrition and self-care, so a relative lack of energy follows directly from a lack of resources. In other cases, the chronic behavioral inertia associated with the illness causes a state of deconditioning to occur; the person feels anergic and fatigued because there is a loss of muscle tone and autonomic responsiveness after a period of weeks on the couch.

The form of fatigue directly related to mental illness is the feeling of anergia that comes with little or no exertion. In mental fatigue, the problem is not in the muscles or energy stores, but in the failure to become aroused to action by need or desire (Boksem and Tops 2008). Failure of tonic arousal leaves a person sleepy and inattentive. Failure of phasic forms of arousal hampers the capacity to pursue pleasure or react to threat. A complaint of feeling tired or fatigued in this case corresponds to the difficulty mobilizing effort when the spur of phasic arousal has been dulled (Eriksson and Wallin 2004). We return to this latter form of anergia in the section on motivation, and discussions of apathy and anhedonia.

Normal fatigue induces a behavioral drive to rest, which resolves the drive and restores the energy in both objective and subjective aspects. Mental fatigue frustrates a person because the pursuit of rest it inspires fails to accomplish its goal; repose serves no purpose. And yet there is no arousal of interest to do anything else (Smith 1981). Although physiologic needs in this case fail to engage the mechanisms of arousal, they may still demand satisfaction. For a person stuck in an anergic state, the impetus to get out of bed to shower or eat or dress may require arousal by motivations other than a desire to be clean, well fed, or socially presentable. The impetus may arise instead from the sense of alarm or disgust at the adverse consequence of not acting. Thus a person in an anergic state describes mundane activities of daily living as a series of grim struggles to "push" to get things done.

Anergia is a component of psychiatric diagnoses such as depressive disorders (major depression and dysthymia) and is a frequent complaint in somatoform disorders and a common side effect of some psychotropic medications.

## Agitation

In states of agitation, the arousal is high but the ability to connect the arousal to a salient goal is weakened (Berkowitz 1989). Physical and mental restlessness, as well as emotional volatility, produce an uncomfortable state: arousal without purpose. The arousal induces behavior such as pacing, a form of movement without purpose. A caged and angry animal, or prisoner, highly aroused, impotent to find a salient course of action or object on which to act, can do naught but pace and growl at passersby.

Disturbances in tonic versus phasic hyperarousal may produce different varieties of agitation (Lindenmayer 2000). In states of delirium or intoxication, the hyperarousal affects behavior globally; there may seem to be no meaning to the stimuli that trigger an eruption of violence. In contrast, someone primarily in a state of high phasic arousal may be able to identify from moment to moment the connection of the state of arousal to some actual goal or purpose.

Agitation can be a dangerously explosive state, as the agitated person experiences no ready relief from action or reduction of arousal from completing an action. The person may seek out increasingly aggressive and reckless means to find some satisfying activity and is at risk to execute unpredictable, possibly violent action. The pattern of "escalation" is a familiar one in psychiatric wards where severe mental illness is treated. As a patient grows more agitated, a mildly perturbed response to being asked to get dressed for breakfast in the morning may grow to the hostile refusal of occupational therapy by lunchtime, a loud argument with another patient by mid-afternoon, and placement in locked-door seclusion by dinner, after the patient has punched a fist through a wall and threatened a nurse.

This pattern may also explain why a prior history of violent acts may have a permissive effect on agitated violence. If prior experience has taught that only a significant act of violence will provide some sense of relief from the state of arousal, then the progression to violence may occur more rapidly in the future. This is a familiar pattern in domestic violence as well, where alcohol-fueled agitation may lead ultimately to a shocking (to both parties) outburst of violence early on, but later become a commonplace experience, part of the standard repertoire of destructive interactions within the relationship.

Agitation is a symptom commonly seen in mood disorders, schizophrenia, alcohol and drug intoxication and withdrawal, and delirium. A propensity to agitation may also be a maladaptive behavior associated with emotional volatility and consequently frequent interpersonal conflict.

## Delirium

Delirium encompasses the many varieties of severe mental disturbance that arise from disrupted regulation of arousal (Ross 1991). A person who has delirium may be disoriented to place and time and is characteristically disoriented to context. Delirium in this sense encompasses disruptions in tonic arousal that occur in gross brain dysfunction or encephalopathy and in severe states of intoxication, as well as extremely high states of phasic arousal, as seen in manic delirium. A delirious person experiences inappropriate and incongruous patterns of activation and somnolence. The person's confusion about space, time, and context reflects, sometimes vividly and sometimes incomprehensibly, the person's aberrant internal state of arousal, which interferes directly with memory processes and warps the apprehension of facts and context.

The common causes of delirium—drug or alcohol effects, metabolic disturbances, fever and other systemic illness—push a person through phases of agitation and lethargic stupor, disconnected from the normal sensory cues that signal the need for high or low arousal states. A patient in the grip of incongruous arousal states, unable to interpret information accurately or to behave coherently, appears to others to be grossly insensible to reason. The delirious person sits safely in a hospital bed but is overcome with apparently nonsensical fears. Their mutable nature sets these fears apart from hallucinations and delusions that occur without systemic illness, which tend to follow a theme.

Many medications prescribed by physicians have mixed effects on alertness. The most common offenders, used for a wide variety of medical illnesses, have anticholinergic properties—they block the effects of acetylcholine in the brain (Campbell et al. 2009). Cholinergic neurons maintain tonic arousal; blockade may have complex effects, however, as the systems engaged by acetylcholine receptors include neurons that inhibit as well as activate brain processes. Blocked inhibition leads to overactivation, that is, blockade of cholinergic stimulation may unleash brain processes normally inhibited indirectly by cholinergic neurons that stimulate inhibitory neurons. Delirium occurs in the context of withdrawal of some pharmacologic agents, especially "depressants" such as alcohol and drugs like benzodiazepines and barbiturates. The state of uninhibited hyperarousal that results from the abrupt removal of depressants can produce great alteration of consciousness, as well as physiologic reactivity.

Encephalopathic delirium (confusion as a result of gross brain dysfunction) follows from severe systemic illness and thus marks a bad prognosis (Siddiqi et al. 2006). In these cases, the systemic illness has advanced to a degree that it has affected the brain's own metabolism—as seen in states of low oxygenation in lung diseases, electrolyte imbalance, septic shock, and hypoglycemic reactions to insulin overdose.

Encephalopathic delirium poses a particular challenge in patient management, as the same patients who most need to be able to report subjective symptoms, and to cooperate with treatment, become behaviorally unable to do so. Patients who have delirium unwittingly engage in dangerous behavior, like pulling out intravenous lines or trying to walk while in a weakened state and risking a fall. However, medicating encephalopathic agitation carries its own risks. If patients are sedated to attempt to constrain dangerous behavior, the resulting intoxication can make the delirium even worse; if they are restrained physically, they tend to interpret the situation as threatening, hence they may become more combative.

Diagnoses primarily associated with delirium are systemic illness and alcohol or drug intoxication or withdrawal syndromes.

## 2.2. Sate Ain't So: Immoderate Appetites

The body makes its specific needs known to the brain, and hence affects behavior, by triggering specific appetites. Abnormal appetitive behaviors can produce problems on their own and are an indirect source of many of the problems experienced by patients who have mental illness.

The hypothalamus and the amygdala mediate the cortical processes associated with internal signals of physical need, sensory perception, and programmed actions to satisfy the need. The cell clusters or nuclei of the hypothalamus receive and process information about the physiologic state of the body and communicate with both cortical and subcortical structures (Hoebel 1997). Communication with the amygdala adjusts the state of phasic arousal, as described previously (Lang and Davis 2006).

The hypothalamus receives information in three major forms, described in Table 3. Autonomic neurons provide information about the status of visceral organs. Hormonal signals provide information about metabolic and homeostatic states of appetite and satiety for sleep, sex, and food. The biochemical and physical properties of the blood provide data on the general state of health directly to hypothalamic cells, including serum osmolality (salt content) and body temperature. The hypothalamus informs the amygdala of these needs, which in turn translates the information into the neuronal signals required for the regulation of motivated behavior (Critchley 2005).

*Table 3.*   Major Input Sources and Output Paths

| Function | Signal | Route |
|---|---|---|
| *Interoception* | | |
| Thirst | Serum osmolality | Hypothalamic sensors |
| Air hunger | Hypercapnia (hypoxia) | Carotid bodies to brainstem respiratory centers |
| Hunger | Ghrelin, orexins, others | Hypothalamic receptors |
| Gastric satiety | Leptin, insulin, cholecystokinin, gastric stretch receptors, others | Hypothalamic receptors; subcortical and brainstem nuclei |
| Lust | Vascular engorgement of stretch receptors in sexual organs | Autonomic nerve signals |
| Visceral discomfort / pain / urgency | Stretch receptors in smooth muscle organs | Autonomic nerve signals |
| Sleepiness | Melatonin; retinal light receptors | Hypothalamus |
| Phasic arousal | Monoamines | Various subcortical nuclei to cortex and other subcortical structures |
| *Perception* | | |
| Vision | Neuronal signals induced by photons | Optic nerve to occipital cortex via thalamus |
| Hearing | Neuronal signals induced by sound waves | Auditory nerve to temporal cortex via thalamus |
| Touch | Neuronal signals induced by pressure sensors in the skin | Various peripheral sensory nerves to parietal cortex via thalamus |
| Smell | Chemical activation of neurons | Specialized chemoreceptors in olfactory bulb to cortex |
| Taste | Chemical activation of neurons | Specialized chemoreceptors in tongue to cortex via thalamus |
| Equilibrium | Rotation and motion of semi-circular canals in the ear | Vestibular nerve to cortex |
| Proprioception | Stretch receptors in muscles | Peripheral nerves to cortex |
| Pain | Specialized receptors in skin and mucosal tissue | Peripheral nerves to insula cortex |
| *Output* | | |
| Motion | Neuronal impulses to skeletal muscles | Corticospinal tracts |
| Endocrine | Hormone release in peripheral glands (adrenal, gonadal, thyroid) | Hypothalamus to pituitary |
| Autonomic | Allostatic regulation of visceral function | Subcortical and brainstem nuclei to autonomic ganglia |

The various sources of physiologic information represent the state of the body in its particulars. Low blood sugar induces specific *appetitive* neuropeptides that, in turn, activate specific hypothalamic centers. When we eat, and blood sugar and fat content of blood rises, the brain no longer emits appetitive neuropeptides and a new set of polypeptides signal *satiety* to the hypothalamus (Broberger 2005). Bladder distension stimulates stretch receptors that convey autonomic impulses to other areas of hypothalamus; emptying the bladder eliminates those signals and replaces them with signals denoting relaxation. Hypotension-induced hormone release and overly concentrated serum stimulate yet other hypothalamic cells that, in turn, convey thirst signals relentlessly until one drinks and corrects the blood chemistry (Johnson and Thunhorst 1997).

Hypothalamic signals, processed in the amygdala and translated to other parts of the brain, form the basis of motivated behavior (Stellar 1954). The signals from specific hypothalamic nuclei, representing specific physiologic domains, motivate specific appetitive behaviors. Once a sequence of appetite and satiety signals has become linked to a sequence of actions, encoded in the cortex, the reemergence of the same appetite later engages the same cortically encoded actions. For similar reasons, they also selectively activate cortically encoded patterns of perception that correspond to patterns that were perceived in past episodes of appetite and satiety. Thus, the appetite guides us to what we need. The connection of appetitive arousal to associated actions and perceptions constitutes the essence of a behavioral *drive*.

In parallel, general signals of physiologic need, as occur when an appetitive drive goes unmet for a prolonged period of time, generate a general state of arousal to fuel whatever drive has been selected by the specific signals of appetitive need (Pfaff et al. 2005).

Sensory and autonomic feedback thus plays a major role in the regulation of drive (Esch and Stefano 2004). If we eat until our bellies are full and drink until our whistles are wet and smoke until the tension wafts away, we will have, in the ideal, consumed the optimal amount to correct the physiologic need, or to produce the desired pharmacologic response. However, one may obtain and consume the object of a drive but fail to experience a rapid resolution of the drive. This disconnection between sensory registration of an appetitive goal, and the neurohormonally mediated experience of satiety (Rolls et al. 1988), creates some problems in the modern world. Many of the substances humans ingest for food or for pharmacologic properties, such as sugar, fat, tobacco, alcohol, opium, cocaine, cannabis, and coffee, have been engineered to deliver larger effects in ever-smaller volumes. Humans in the time before refined sugars and deep fat frying, for example, could rely to a greater degree than at present on gastric distension to signal adequate intake of calories. Now, by the time a person feels full, he or she may have taken in many times the amount of calories needed for sustenance. Rampant obesity results. By the time a modern person is aware of the subjective, autonomically mediated effects from a bacon cheeseburger, a double espresso, a martini, a cigarette, crack cocaine, or heroin, enough has been taken in to do damage or fuel addiction (Orford 2001).

Disruptions in the arousal and regulation of drives manifest in disturbances of sleep, feeding, and sexual activity.

## Sleep

Sleep restores body and mind. The sleep cycle includes two components: the homeostatic component, which drives us to sleep about a third of every 24-hour cycle, and the circadian component, which links the desire to sleep to daily fluctuations in hormones timed to the body clock. Melatonin hormone, secreted by the pineal gland in daily surges, promotes sleepiness. As long as the daily surges in such hormones are well timed, and one keeps to a predictable schedule, sleep is initiated at bedtime and sustained until morning (Saper et al. 2005).

Narcolepsy, a disorder in which a person has frequent plunges into sleep, disrupts the neural/hormonal regulation of sleep (Sutcliffe and de Lecea 2002). Mood disorders, drugs, alcohol, and delirium, all of which affect the general state of mental arousal, disrupt the physiologic regulation of sleep in a variety of ways. It might seem that sleep results from a process of shutting down the brain, but in fact sleep requires an alternative set of active brain processes to maintain slumber, so the system has vulnerabilities at a number of points (Neubauer 2003).

Lack of sleep affects not only the drive to sleep, but also arousal in general. In the initial phase of sleep deprivation a person often experiences excessive arousal, followed by erratic arousal and lethargy throughout the day. Ongoing forced sleep deprivation diminishes the capacity to sustain attention or to modulate emotional arousal. Ultimately the drive to sleep overwhelms other salient drives. Normally one would not want to go to bed hungry, but if one stays awake long enough, one will sleep no matter how long since one's last meal. Extreme forced sleep deprivation causes such strong and reliable distress that it has frequently been employed as a method of torture.

Sleep apnea syndrome causes chronically deficient sleep. The mechanism for the inability to maintain a deep sleep in sleep apnea begins with airway constriction that emerges when the muscles surrounding the airway relax with the onset of deep sleep. With the airway constricted, carbon dioxide accumulates and stimulates arousal, waking the person before the benefits of sleep can be enjoyed.

Sleep is a motivated behavior. People have not only a need for sleep, as they have for breathing, but also a desire for sleep and a fear of not being able to sleep. Both states motivate complex behaviors beyond simply lying down and shutting one's eyes. Good sleep depends on a desire for sleep. Satisfying sleep rewards and reinforces behavior that leads to it. The anticipated pleasure of comfortable rest facilitates sleep by inducing a state of relaxation.

Conversely, in a state of mind where the pleasure response is impaired, as in a depressive syndrome, the failure to anticipate satisfaction and to induce the pleasure response contributes to the common symptom of chronic insomnia. Other people with depression alternatively, feel drawn to stay in bed long hours, anergic, lacking sufficient arousal by the prospects of pleasurable activity to motivate full awakening. Sleep may occur on and off for a large portion of the day, but fails to satisfy, that is, it rarely restores any interest in getting up.

A person may become conditioned to experience insomnia if bed becomes a trigger for arousal, not relaxation. This can be a product of habit when a person conducts intensive, high-stakes work on a laptop just before turning off the lights or enjoys watching action movies late into the night. When a person has, for whatever reason, struggled to fall asleep for some time, bed no longer suggests pleasure. Without the pleasurable anticipation of sleep, it is more difficult to induce the state of relaxation and diminished arousal that brings it on. The result is a self-perpetuating problem with insomnia.

Psychiatric diagnoses commonly associated with sleep disturbances include delirium, dementia, major depression and mania (bipolar disorder), and generalized anxiety disorder. Dyssomnia as a primary complaint may also be addressed by internists and neurologists.

## Eating

An intricately choreographed play of blood chemistry, polypeptide hormones, and autonomic tone drives eating, by an equally complex set of conditioned behavioral preferences with respect to the type, quality, and quantity of food (Saper et al. 2002). In addition, there are other critical motives for eating that have little to do with nutrition.

Eating is commonly a rewarding social activity; to consume the same foods for the same period of time as tablemates facilitates bonding. Eating also produces a pleasure response, even without a biological drive to eat (Lowe and Butryn 2007). Many foods consumed in developed societies have little value other than to induce pleasure. Eating may relieve boredom when one becomes restless, and dull the pain one may feel when isolated from others. For these reasons, and because calorie-dense, fatty food is cheap and plentiful and the needs of life can be obtained with little caloric expenditure, non-nutritional eating and obesity are epidemic in developed societies.

Although not as common, other disorders of ingestive behavior can present with dramatic manifestations in a clinical setting. Pica affects children and pregnant women in whom there is a strong compulsion to eat nonfood materials like dirt and paint chips. Presumably the apparatus to detect salient properties of food erroneously perceives such materials, some of which may have a pleasant taste, to have the potential to relieve hunger. The child may endanger herself or himself by ingesting poisonous materials; the lead contained in old paint has historically done particular harm to the intellectual development of poorly supervised, often poorly nourished children in older cities with aging housing. Some patients inexplicably consume indigestible objects like coins, hair, or nuts and bolts, for reasons that likely have to do more with false belief than with drive. A "drinking disorder," psychogenic polydipsia, the drive to overconsume water, sometimes leads to dangerous changes in a person's blood chemistry.

Many psychiatric patients gain significant amounts of weight after starting psychotropic medications, especially if the medication is among the second-generation dopamine-blocking drugs. Patients describe an insatiable hunger that can lead to a rapid onset of obesity and complications like diabetes. Besides the adverse impact on health, the negative effect on a patient's self-image often contributes to therapeutic ambivalence and non-adherence.

Many medications reduce weight by inhibiting appetite, but as of this writing none do so safely and reliably. Drugs that enhance catecholamine transmission, such as amphetamines, reliably inhibit appetite but also induce dependence and cause irritability and paranoia. A safe and reliable weight loss drug remains the holy grail of behavioral psychopharmacology.

Diagnoses commonly associated with eating problems include major depressive disorder—in which disturbance of appetite can increase or decrease feeding—as well as mental retardation and dementia. Eating disorders like anorexia nervosa and bulimia do not imply a change in appetitive drive, and are described later as forms of addiction.

## Sex

Sex distracts people from activities that might be far more constructive; however, few would want to give it up (Seidman and Riede 1994). Many thinkers throughout history have echoed the words of the famous prayer by St. Augustine of Hippo, "Give me chastity and continence, but not yet." Sexual behavior, unlike other biologically driven human behaviors, is not necessary for individual survival, and requires cooperation with other people to be fully satisfying. A person may have sexual problems not because of an abnormal sexual drive or desire, but because no compatible partner is available.

Sexual dysfunctions can derive from normal human variation (Meston and Frohlich 2000). Some individuals have a relatively high sexual drive, and some a relatively low drive. These trait variations generally pose no problem unless there is incompatibility between committed life partners, in which case it can become a source of conflict. Having a high sex drive can also be a source of problems if it gets in the way of other necessary activities. Whether or not humans are "wired" to be monogamous, monogamy prevails in most societies, so a strong drive to stray from it carries heavy consequences.

A significant change in sexual drive can be a source of distress. In some cases, drive remains unchanged, but inhibitions weaken; this often occurs in health care settings, disconcertingly, among previously well-behaved patients who have dementia and begin to grope the nurses. Excited, manic mood states inflame sexual drive and incite hypersexual behavior and preoccupations. Loss of libido, conversely, accompanies anhedonia. It can also be symptomatic of deficits in sex hormones, such as testosterone, and an unfortunate side effect of drugs often used in psychiatry, in particular, those that raise synaptic serotonin levels. When an apparent loss of libido relates only to the existing partner, it suggests deeper conflicts within a relationship.

Other sexual dysfunctions primarily impair performance. Stressful arousal ("performance anxiety," worry about finances or other life issues, and relationship conflicts) inhibits sexual arousal. So do damage to nerves and blood supply to erectile tissue in the genitals, certain medications, and excessive alcohol. Female performance dysfunctions include vaginismus (a contraction of smooth muscle around the vagina), which can produce dyspareunia (pain during sexual intercourse). To resolve sexual dysfunction between partners, one may need to tease apart biological, psychological, and interpersonal factors. Even if the source is purely biological, the cumulative effect of impaired performance within a relationship can be the emergence of tension and conflicts that then add an emotional dimension to the problem.

One other form of dysfunction worth mentioning is not a matter of sexual performance, but of limited capacity to navigate sexual relationships. For some individuals, particularly those who have neurodevelopmental problems, the physical aspects of sexual maturity proceed on a normal schedule, while the mental capacities needed to find and maintain relationships with appropriate sexual partners can be severely impaired. A person in this unfortunate situation may not be able to articulate the source of frustration, but in acting on the urgent erotic drive may become dangerous to others. Some serious behavioral difficulties seen with young institutionalized, developmentally impaired adults can be attributed to powerful desires for unattainable sexual partners.

Diagnoses in which sexual dysfunction may be a factor include mood disorders, impulse control disorders, personality disorders, sexual disorders, mental retardation, and dementia (Fagan 2004). "Deviant" sexual behavior is addressed later, in the section on habits.

### Visceral Functions

Behaviors regulated by the autonomic nervous system, such as those concerned with evacuation, breathing, and swallowing, recur with great frequency and tend to be expressed in highly stereotyped actions. They can be considered as appetitive in the sense that they follow the same dynamic of urge, action, and relief that characterizes other appetites. Similar to autonomically regulated actions like digestion and cardiac circulation, these functions can and do occur without conscious control, but unlike digestion and circulation, they may readily be overridden by conscious control. Disruption in evacuation, breathing, and swallowing may follow from serious mental impairment, and may produce dire consequences.

Development of bowel and bladder control marks the beginning of sentient life, as the loss of control often signals its wane. At various times in recent history bowel habits in particular have become a focus of intense theoretical interest (Szasz 1951). Most famously, or infamously depending on one's point of view, the early psychoanalysts proposed that much human suffering, or neurosis, devolved from conflicts between parent and toddler over potty training. Parents, being highly motivated to encourage a child's completion of this essential developmental task, at times find that their expressed disapproval over failures becomes highly motivating for the child. In some cases of overzealous parents or an oversensitive child, the child may fight off all urges to defecate, to the point of impaction, in order not to risk suffering the shame of failure. One may still hear a particularly rigid person described as "anal-retentive" for this historical reason.

Once a child has developed excretory control, loss of control may signal a problem in mental life (Bongers et al. 2007). The occasional loss of bladder control—enuresis—is a highly common event that may signify only an overtired or emotionally stressed child (Glicklich 1951), whereas recurrent loss of bowel control—encopresis—often suggests a severe childhood mental illness.

Total loss of control over excretory function rarely becomes an issue for neurologically intact adults, unless they are delirious or intoxicated or have dementia, but concerns about excretory functions frequently arise in medical settings. Complaints of loose stools, bowel urgency, constipation, and so on are so common that they now comprise a diagnostic entity: *irritable bowel syndrome* (Thompson 1984). Similarly, symptoms of bladder discomfort and urgency, in the absence of a detectable pathological entity, comprise another set of loosely defined *cystitis* syndromes. Because both excretory systems respond to alterations in the quantity and quality of a person's intake of food and drink, and both are under the control of autonomic systems that may increase or decrease smooth muscle activity, excretory symptoms can often be associated with emotional distress.

With respect to breathing, it has long been thought that chronic hyperventilation may be associated with anxiety attacks, in which sudden feelings of breathlessness are a common symptom (Bass and Gardner 1985). The experimental manipulation of respiratory drive by inhalation of carbon dioxide has demonstrated that hyperventilation is more likely a result rather than a cause of acute anxiety, and suggests that one possible explanation for the visceral symptoms common in anxiety states involves an oversensitivity in some people to interoceptive signals of physiologic distress, such as breathlessness and heightened bowel activity.

Swallowing problems occur with less frequency, and often reflect anxiety as well. The feeling of a lump in one's throat, or "feeling choked up," is a common manifestation of emotion, but when it escalates to a persistent feeling of throat obstruction, in the absence of a pathological cause, clinicians call it *globus hystericus*.

Disturbances in visceral sensation are a hallmark of generalized anxiety disorder and panic disorder. Loss of excretory control in children tends to denote some degree of emotional distress or behavioral maladjustment. In adulthood, it suggests delirium or dementia.

## 2.3. Sense Insensibility: Misperceptions

Neurobiologists do not yet fully understand the biology of perception, but one may construct enough of a model of its mechanisms to conjecture how, in mental illness, our senses may mislead us. Hallucinations, hysterical blindness, and other mental problems of perception demonstrate the hierarchical nature of perceptual organization and its susceptibility to influence by errant signals and intense states of arousal.

We experience perception passively, as if the world projects itself into the theater of consciousness. In fact, the brain analyzes and adds information to every unit of sensory input *before* it becomes part of conscious perception (Mesulam 1998). All sensation begins as a quality of objects in the environment and of bodily processes: electromagnetic radiation in the visual spectrum; waves of sound pressure in the atmosphere; hardness, temperature, and contour of objects; bioactive chemicals in the air and on the tongue. Churning of the gut, pressure in the bladder, fever and chill, and other visceral events likewise become sensory data for the brain. Receptor cells translate these properties of objects and the body into neuronal signals, and transmit these signals to the thalamus.

Circuits between thalamus and cortex process raw sensation into useful information (Livingstone and Hubel 1988). Neurons radiate to and from specific subunits of the thalamus to specific regions of the cortex. Via this feedback loop, a unit of sensation acquires definition by its relationship to signals from the sensory units immediately surrounding it. Thus, the information content of an individual point of light, a star, for example, is significant when it is surrounded by a field of darkness in the night sky, but miniscule within a field of similar luminosity during daylight hours.

The cellular organization of primary sensory cortex maps the physical properties of the world. Occipital neurons that receive visual input sit relative to one another as they are in the retinas; hence they constitute a virtual map of the visual world. Somatosensory (for example, tactile) input, organized on a virtual map of the body, feeds a strip of parietal cortex that borders on the frontal lobe. Auditory information reproduces a tonal map on the top of the temporal lobe. The logical organization of gustatory, olfactory, and visceral maps in the cortex remains elusive, but similarity across individuals suggests some innate capacity to detect a finite set of qualities.

By the time a unit of sensory stimulation reaches the cortex, it conveys at least three dimensions of information: the signal itself, its location on a virtual map, and thalamic enhancements to the signal. Meaning is derived from these data, and context applied, as co-occurring combinations of these enhanced signals converge at points in the surrounding cortex to form higher-order units of information. Thus, visual data about a circle we see in the center of our vision project to the occipital cortex, where these signals map to a ring of cortical neurons that corresponds to light receptors in the retina. Neurons in this pattern combine to signal another neuron or set of neurons that condenses the unique information encoded on this map. A set of several units that define a small section of a curved line in the upper right quadrant of the visual field, for example, may converge to a neuron that registers "arc at two o'clock." At the same time, other units converge to a point that detects radial symmetry in objects with similar coloration, while yet another localizes these sensory signals to a point in space relative to the viewer. Any time a sensory input stimulates that particular set of primary visual neurons, these same, smaller, secondary sets of neurons will also be activated. When a set of these secondary visual processors line up together to define a circle, the neuron that receives this collection of inputs becomes the final common cortical pathway for all circles.

This explains how unique patterns of sensory information can be encoded hierarchically, but not how we see this pattern as a "circle" rather than one of a near-infinite number of unique shapes. We may be born with a particular sensitivity to radial symmetry in visual objects, but not with the abstract concept of round shapes. How does the quality of roundness expand from the property of specific objects, to a general quality of many objects? The formation of an organized perception begins early in life. The first circles we encounter exist in objects that have some quality of radial symmetry: balls, teething rings, nipples (natural or man-made), and household items (plates, cups). These all look round from some angle, but most important to an infant, they have a unique tactile uniformity (that is, they have no sharp corners) when held in the hands or placed in the mouth. In order for an infant to experience the qualities of a round object, it must be held, gummed, or rolled on the ground. These actions provide simple tactile data, and also complex feedback about the sensory consequences of acting upon the object.

A set of secondary visual neurons comes to encode the concept of "circle," not simply because circles are intrinsically interesting or their patterns are hard-wired in the cortex, but because what looks like a circle tends to behave in a particular, round way when acted on. The circle's tactile properties resonate with its visual properties. Because one encounters round objects frequently, the neuronal circuits denoting circle become fixed in the cortex, while the neuronal circuits denoting an irregular, asymmetric myriagon, do not. Similar processing occurs throughout life, albeit the relationship of an object to how it feels in the mouth grows less salient as one grows older. At that point, objects of perceptions become fixed through sensory repetition and active play, and actions become fixed through performance. With increasing sophistication, language, and literacy, objects that cannot be directly perceived and acts that cannot physically be performed are fixed by "playing" with them as ideas.

Note that the organization of the cellular elements of perception, at least in some sensory modalities, is understood in far more detail than has been laid out here (Katz and Crowley 2002). For example, the individual unit of visual perception is not a point of light, like a pixel on a video screen, but a column of cortical neurons that react specifically to gradients of light oriented in a particular direction. The point of this rough sketch has been to highlight the logic of information flow from world to mind, not to delve into the mechanisms.

## Hallucinations

True hallucinations—perceptions without a stimulus—occur in any sensory modality. Hallucinations can occur in the absence of confusion, poor lighting, or background noise and have about the same quality as a true perception. An auditory hallucination seems like it is coming from some direction in the environment. A true visual hallucination appears to be fixed in the field of vision, in daylight, and does not merely slip through peripheral vision. The power of hallucinations to intrude on actual perceptions in the same modality suggests that the mechanisms of sensation itself are intact.

*Elemental hallucinations* are simple and amorphous: a buzzing sound or a light, for example. *Formed hallucinations* with identifiable content are also common. The fact that some false perceptions appear to be fully formed objects—visual images rather than points of light, voices rather than tones, the distinct feeling of bugs under the skin as opposed to mere itching, identifiable tastes and smells—suggests a potential, general mechanism of hallucinations. Elemental hallucinations likely occur from aberrant activation of primary sensory cortex, in regions where perception conforms more closely to the raw data of sensation, whereas formed hallucinations arise from activation of areas of cortex that encode complex, organized perceptions.

One clue to the possible source of hallucinations comes from studies performed by Wilder Penfield, a neurosurgeon who applied mild electrical stimuli to the cortex of patients whose brains were opened for surgery (Penfield 1975). He used this technique to localize the focus of a seizure, so that patients who have intractable epilepsy could be cured surgically. Penfield found that patients would experience hallucinatory experiences when stimulated at many points on the sensory cortex. The specific cortical location predicted the modality of the hallucination, which lasted only as long as the electrical stimulus. Therefore it is reasonable to assume that in a pathological hallucination, whatever aberrant stimulus evokes the hallucination must be persistent and specific to a cortical locus. Such a process suggests a deficit in the modulating capacity of monoaminergic neurons, either in their direct effects on cortex or indirectly through their influence on the subcortically mediated mechanisms of tonic arousal (Behrendt 2006). Neuroimaging studies of hallucinations suggest generalized abnormalities in brain function (Allen et al. 2008), consistent with the idea that a general failure to modulate perception predisposes one to hallucinations.

The aberrant arousal of a particular center of voice perception does not necessarily stimulate each specific detail of the hallucination. If the brain is fooled into believing that it is hearing a voice, it may attribute the thoughts generated concurrently by other brain activity to the aberrant voice. Therefore, the common hallucinatory experiences of hearing voices commenting on ongoing, mundane activities unites the false sense of hearing the tones of a human voice with the normal, ongoing sensory feedback processes involved in the regulation of motor activity (Strik and Dierks 2008). In other words, as the brain selects, activates, and regulates sequences of motor activity, the simultaneous stimulation of a voice-detection region in temporal cortex provides the narration. Command hallucinations, in which a person reports that voices direct him or her to act in a certain way, often instruct people to perform acts that produce a high level of arousal, such as suicide, either because the person much desires to perform them or much fears to perform them. Either way, these thoughts contain extremely high emotional salience. The voice simply narrates whatever information the strong arousal state renders salient.

Auditory hallucinations are a common element of schizophrenia and, to a lesser degree, mood disorders. Visual hallucinations are common in both delirium and dementia.

## Illusions

An illusion is a false perception, produced by a real sensory stimulus (Norton and Corbett 2000). Illusions tend to occur when signals to sensory cortex lack contextual information from the environment or from memory. Thus, a visual illusion occurs most commonly in a semi-darkened room, in someone who is visually impaired, has dementia, or is delirious. Auditory illusions tend to occur in the context of active white noise, like the whirr of an air conditioner.

The concept of illusions encompasses normal imaginary ideas (pareidolic illusions), like seeing shapes in the clouds or hearing music in traffic noises. These remain mere flights of imagination as long as the capacity remains to place them in their proper context. Completion, or inattentive, illusions occur when ambiguous sensory information or a lack of cognitive focus on sensory stimuli leads to erroneous interpretations. Affective illusions tend to cause the most distress. In these cases, the combination of imagination, ambiguous or incomplete sensory input, and an activated emotional state may impel agitated, defensive behavior, if the illusion is perceived as menacing.

Illusions occur in delirium, alcohol and drug intoxication, and withdrawal.

## Pseudosensory Symptoms

Although not as seemingly widespread now as in Freud's day, "hysterical," or "conversion," symptoms of sensory loss are still seen in practice. They differ from true lesions of sensory organs, nerves, or cortex by their atypical features. For example, a person may truly have diplopia—double vision—if the visual data from the two optic nerves fail to mesh in the cortex, but there is no way to understand "triple vision" as anything but an hysterical symptom.

A claim of a loss of sensation in a section of body inconsistent with the distribution of peripheral nerves or the representation of the body map in the cortex also suggests a pseudosensory symptom. For example, abrupt onset of numbness in the hands but not the arms or feet cannot readily jibe with a likely pathology of peripheral nerves, spinal cord, or brain.

Emotional factors may also mark a pseudosensory symptom (Harvey et al. 2006). The person may express either an exaggerated emotionality or odd indifference to the symptoms. A person might frantically report being unable to see though clearly able to walk through a well-furnished office without stumbling. Others exhibit an odd absence of distress: *la belle indifférence*. Where a person who had a true sudden loss of vision, hearing, or tactile sensation ought to be concerned about the possible permanence of the symptom and lethality of its cause, people who have pseudosensory symptoms often seem fairly comfortable with the idea that their deficit is stable and with the expectation that others will now care for them in their time of need.

How can a neurologically intact person doubt the evidence of the senses? Clearly, a person who has hysterical blindness can receive visual stimuli. The pupils respond to light; the person exhibits defensive reflex responses to abrupt motion in the visual field. In what sense can the person not see? Leaving aside cases of frank misrepresentation, there seems a disconnection between sensory information taken in and perceptual awareness of that information. That is, the person who has a pseudosensory loss can take in, but not make use of, sensory information.

One may conjecture that the person with a pseudosensory loss has come to fear certain modes of sensory awareness. Dread of encountering objects in the environment leads to the neglect of perceptual information—a kind of defensive flight from perceived danger performed automatically, without conscious reflection or intent. A suggestible person might convince himself or herself that a danger not perceived is a danger not real, and report it as a failure to see, whereas another, more insightful patient who has the same level of distress might describe the feeling of dread directly and not feel the need to avert the mind's eye. Pseudosensory loss thus implies an inhibited capacity to entertain perception in working memory.

Hysterical, or pseudosensory symptoms are central to a diagnosis of conversion disorder and are seen in dissociative disorders. We revisit the topic in the upcoming section on pseudomotor symptoms.

### Pseudohallucinations

True hallucinations signify severe mental dysfunction. One often encounters patients who claim to hear voices "inside" their heads. These differ from true hallucinations, in which the false perception has the quality of a true perception. A true hallucination seems specific to one of the primary senses and has the quality of a sensory experience; when one hears a voice speaking intelligible words, one can repeat them as if one were listening to a conversation. When pressed about the details of a pseudohallucination, the patient often has trouble answering convincingly whether, for example, the voice spoke in the first, second, or third person (for example, whether the voice said to "kill myself," "kill yourself," or "kill him"). Pseudohallucinations generally signal intense emotional distress, which suggests that the heightened arousal associated with distress enhances the attention paid to the "inner voice" of working memory to the degree that it seems as if it had taken on the qualities of a true perception, though one may more accurately consider it a strongly emotionally tinged thought (Bishop and Holt 1980).

No particular diagnostic entity is associated with this symptom, but adjustment disorder is a likely diagnosis, as is malingering, if the patient's intention is to pretend to have a severe symptom in order to gain something.

## 2.4. Nominal Anomaly: Confounded Cognition

Having formed primary sensory stimuli into organized perceptions, how does one use the perceptions? In the course of development the primary components of perception—shapes, colors, tones, qualities of touch, and so on—somehow define meaningful objects and concepts. Intelligent and adaptive human behavior requires objects and concepts to have nuanced, accurate, and socially shared significance. The process by which perceptions acquire significance constitutes cognition.

Inadequate cognitive capacity can be innate or acquired. Subnormal intelligence thus results from an innate, relative inability to name and discriminate objects. Disorganization of thought and behavior represents an acquired loss of coherence, as an increasingly idiosyncratic interpretation of reality leads to incomprehensible speech and behavior.

The previous section described how perceptions become organized by qualities as one encounters objects over time, and plays with or manipulates them.

Thus, the patterns that commonly occur in one sensory modality become linked to patterns in other modalities. In an analogous way, perceptions assume significance because they link to properties of the things they do, or that we can do with them. When we first encounter the world in infancy, it is not a matter of innate knowledge that the ball we like to play with is a member of a class with all other spherical playthings. An infant comes to know that all the spherical objects in his or her playpen are balls because they have no sharp edges, they all roll, and the older people in his or her life utter the same sound to refer to them.

After we identify a class of objects, we learn to discriminate within that class. The concept of a "ball" arises in an expanding range of contexts, and acquires modifications: baseball, basketball, gumball. The functional attributes of the concept "ball" also expand. A gumball is round but may not be thrown or bounced; a football is not round but is thrown like other balls. Ping pong balls are okay to play with in the house; basketballs are not. And to add to the complexity, the word also connotes dancing and part of the foot. In time we may cast off the term *ball* entirely when we need precision. In geometry, an ideal ball-shaped object is really a "sphere," synonymous with arithmetic concepts of three-dimensional radial symmetry, but not with any specific physical function.

Abstract or imaginary objects arise by association with other concrete words or symbols and become established to the degree that they inspire similar sets of associations in the minds of other people. For example, the fabled purple cow exists only as an imaginary object. No one has ever seen one (not a real one, at any rate). But I can have a colorless visual concept of a "cow" and formless concept of the color purple, and readily imagine a purple cow presumably when the neuronal networks associated with those concepts are active at the same moment. Your image of a purple cow probably differs from mine, but if we communicated about our ideas, through artistic rendering or detailed verbal description, we could converge on virtually identical concepts. To the extent that we can expand the number and sophistication of qualities that define an object or concept, we have intelligence.

In its simplest, operational definition, intelligence is merely the factor that accounts for relatively high or low scores on various tests of mental performance. Correlations between test performance and life achievement validate the concept to some degree. Controversy emerges over the way tests are conducted and interpreted (Gould 1981). Obviously, a test question that assumes knowledge of the anatomy and behavior of horses is unfair to underprivileged city kids. Less obviously, perhaps, tests of vocabulary and analytical skills favor those raised in enriched environments and provided with excellent training. Useful information or not, a measure of performance on such a test gauges not an innate quality, but a level of exposure to experiences. Even when test makers try to minimize cultural biases, the question has remained controversial whether intelligence has primarily a genetic basis (Neisser et al. 1997). Alternatively, as in other qualities like height, genes and environment may interact, so low intelligence, like low height, can occur in someone who has a normal genetic endowment but is deprived of nutrition and stimulation.

Although the breadth and depth of vocabulary does not define a person's level of intelligence, in practical terms, and with the caveats outlined in the previous paragraph, it provides a reasonably good proxy. College admission tests rely on vocabulary as a predictor of academic success; psychologists estimate a person's degree of intelligence before the onset of a brain injury from the depth of vocabulary that persists post-injury. Vocabulary as a proxy measure of intelligence perhaps tells us something about the nature of intelligence. It suggests that an important aspect of intelligence is the capacity to discriminate between objects, both real and abstract, and to apply words that accurately convey these differences. Relatively low intelligence might thus result from delays in cortical development or deficits in the biochemical processes behind associative learning that impede integration between sensory and motor networks (Neubauer and Fink 2009). Similarly, to be deprived of rich experience during childhood is potentially to fail to acquire the necessary informational substrate for complex cross-modal integration.

Intelligence as measured on standardized tests yields a statistic called the Intelligence Quotient, or IQ, that is more or less normally distributed across the population. The average IQ by definition is 100, and the standard deviation is 15, so about 68 percent of the population will have an IQ between 85 and 115, and 95 percent between 70 and 130. By convention, an IQ below 70 is considered "intellectually disabled." What does an IQ test measure? Strictly speaking, IQ tests measure one's ability to take an IQ test. The verbal fluency and capacity for abstract reasoning measured on tests seem to correlate with the capacity to succeed in complex social endeavors. Standard IQ tests do not measure other capacities, or "multiple intelligences," thought by some to be distributed unevenly across the population, and also associated with specific modes of success, such as artistic creativity, athletic talent, and "people skills."

Thus, based on IQ testing, a small proportion of people have superior intelligence, the great majority of people have sufficient intelligence to function competently, and a substantial minority has intelligence low enough to produce problems in everyday functioning. If a person who has a moderately below average IQ finds himself or herself in a situation that requires decisiveness, flexibility, and the capacity to assess and use large amounts of information, many decisions are likely to have unanticipated negative outcomes, and he or she will have limited capability to improve performance or learn from mistakes. On the other hand, if intelligence is well above average, a situation that calls for simple, repetitive action is likely to be understimulating, hence the person's attention may wander and the quality of action may suffer as a result.

## Low Intelligence

Low intelligence is not a mental illness, but it can be the result of a somatic or genetic disease, and may hinder performance and adaptation. Common, severe forms arise from chromosomal anomalies like Down or Fragile X syndrome or metabolic abnormalities like phenylketonuria. Low intelligence may also occur in someone who has a perfectly normal brain, just as short height may occur due to a genetic disorder like achondroplasia or may be the normal genetic endowment in someone who has a perfectly healthy, but diminutive frame. In a similar way, the more drastic the deviation from the mean, the more likely there is a cause related to genetic anomaly or toxic exposure.

Low intelligence tends to contribute to clinical problems when the lack of cognitive flexibility leads a person to experience stress in almost any situation requiring judgment and knowledge, and the stress in turn may result in maladaptive behavior as the intellectually impaired individual often possesses a limited range of options to cope with stress (Eaton and Menolascino 1982).

Low intelligence (that is, mental retardation in the old nomenclature and "intellectual disability" in the future DSM) is diagnosed based on IQ, on Axis II using the DSM system.

## Agnosia

Disruption of specific cortical circuits prevents one from being able to parse sensory experience. A person with agnosia may be able to describe the sensory qualities of the object he or she senses, but fails to assemble these qualities into a recognizable object. In the clinic, these deficits commonly result from general deterioration in cognitive function, as in dementia (described more fully in the section on memory). Study of the rare individuals who have suffered focal injuries to the brain leading to circumscribed deficits in perception has helped to elucidate the structure of cognition.

The principal insight about cognition that can be drawn from the study of agnosia (literally, the inability to know) is the apparent localization not only of primary sensory function, as described in the previous section, but of secondary, associative functions that detect patterns in raw sensory input. These functions are not only specific to a certain sensory modality, but also specific to particular qualities of sensory experience. Thus there are visual, auditory, and tactile agnosias, spatial agnosias, even an agnosia for human faces (prosopagnosia) (Farah 1992).

## Disorganization

People who experience *psychotic* phenomena—hallucinations and delusions—often exhibit grossly disorganized speech and behavior. To an outside listener or observer interactions with such a person can be disturbingly unpredictable. A disorganized person demonstrates idiosyncrasies in the association between words, concepts, actions, and experiences. Concepts lose their shared meaning when one lives in an altered reality; speech and behavior may become incoherent, as the person's motives become increasingly opaque to others.

Disorganization may be an acute symptom of illness. In a state of delirium, driven by pathological arousal that distorts perceptions, a person's words and actions may be incomprehensible to anyone else. Some patients in agitated, hyperaroused states also speak and behave incomprehensibly; however, their problem occurs because their thoughts are only half-developed, as they come and go too quickly to be expressed intelligibly. Or disorganization may arise through abnormal development. For example, in childhood-onset autism, the failure to develop skills in cooperative behavior may interfere with the grasp of the common meanings and usages of words.

Disorganized speech and behavior often accompany chronic psychosis. Poor social function correlates closely with impaired cognition in schizophrenia (Kurtz 2006). So, one may see disorganization in chronic psychosis as the result, over time, of poor communication and social engagement. Severe social isolation combined with idiosyncratic, psychotic experiences leads words and actions to drift away from the common shared meanings that were learned originally. Over many years of social isolation and active psychosis, the person's speech becomes more and more idiosyncratic. In these individuals, meaningful communication disintegrates, so that sentences may lose logic, become filled with jargon, or contain words that are themselves nonsensical (to everyone but the speaker).

The diagnosis chiefly associated with disorganized speech and behavior is schizophrenia. Unfathomable words and actions also occur in autism, delirium, dementia, and manic agitation.

## 2.5. Inaction in Action: Motion Sickness

We are rarely aware of the control of individual muscles involved in movement. The mind's contribution to motor activity is worthy of some description, however, because grasping the elements of the control and regulation of movement helps one envision the more complex orchestrations of movement that comprise the mental aspects of planning, intention, and goal-directed behavior.

Movement originates from large cells in the motor cortex (pyramidal cells) that convey signals down the spinal cord. There they synapse to the final neuronal units in peripheral nerves that send signals to neuromuscular junctions of a unit of muscle fibers, thus directly stimulating muscle fibers to contract. When fibers contract in unison, the whole muscle contracts.

Skeletal muscles exist in reciprocal pairs, like triceps and biceps, so as one muscle contracts, another is stretched. Without reciprocity, one would be unable to modulate or undo an action; this arrangement also allows for fine regulation of muscle contraction. Each skeletal muscle contains stretch detection receptors that signal information about the tension of a muscle back to the spinal cord, to create a reflex arc that stimulates flexion in the now stretched muscle. When that muscle flexes, the opposing muscle is stretched. These opposing forces—the mechanism of the knee-jerk reflex—keep muscle groups in balance. Stretch receptors also send this positional (proprioceptive) information back to the brain. Specifically, they produce signals in brainstem nuclei, which transmit the information to the primary somatosensory cortex. The result is a virtual map of the position of and forces acting on all parts of the body relative to each other in space.

Complex motion requires the sequenced and coordinated stimulation of individual motor neurons. It is as important to control the inactivity of motor

neurons as it is to stimulate them. To bend the elbow, for example, the cortical neurons that signal biceps flexion must fire in unison while neurons to the
triceps inhibit flexion. This active suppression of opposing muscle flexion is
necessary to overcome the stretch reflex described above, and implies a hierarchical system to coordinate organized motor activity.

Coordinated and sequenced generation of action comes from a hierarchy
of encoded instructions (Kakei et al. 1999)—in this text, termed an *action
program*. A program encapsulates these instructions so that when a situation
calls for a specific action, the instruction cascades from only one, or a few
neurons, several levels removed from primary motor cortex, through a network that has been shaped by experience to stimulate and inhibit a particular
set of motor units at particular times in the motion. These simple programs
are in turn linked at higher levels to more generalized instructions that serve
to maintain an appropriate tone for an appropriate duration, in concert with
the coordinated activation of other muscle groups. In the example of biceps/
triceps coordination, these might include muscles that control shoulder ro-
tation and hand closure, if the action is to grasp and raise something off a
surface. The cerebellum and basal ganglia contribute to regulate the timing
and sequence of actions.

The somatosensory cortex provides essential perceptual feedback in the
regulation of motion. To grip a coffee cup and raise it off the desk, one must
make dynamic use of visual information about the cup's spatial location, about
tactile pressure to get a firm grip on the handle, about the stretch of fingers
and forearm muscles to gauge the fullness of the cup by its weight, about
texture and heat as the cup brushes one's lips, and about the olfactory and
gustatory qualities of the liquid as it is sipped and swallowed. The neuronal
components of motion at the lowest level may be contained entirely in the
motor cortex, whereas sophisticated programs that unfold over time and involve objects are encoded in networks across large portions of frontal and
sensory cortex (Rizzolatti and Luppino 2001).

The state of the body also influences the action program (Swanson 2000).
Suppose the lifting and sipping sequences described above are embedded in
a complex action program that governs the consumption of a cup of coffee.
Regulation of a program of *consummatory* action includes sensory evidence of
the immediate presence of the consumable item, in this case, of coffee in the
cup, and autonomic feedback about the physiologic state of the body. The action program for coffee consumption overall may be expanded or repeated if

the result is a pleasurable taste or sense of alertness—one may take longer, savoring sips, or just gulp the coffee down, depending on the level of drive and the general context. Coffee consumption may be aborted if nausea or jitteriness is experienced, or if sensory input suggests the coffee has grown unpalatably cold.

## Catatonia

In catatonia, a person demonstrates a global incapacity for voluntary action (Gelenberg 1976). Catatonia denotes the failure to respond behaviorally and adaptively to environmental cues. Many people in a state of catatonia remain immobile and awake but unresponsive; others engage in repetitive action or hold the body in rigid or odd postures. Parkinson disease, a neurological disorder that is caused by a deficit in dopamine activity and often results in patients being "frozen" or "stuck," bears a superficial resemblance and suggests there are multiple routes to catatonia (Northoff 2002).

Catatonia was more familiar in the era before modern psychopharmacology, and it has been described in the context of several of the most severe mental illnesses. For example, the loss of volitional action may be influenced by pathological emotional states (Moskowitz 2004). Interviewed after being in a state of catatonia, patients often recall little of it, but what they do recall frequently is an internal state of paralyzing, psychotic fear. An immobile catatonic patient may report later having thought that willingly to have moved a single finger would trigger a cataclysmic realignment of the forces of good and evil in the universe. A catatonic patient risks serious harm to health and life from self-neglect. One of the most effective ways to bring about a transient resolution of catatonic symptoms is through the use of pharmacologic treatment (GABA-mediated neuronal inhibition) that modulates arousal, consistent with the putative role of pathological fear in sustaining the catatonic state.

Catatonia is seen most commonly with schizophrenia and sometimes with mood disorders and autism.

## Pseudomotor symptoms

A perceived loss of motor control without pathological cause and in the absence of psychosis occurs in states of acute emotional distress (Aybek et al. 2008). Pseudomotor symptoms, like pseudoparalysis or psychogenic movement disorders, disrupt the connection between intention and voluntary motor activity. The fact that a person who has a pseudomotor symptom can be induced to move the afflicted limb under hypnosis or mild sedation supports the idea that hyperarousal blocks voluntary action, as function returns when the person is less aroused.

As a consequence of a pseudomotor symptom, as with pseudosensory loss and other hysterical symptoms, the person often accomplishes two ends simultaneously. First, if one cannot move at will, one cannot engage with dread-inducing objects, people, or situations. Second, the symptom becomes an excellent reason to seek the caring attention of others: a calm, compassionate, nonthreatening clinician or a family member whose hostility may be negated by sympathy and the caretaking role. Hysterical pseudoneurologic symptoms in this way often are overdetermined; they are sustained by multiple, complementary motivations.

As a clinical aside, some clinicians have been known to diagnose hysterical or pseudoneurologic or, in the official lingo, conversion symptoms when the patient presents with unexplained neurologic symptoms, especially when the patient seems emotionally labile or "difficult." In these cases, the clinicians may have erroneously placed the diagnostic focus on the absence of a pathological explanation rather than on the patient's behavioral motivations. In the absence of positive evidence for a behavioral motivation to experience pseudoneurologic symptoms, one should always favor the hypothesis that the patient has an atypical or obscure or emerging neuropathological condition that remains to be diagnosed (Stone et al. 2005).

Pseudomotor symptoms are the core feature of the diagnosis of conversion disorder.

## Dyskinesias

Impaired kinetic function—that is, abnormal, involuntary movements such as tics, tremors, limb twitches, and gyrations—commonly occurs as a consequence of neurodegenerative illnesses and medication side effects. A variety of subcortical structures coordinate motor regulation. Perturbations of cholinergic and monoaminergic neurotransmission, in particular dopamine-mediated pathways, can interfere with it. These symptoms are more in the purview of neurologists than psychiatrists, but are common enough in psychiatry to warrant mention. Thus, Parkinson disease, and Parkinsonian side effects of dopamine-blocking agents used for psychotic mental illness, impair dopamine's role in generating and modulating action. Additionally, dopamine inhibitors, and occasionally serotonin reuptake inhibitors as well, can provoke a form of restlessness known as akathisia, in which a person has a difficult time staying still. Parkinson disease, as well as Huntington disease and several other, less common, so-called subcortical dementias, involve amotivational states as well as problems in motor initiation, control, modulation, or regulation. Motivation and the management of the mechanics of coordinated, sequenced action thus appear to use similar subcortically mediated processes.

Tics, which are the characteristic feature of Tourette syndrome, present as frequent, stereotypic, simple gestures or vocalizations. A person who has tics often feels a powerful urge to perform an action—to grimace, or say a word, or twitch a limb. The urge is discharged upon performing it, but the urge recurs repeatedly. The symptom is consistent with the aberrant firing of a low-level action program that encodes a unitary or extremely simple action sequence. As it is activated at a low level, it is apparently beyond the reach of the normal mechanisms of motivation and sensory regulation, hence difficult to control by conscious effort.

Dyskinesias of various kinds are common in some forms of dementia, in the stereotypic movements of some patients who have schizophrenia, in Tourette syndrome, and in medication side effects.

## 2.6. Order Disorder: Dysregulated Actions

Simple motion such as standing, scratching, or shifting position can be controlled by internal signals generated by stretch receptors, somatosensory input, and visceral feedback. To move effectively through the environment, one must regulate one's actions using constantly updated proprioceptive, interoceptive, and perceptual information, both to select action germane to one's drives (hunger impels a person to reach for an apple and not a hammer) and to ensure that the environment guides the action (for example, sidestepping that debris on the sidewalk). The integration of environmentally informed action with sensory and autonomic feedback ensures that one's actions competently achieve their goals and that action stops on achieving them. Failure to fully integrate drive and environmental context can result in phenomena such as obsessions and compulsions, in which there is evidently a low-level failure to regulate goal-driven thought or action despite receiving signals that the objective of the action either has been completed or would be unnecessary.

Goal-driven action emerges from programs sequenced hierarchically into meta-programs that translate broad aims (eat!) into smaller steps (reach! grasp! lift! bite! chew! swallow!) (Botvinick 2008). Physiologic signals relayed via the hypothalamus to amygdala and ventromedial prefrontal cortex select the appropriate program. Whether or not one acts to execute a program hinges on the degree of phasic arousal available to trigger the "go" signal.

The simpler the program, the more it depends on sensory cues and the less on sustained arousal and goal-directed planning (Corbetta and Shulman 2002). People-watching on a park bench on a warm spring day, with no higher goals in mind, only the pull of novel or attractive sensations arouses the simple motor programs to adjust head, neck, and eye position to follow the sensations. Unless some stronger motive emerges, like waving to a passing friend, one remains on the bench, lost in thought.

Consummatory behavior requires a somewhat higher degree of arousal and specificity of salient stimuli (Berridge 2004). Scratching an itch takes more arousal and regulatory control than does people-watching. An itch provokes arousal and provides a target for goal-driven action. The itch stirs a sequence of actions (reach, curl fingers, move hand back and forth), and sustains them until the itch is gone. Arousal of a drive for consummatory behavior may stimulate attention, rather than action, when the object of the behavior is unavailable. Mild thirst makes a person attentive to signs of water for as long as the drive persists, even while actively engaged in other goal-driven actions.

The stronger the drive, the more likely one will engage in complex behavior to obtain the needed object. In general, this means either searching for it or synthesizing it—in other words, performing a *procedure*. Procedures involve a series of steps, each aimed at an intermediate goal that moves one closer to a behavioral objective. In the process of learning a procedure, one essentially ascribes salience to objects for which one otherwise has no specific use; the subroutines that include these intermediate objectives become written into the neuronal architecture of the complex action (Polk et al. 2002). Thus, one's interest in a specific jigsaw puzzle piece reaches a peak before one finds it; afterward the piece blends in with the rest of the puzzle. Or, as one mixes up eggs for an omelet, one works to attain a desirable consistency, though the raw egg itself is unappetizing.

To consume something at hand requires a less potent drive than to get up and find or make it. To *not* consume or pursue an object of desire requires an even stronger drive—that is, an action program invested with salience to a broader spectrum of appetites and drives. Going to professional school, for example, may force a student to forgo immediate desires (like buying a house or watching a football game on a Sunday afternoon) in anticipation of greater satisfaction in the future. Raising a child, similarly, forces deferment of many more immediate desires, over an even longer period of time, but does expand the potential to reap greater rewards over the entirety of life.

Simple and sensory information guides the use of an object already in hand. A hungry person sees an apple, grasps it, raises it until it almost touches the teeth, then bites. Information becomes more critical when the object of a drive is not available; one must comb one's memory to recall where and how to get an apple. But if there are competing motives—two different appetites or a constraint on appetite—experience may be unable to break the impasse. To eat an apple or a banana or a cookie or a celery stalk? Or skip between-meal snacks to lose weight or to have a greater appetite for dinner? Or avoid the apple because it was genetically engineered or treated with pesticides or because of being on a hunger strike? All such decisions include predictions about the likely value of the outcome of competing objectives, and none can be fully informed by direct experience. The brain processes that weigh the expected value of future rewards occur separately from those that gauge the value of immediately consumable objects (Montague and Berns 2002). Conceptual considerations about the mental processes that calculate these decisions are discussed in the section on executive function.

Figure 3 illustrates, in comic form, the diverging courses of action a man might take, from simplest to most complex, in accord with the man's degree of motivation to possess, acquire, or improve on a lost item.

### Obsessions/Compulsions

An obsession is an intrusive, sometimes repellent thought or image that one wishes to resist. Examples include fears that one has become contaminated by germs or toxicants, or that one has run over someone with a car, or that one will do some socially outrageous thing like shout obscenities in public, or that loved ones are going to be killed. Obsessions seem too strong to ignore and persist despite distraction or attempts at suppression.

Compulsive actions feel driven by forces other than desire or appetite or other adaptive motivations. One expects no gain or satisfaction from a compulsive act, just relief. Common examples include repeated hand washing, repeated checking of doors and appliances, counting rituals, and hoarding

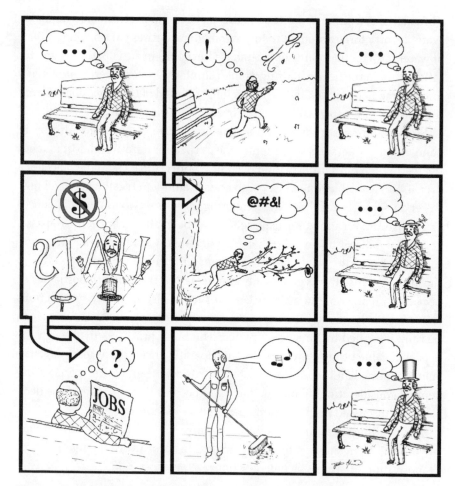

*Figure 3.* Complexity of action is a function of both the strength and persistence of a drive. *Top row:* an acute, stimulus-driven action may be self-limited if the drive is strong but transient. Our man's hat blows away, and he will expend energy to chase it, but once he loses sight of it he finds he doesn't miss it all that much. *Second row:* a persistent drive fuels a simple procedure, or simple sequence of procedures. In this example, he really wants his hat back. The attempt to purchase a new hat fails due to lack of funds, but the attempt to retrieve the hat from a tree succeeds. *Third row:* a strong and persistent drive fuels complex procedures, involving planning and uncertainty. In this case, he not only wants a hat, but he wants to upgrade his headgear. The lack of funds prompts an open-ended search for employment, which leads to labor, which leads ultimately to the purchase of a new hat. Drawings by Jack MacKinnon.

(that is, refusing to throw away worthless items like old newspapers). Such behaviors done in moderation can be normal. To feel a need to double check the door is within the bounds of careful behavior, but it is not normal to quintuple-check, and likely to produce significant problems in life if one feels driven to check 50 times. Careful behavior differs from pathological compulsion because, with careful behavior, action reduces the salience of the drive.

Obsessions and compulsions evade the normal regulatory constraints on action (Cavedini et al. 2006). As procedures, obsessions and compulsions tend to be simple. Most obsessive thoughts center on elemental worries: not the existential angst that one has chosen badly in life, but the simple fear that some singular, bad thing has occurred or may occur. Obsessions about social transgressions, like committing blasphemy, reflect a complex grasp of social appropriateness, yet involve fears of performing simple, rather primitive vocal acts. Similarly, compulsive behavior tends to be a procedure with only a few, stimulus-bound steps: turning a key or knob, washing hands, adding something to a pile, and so on. Compulsive behaviors are so simple, in fact, that they have been observed in other animals—dogs sometimes manifest a paw-licking syndrome that resembles compulsive hand washing (Eilam et al. 2006).

People who have obsessions and compulsions often have other forms of repetitive, simple behavior as well, such as tics (Graybiel 2008). But they tend not to have a global problem with all behavioral regulation; rather, they feel driven to perform only certain kinds of actions. That is, a person who performs compulsive checking generally does not also have an equally strong compulsion to count, clean, or hoard (Mataix-Cols et al. 2002). It appears plausible that the mechanism behind obsessive and compulsive phenomena must involve the errant selection and activation of simple action sequences encoded in frontal cortex. Because the action is aroused via an abnormal route beyond the sensorimotor feedback control of normal goal-directed action, completion of the action does not quench the impetus to act, hence the urge to act remains.

The common themes in obsessions and compulsions may yield insight into their nature. They rarely if ever involve a fear of direct harm, but rather of being exposed to the risk of harm (Abed and de Pauw 1998). Typical concerns reflected in obsessions and compulsions include the fear of being exposed to disease or dirt or dangerous chemicals, the fear of being exposed to danger from fire or home intruders, the fear of throwing out something that might be urgently needed someday, the fear of committing an unpardonable social offense. The fear of contracting an actual disease or being actually burned or invaded or socially ostracized is secondary, a step removed from the center of concern, and sometimes merely an afterthought. Nor does the person who has an obsessive preoccupation or compulsive behavior believe that the preoccupation or behavior is warranted by the circumstances. There is no excessive fear of disease or fire or ostracism. The obsessive-compulsive concerns make sense as expressions of an unusually intense fear of fear itself, of being left vulnerable to the risk of some specific form of physical, economic, or social harm, but not to actually suffering from harm. Whereas a person who has a paranoid delusion might bar the door from fear that danger lurks right outside, a person who performs compulsive checking examines the door repeatedly because failing to do so *might* allow an intruder to come in. However, no intruder is expected.

Many children express obsessive-compulsive phenomena in the normal course of development. Obsessions and compulsions are core to the diagnosis of obsessive-compulsive disorder and may also accompany mood disorders and the prodromal phase of schizophrenia.

## Extravolition

Some patients describe a disturbing feeling of the removal of volition; that some external force is directing their actions. This is not the same as the feeling of acting under the coercive influence of another person. There is no sense of wanting to do something or even of acting with reluctance. With extravolition, also known as a passivity experience, the person feels his or her actions are literally conducted without will. However, the person's actions may seem to the observer neither unusual nor uncharacteristic (or, at least, no odder than the volitional acts attached to the usual states of illness), and unlike truly avolitional actions like seizures, they are regulated by environmental stimuli.

This symptom of schizophrenia, as well as interruptions in the flow of thought (described as avulsions/intrusions in the section on attention), and telemission (the sense that one's thoughts are shared, involuntarily, with others, described under communication), share the remarkable property that they are purely subjective (Moscarelli 2009). There is nothing in the behavior of a person with such a symptom that validates its existence to the observer; the individual's private sense of being manipulated or of not owning his or her thoughts is all there is to it. Thus to speculate on the nature of these symptoms is to speculate on the nature of consciousness itself. In this case, one might speculate that there are feedback circuits of motor activity that relay information from prefrontal cortex to other parts of the brain about what action a person has just taken, and that this information fails to become integrated with the signals to prefrontal cortex that motivate genuinely volitional actions. This might create the unusual situation of a disconnect between the normal mechanisms that still motivate a person's actions, and the conscious self-awareness of that motivation.

### Apraxia

Like agnosia, apraxia—the inability to conduct organized, goal-directed behavior—can emerge from general cognitive deterioration, or occasionally as the result of a focal lesion. A variety of apraxias are recognized, classed by the nature of the function disrupted—for example, localized to face or limbs, or to gait (Gross and Grossman 2008). Overarching impairment in the organization and performance of goal-directed tasks, known as ideational or ideomotor apraxia, may render a person unable to demonstrate how to use an object (Wheaton and Hallett 2007). For example, asked to show the exact hand movements involved in shooting a pistol, a person with apraxia might point his or her finger in mimicry of a gun, but not know to flex the index finger as if actually pulling a trigger. Some forms of aphasia (inability to produce meaningful speech) are thought to reflect a specific form of apraxia (Kertesz and Hooper 1982).

## 2.7. Summary: Elementary Mind

The transformation of internal signals and external qualities into useful information begins with interoceptive and perceptual processing. The end result is *information*: the qualities the mind adds to a raw sensory experience that make it useful as a goad and guide for action. The utility of information may be measured by the adaptive quality of the actions it modifies and controls.

Interoception informs arousal and appetite. Tonic *arousal* denotes the general state of alertness, mediated primarily by acetylcholine-secreting neurons and reflected in the rapid, synchronous waves of brain activity one can see on an electroencephalogram of a wakeful person. Phasic arousal refers to changes in the state of brain activity in response to signals of threat or need. Phasic arousal is mediated by monoaminergic neurotransmitters—dopamine, nor-epinephrine, and serotonin—which radiate across the cortex to alter the localized intensity of neuronal activity, in response to demand. Insufficient arousal leaves one with anergia, or symptoms of fatigue and lethargy. Arousal in excess of demand renders one agitated, and potentially violent. Arousal disconnected from normal biorhythms produces delirium, as it interrupts cognitive processing, alters the significance of perceptions to the delirious person, and thus perturbs behavior unpredictably.

The mind gathers information about its specific needs largely from *appetitive* signals. Each system informs the mind when relief is needed, and again when satiety has been attained. Disruption of appetitive processes can be physiologic or voluntary, as one can choose when, by what method, and how thoroughly to satisfy an appetite. Sleep can thus be affected by alterations in the mechanisms of arousal, by external factors that impose on healthy sleep, and by behavioral influences. The drive to eat can be profoundly increased or decreased by purely biological disorder, or by maladaptive choices that may have a significant impact on the quality of life. Adaptive and satisfying sexual behavior generally requires a partner whose desires are in synch with one's own. The satisfaction of visceral functions may go awry when their auto-nomic regulation conflicts with other behavioral goals.

*Perception* extracts usable information from raw sensory data about the environment. The capacity to find order in raw sensation depends on integra-tive processing across multiple sensory modalities. One learns to identify shapes, for example, because their visual qualities match certain tactile prop-erties. The phenomenon of hallucinations, or aberrant perceptions in the ab-sence of sensory input, illustrates how a misfiring neuron (or set of neurons) can produce complex but false information. Illusions also provide false infor-mation, but tend to arise from abnormal states of arousal, like delirium or intoxication. Hysterical pseudosensory symptoms and pseudohallucinations demonstrate the potential for the perceptual function to be influenced by emotion and to be affected by behavioral motives.

In the development of *cognition*, one comes to learn how to differentiate one object of perception from another, and how to find common concepts that link them. Intelligence is a measure of the capacity to do so. Poor capacity for intelligence, whether due to natural endowment, environmental depri-vation, or biological dysfunction of the brain, may pose clinical problems. A person who has low intelligence may have a diminished ability to adapt to complex environments and challenges. When one has once possessed but lost the ability to recognize the full, accurate, and shared meaning of things, this implies not poor intelligence, but agnosia when a structural deficit affects entire cognitive domains, or disorganization when cognitive function is adrift, but not lost completely.

*Motion* can be understood hierarchically. At the foundation, the simplest neuronal elements convey signals to individual muscle groups, to produce motor activity. Effective motion requires the orchestrated activation of these motor elements. Action programs thus serve to unite a set of cortically encoded motions into a goal-directed activity. Purposeful action differs from mere motion in that action requires regulatory input from the perceptual parts of the brain. Some suggestible individuals experience a transient, circumscribed pseudomotor symptom under conditions of severe stress. One might see it as an inhibition against motion, motivated by the care, concern, and freedom from painful responsibility that ensues. Catatonia inhibits all volitional movement, and accompanies states of delusional terror. Both states respond temporarily to GABA-mediated tranquilization. Unlike pseudomotor symptoms, catatonia may persist despite taking a serious toll on the physical health of the patient. Abnormal movements—dyskinesias—like tics, tremors, rigidity, and so on present primarily in the domain of neurology, but bear mentioning because they occur commonly with mental illness.

Effective action requires constantly updated information about the environment. In a regulated *action* perceptual input starts, stops, and modulates the intensity of an activity according to environmental conditions. Obsessions (intrusive intentions to perform a simple but unwanted action) and compulsions (the needless but driven repetition of actions that fail to bring satisfaction) illustrate another failure of the control of action. In obsessions and compulsions, the failure of regulation occurs at the point where completion of an action (or of a thought process) would normally trigger release from the drive to perform it. Failures of action regulation also occur in psychotic extravolitional, or passivity experiences, in which the forces that arouse one's behavior become detached from one's recognition of any motivation to perform them. Brain insults can also cause a person to lose the ability to plan and organize simple actions, that is, to become apraxic.

# CHAPTER THREE

# Integral Mind

The primary elements of mental life—pure perception, programs that direct action, raw arousal, undirected appetite—barely register in the subjective world, but the results of their integration are more familiar: thoughts, intentions, and feelings. These subjective states emerge from the system that transforms their elements into useful information. Information about the body state defines the value, or *salience*, of objects of perception and action, with respect to our interests (Damasio 1999).

When we perceive a salient object or perform an action that alters the body state, the neuronal networks that encode the traces of the perceptions and actions remain active in real time, unlike a computer circuit that does its business instantaneously. For some time after a perception or an action, residual activity in the associated neuronal circuits allows them to become associated with prior and subsequent cortical activity. One may understand *thought* as this entrainment of live cortical activity one instant into the flow of cortical activity an instant later. That is, if one can understand conscious perception of the environment as a cascade of neuronal events triggered by external stimuli over time, one can understand a thought as a cascade of neuronal events stimulated internally, over time, by the neuronal events that happened just before. Thought begets thought, as the residual activity in a neuronal network activated in one thought becomes part of the input of the next thought. A train of thought thus represents the uninterrupted succession of network activating network, back and forth and round and round across the brain, until interrupted by something more salient, or until the state of arousal diminishes and attention wanders.

*Intention* links thought to drive. It marries an aroused appetite, defensive impulse, or conditioned desire to a specific program of action to satisfy it. Satiation quells the drive, but when time has passed and the drive returns, the appetitive or arousal signal automatically re-engages this established complex of drive, object, and action. Conversely, when one encounters a sensory stimulus that tickles the cortical representations of something one found salient in the past, a previously unfocused urge gels into a specific intention. In this way a thought about an object that has some salience to our drives automatically activates thoughts about the procedure we would undertake to obtain it, and vice versa. Linked to an active drive, these create a fully formed intention. At any given time we may harbor a number of intentions that may be compatible, unrelated, or in conflict.

A *feeling* unites thoughts with physiologic signals. Feelings and intentions share the property that they include information about the world and the state of bodily arousal. Feelings differ from intentions by the lack of a specific object or objective attached to them. Some feelings fall short of intentions simply because the drive has not yet ripened into a need or desire; others, such as the feelings of boredom or helplessness or desperation, have no specific object attached to them, by definition. If we knew what we wanted, or needed, or needed to get away from, we would have a different state of mind from a feeling, we would have an intention.

Do these subjective aspects of mental life have a function? Subjective life emerges from the melange of perceptions, thoughts, feelings, intentions, predictions, and memories that emerge from an awake brain (Tononi 2004). These elements of our subjective world correspond to specific, adaptive activities of the brain. When the brain derives information from its own activity, it essentially provides the mind with data about the internal effects of one's external experiences.

Mind need not, and perhaps cannot, be reduced to brain structure and activity. The content of mind courses through the neuronal networks of the brain

*Table 4.*    Integral Mind: Integration, Storage,
and Basic Use of Primary Mental Input and Output

| Function | Description | Disruptions |
|---|---|---|
| Attention | Integration of elements of mind in anticipation of possible goal-driven action | Distraction, avulsion/intrusion |
| Memory | Retention of perceptions following salient experience | Amnesia, flashbacks, pseudo-memory/pseudoamnesia |
| Habit | Goal-directed behavior conditioned by prior experience | Addiction, restricting/bingeing/purging, sexual deviance, self-injurious behavior |
| Value | Executive function: prediction of the relative value of the outcome of goal-directed activity | Disinhibition, suicidality, demoralization |
| Motive | Prediction of the quality and intensity of the immediate consequences of anticipated action | Anhedonia, apathy, territoriality |
| Desire | Quality of motivation to attempt to acquire an object because of its anticipated value | Dejection, excitement, irascibility |
| Alarm | Quality of motivation to attempt to avoid being surprised and startled by danger | Dread, paroxysms, guilt, paranoia |

as water flows in a river. The river remains constant, but from moment to moment the water molecules are never the same. Their movement over time, not their positions at any given time, carries boats and turns millwheels and powers hydroelectric plants. With mental life, the neurons and network circuits are always there, but they have no informational significance apart from their dynamic interactions with each other and with the environment.

Mental illnesses that derive from the elements of mental life tend to produce isolated symptoms. Forms of mental illness among the integrative processes of mind affect cognitive, executive, and affective functions. Many integrative dysfunctions derive from disease processes, but manifest clinically as maladaptive behavior. Addictions of all kinds and the core symptoms of major psychiatric syndromes arise from these integral functions of mind: depression and bipolar disorder, anxiety disorders, and dementia. The integrative functions of the mind as portrayed in the following chapters are charted in Table 4.

## 3.1. Off-Track Vetting: Disrupted Attention

The term *attention* calls to mind—brings to attention—the image of a spotlight illuminating one part of our mental activity, or zooming in and out of our inner map of thoughts, feelings, and intentions, or turning over an idea to examine its many facets. These images all assume a virtual observer who conducts the illuminating, zooming, and examining. If a model of attention depends on a virtual observer, implicitly or explicitly, it begs the question: who controls the virtual observer? If there is no virtual observer directing attention—if our minds are self-directing—then does this mean we have no free will to influence what we may choose to do or think? Philosophers have struggled over this problem for eons.

Rather than become sidetracked by philosophical problems, let us define attention by its function rather than by our subjective experience. Attention may be linked to action, or the readiness for action, but it seems not to be a requirement for action: one may act without paying attention and attend without acting. Acts that can be performed inattentively, if they are not simply mistakes, tend to be automatic and repetitive, requiring no new information. Attention paid without acting tends to characterize apprehensiveness; we suspend action while we gather more information. One can thus define attention as a state of readiness for action contingent on the appearance of a perception that cues one to act (Robbins 1997).

Attention is one aspect of *working memory* (Knudsen 2007). Working memory buffers the constant churn of perceptions, thoughts, feelings, intentions, and possible actions, to maintain the potential to engage them in action. A mind at attention resembles a car at a stop light, engine idling. The pistons pump, the driver aims the wheels in the direction she or he intends to go, but keeps a foot on the brake, awaiting the green light. In a similar way, the suspended state of arousal engages thoughts and aims intentions, and thus maintains attention until stimulated to act.

Some have argued that the idling consciousness that exists in a state of attention rehearses whatever action might come next (D'Esposito 2007). The prefrontal networks that coordinate action communicate with the higher-order sensory networks that guide action, as if the action were ongoing, rather than contemplated. Tonic arousal keeps the attention idling; phasic arousal revs the engine now and then. If the purpose of action wanes in importance, then the focus may shift elsewhere; deprived of fuel, the idling engine stalls.

Inattentiveness can result from alterations of arousal in either direction. In a state of low arousal, lost in a daydream, attention wanders as working memory drifts along with it. Pulled out of a reverie one may find it difficult to relate what exactly was on one's mind at that moment because the disparate elements hang together weakly. In a state of high arousal, the failure to hold salient perceptions, intentions, memories, and feelings in working memory reflects distractibility. A distractible person may focus laserlike on a train of thought only up to the point that other environmental stimuli of seemingly equal salience shift working memory to other trains of thought.

### Distraction

Attention to one task tends to weaken when a more stimulating opportunity beckons. Lacking motivation, and in states of intoxication, delirium, sleepiness, or fatigue, ineffectual drive fails to maintain focus on any one thing, so attention may wander freely, to become distracted, to alight on random associations or become stuck in ruminations.

Lags in cortical development can produce deficits of attention in learning-disabled children. That is, neuronal networks mature later than average. Lacking fully formed myelin sheathes, the axons transmit their impulses slightly more slowly than they should. Such children have more difficulty integrating activity across disparate areas of cortex (Castellanos and Tannock 2002). The capacity to maintain focus on abstract concepts that require complex cortical processing thus lags relative to that of peers. Immediate sensory stimuli overpower abstract thoughts and thus lead the child's attention astray. The child's performance at tasks calling for sustained attention might be adequate for a child several years younger, but inadequate at grade level. Although the cortical development in such children eventually catches up, the damage may accumulate if the inattention blocks the optimal development of age-appropriate cognitive skills.

A moderate degree of arousal enhances attention; excessive arousal tends to detract from it. Fearfulness or excitement helps focus attention up to a point, but other cues may redirect attention chaotically. People often describe themselves in these states as having "racing thoughts." Fearful racing thoughts characterize panic when they occur in the midst of crisis, and rumination when they occur in bed in the dark with nothing but worry to occupy the mind. Frustrated or angry racing thoughts, so intense and vivid that they overwhelm other cognitive affairs, may take the form of pseudohallucinations, as described in the section on perception.

Excited hyperarousal, seen in manic states, leads to intense focus on whatever thoughts or environmental stimuli happen to appear in working memory from moment to moment. Because any given idea seems so potentially exciting, attention tends to light on new stimuli, for brief periods, before moving on to the next irresistibly attractive stimulus. The person who has this type of excitement describes "too many thoughts"—ideas following quickly, one after another, in many different directions.

Attentional impairment is the core feature in the diagnosis of attention-deficit/hyperactivity disorder, and a common feature in mood disorders and delirium. Panicked thoughts along with symptoms of sympathetic arousal characterize panic attacks; pseudohallucinations and anxious ruminations occur in many states of high emotional distress.

### Avulsion/Intrusion

We take for granted that our thoughts are our own. Avulsion, or thought withdrawal, is the experience of feeling deprived of thoughts, as if some force had somehow reached in and removed them. Intrusion, or thought insertion, is the experience of feeling that thoughts have been placed into the stream of consciousness by some external force. They are working memory deficits in the sense that they are interruptions in the flow of awareness of one's own mental activity.

Avulsion and intrusion can be understood as expressions of the same general, pathological phenomenon. When a person experiences a normal interruption in the flow of thought, it is because attention has drifted or one has become distracted momentarily by other stimuli, but there is no sense of discontinuity; one can always paddle back upriver to re-enter the mainstream. In contrast, an avulsive or intrusive fragment of consciousness cannot be traced to its source. Like extravolitional experiences, described in the section on the control of action, the phenomenon is wholly subjective, a matter of how the person integrates the present train of thought into the general flow of working memory. What could account for the entry into working memory of a thought unlinked to other thoughts, or an action unlinked to intention, or a perception unlinked to sensory stimulus? As suggested in the discussion of hallucinations, it seems plausible to suppose that all of these phenomena could arise from aberrant activation of networks outside the circuits active in working memory at a given moment. Imagine the normal flow of thought as a symphony, and the psychotic symptoms as the dissonant music that would result if a group of rock musicians were to sneak on stage behind the horn section, plug in their electric guitars, and begin a simultaneous concert.

Avulsive and intrusive experiences are seen primarily in schizophrenia.

## 3.2. Forget-Me-Not, Not: Faulty Memory

All memory is selective. We retain information about things that arouse, excite, puzzle, frighten, relieve, or satisfy us. Memory requires neuronal plasticity—the changes in synaptic function that unite neurons into networks. There are two main phases of memory. Hippocampal associations mediate short-term memory. Neuronal associations within the cortex encode the most salient short-term memories and etch them into permanent, or long-term, memory (Squire and Zola-Morgan 1991). Less salient short-term memories fade in time, which is a good thing (Schacter 1999).

Memory denotes the functions of retention and recall. Memories denote something else: the subjective end result of the memory process, filtered through present thoughts, feelings, and intentions. The inability to retain information in memory devastates patients. The apparent inability to bring up old memories, and the experience of recovery of supposedly lost or "repressed" memories has more to do with present thoughts, feelings, and intentions than with the process of information retention and recall (Zola 1998). Table 5 compares the varieties of learning and memory.

How does the brain select what to retain? How does it access what it has retained? We retain memory traces of an experience *because* we access it frequently. The neuronal patterns active at a given instant in working memory can be fixed, at least temporarily, if they are bundled in a potentiated network linked together in the hippocampus (John 2001). If one is aroused by need or desire, the accompanying monoaminergic activity enhances these specific neuronal patterns preferentially over the less salient, mundane patterns that occur most of the time. Moreover, if an experience is important to survival, one will be more attentive to perceptions, interoceptions, and opportunities to act—hence there are more tags to ensure the experience sticks in memory. We retain the residues of significant experiences preferentially because they occurred when we were aroused, excited, puzzled, frightened, relieved, or

*Table 5.* Modes of Learning

| | Function | Structure | Utility |
|---|---|---|---|
| *Memory* | | | |
| Working | Integrate present perception and interoception with pre-existing thoughts, feelings, and intentions | Cortex-wide neural circuits incorporating sensory input | Maintain focus on environment and context simultaneously |
| Short-term | Retain the perceptual aspects of salient experiences for future reference | Hippocampus-dependent cortical circuits | Adjust to new or changing threats and opportunities |
| Long-term | Retain often-used and highly salient facts and experiences for permanent reference | Hippocampus- and sensory-independent cortical circuits | Readily reference frequently encountered or extremely important past experiences |
| *Skill (procedural memory)* | Retain the sequences of coordinated motion involved in skillful action | Cerebellum, motor cortex, basal ganglia | Perform tasks learned through practice, without the need to retrain |
| *Conditioning* | | | |
| Classical | Connect reflexive reactions to salient environmental stimuli | Plasticity in various subcortical circuits | Detect signs of immediate threat or opportunity |
| Operant | Retain sequences of actions involved in successful attainment of goals | Incorporates elements of short-term, long-term, and procedural memory | Similar to procedural memory, but includes cognitive skills and tasks |
| Fear | Prime autonomic nervous system for defensive reaction when threat is perceived | Circuits incorporating amygdala, bed nucleus of stria terminalis | Rapid defensive response, unimpeded by startle reflex |
| Reward | Associate drive-salient stimuli with goal-directed behavior to pursue drive satisfaction | Circuits incorporating ventral tegmental area, nucleus accumbens, VMPFC, amygdala | Ensure behavioral activation when a needed or desired object is near |

satisfied, and because we access them frequently in new contexts (LaBar and Cabeza 2006).

One may speculate that memories become permanent because their associated neuronal networks become self-sustaining. When a significant experience leaves traces in short-term memory—that is, triggers a hippocampus-mediated association—activation of any cortical element of that memory stimulates a chain of associated neurons downstream. Some of these neurons loop back from the hippocampus to the regions of cortex from which the activating neuron originated. When the original neuronal element of the experience is reactivated in this way, the circuit begins anew (this was illustrated in Figure 2). Thus an activated neuronal element within the network representing a short-term memory ultimately restimulates itself. The more salient a memory in everyday life, the more likely the reactivation of any of the neuronal elements that comprise the memory will find a path back from the hippocampus to their point of origin, and so create a self-sustaining loop. Thus the memories we ultimately retain in long-term memory never completely lose access to working memory because somewhere in the background they keep going and going.

The more momentous the event, the more likely it will become cross-linked to other life events, if only because it remains active in the background of working memory longer while one gets on with life. When a memory has been around long enough—on the order of months—and frequently accessed, the cortical network in which these neurons reside assumes a privileged place in mental life as part of permanent memory, and no longer requires the hippocampus to bind together its elements.

The quality of most memories changes as they make the transition from short-term imprint of a single experience to permanent memory (Moscovitch et al. 2005). The recursive process of activation and reactivation of short-term memories, across many different contexts, can explain how a richly detailed autobiographical narrative can be condensed to a simple fact in one's knowledge base. As the original memory tracing is rolled repeatedly through working memory, some core aspect of the original experience resonates with new information in active working memory, and some unique aspects of it remain apart from present experience. The unique aspects, if they rarely or never are reactivated in ongoing experience, fade relative to the aspects that are engaged and re-engaged.

For example, if you have taken a human anatomy course recently, you can probably recall many vivid and specific recollections of your individual sessions in the lab, including the joke you told your lab partners about the law of conservation of omentum, your inspired dissection of the brachial plexus, and so on. If you had a life-changing event in anatomy lab—say, you became engaged to your fiancé during a dissection session—you would never forget that day (Tulving 2002). Otherwise, all of those anatomy sessions will eventually recede in specificity, leaving mainly an impression about what anatomy was like, perhaps peppered with a few specific sensory details. Yet the sessions will also leave behind a firmly fixed knowledge of human anatomy.

Once one has studied anatomy, one never stops to think about where to locate the spleen, one simply knows it; but it may be hard to recall where one first heard about the spleen. Useful *knowledge* finds many applications. With each use, the unique but unimportant details attached to its acquisition wear away from disuse, while the useful bits are retained as a part of a permanent knowledge base. Unless some extraordinary thing happened in class one day, the long-term memory of the learning experience is likely to be nonspecific and impressionistic, while the core of the knowledge lives on.

Enriched memories for events survive this winnowing process as they are told and retold. The narrative itself becomes the fact of the matter. Communicated from one person to another, narratives have a power beyond that of mere fact to enlist the full apparatus of thoughts, feelings, and intentions in their reconstruction. Narrative memories both true and fictional, once entrenched in the cortex, can become impervious to change, even when new facts emerge that might alter the original narrative.

## Amnesia

In the absence of a functioning hippocampus, a person loses the ability to form new memories about facts and personal experiences; he or she has a form of *anterograde amnesia*. The person may be able to converse intelligently about things that happened in years long past, dress and eat independently (given the clothing and food), and live out a limited existence fully alert to present surroundings, but remain unable to hold on to any new information for more than a few moments (Zola-Morgan et al. 1986). This kind of amnesia does not preclude learning new skills, just new facts and experiences. If a person who has amnesia does learn a new skill, such as how to solve a pegboard puzzle or read backward in a mirror, he or she may have no recollection of the training experience or the fact that the task had ever been attempted before. In technical terms, *procedural memory*, which is largely a function of plasticity elsewhere in the brain, remains, whereas the hippocampus-mediated capacity to establish new memories based on *episodic*, or experiential memory, fails (Squire and Zola 1996).

Bilateral hippocampus lesions are fortunately relatively rare, but short-term memory loss frequently occurs as a side effect of electroconvulsive therapy (ECT). In ECT, patients—usually those who have severe depression—receive a series of treatments in which an electrical current is passed through the skull to produce a generalized seizure. Seizures induced by ECT interfere with the consolidation of short-term into long-term memory. Experiences during the course of ECT fail to become part of permanent memory. Once the course of ECT is complete, the capacity to retain new events returns to normal, but there may remain a permanent gap in autobiographical recall of the weeks before and during the treatments (Squire 1986).

The common forms of progressive dementia begin with subtle memory deficits. Because many older people have established stable habits, and have retired from active work responsibility, the deficits may not be readily apparent. But they tend to progress over many years to loss of other cognitive faculties, including the capacity to perform previously habitual actions (apraxia), to identify previously familiar objects (agnosia), ultimately, to speak (aphasia) or perform any coordinated action. These progressive dementias differ from focal dementias caused by a discrete stroke, for example, because of the cumulative loss of connectedness between cortical areas. Accumulation of protein (amyloid) plaques in cases of Alzheimer disease, or a series of small strokes in cases of vascular (multi-infarct) dementia, impede intercortical communication more, the more these pathological processes progress. Thus the severe failure of memory in end-stage dementia follows from a general inability to perform integrative cognitive functions.

## Flashbacks

Intrusive memories, or flashbacks, occur frequently to individuals who have experienced a threat to life or bodily integrity, that is, to individuals who have experienced trauma (Ehlers et al. 2004). Arousal enhances the salience of an experience and promotes the association of neurons into the potentiated networks that constitute the components of memory. A traumatic experience triggers the release of large quantities of norepinephrine (sympathetic activation, or "fight/flight"), which arouses the sensory regions of cortex (Southwick et al. 1999), and thus enhances sensory awareness and memory retention.

A truly salient traumatic event will be revisited in mind repeatedly for a variety of reasons. Fearful arousal stimulates mental activity aimed to find, in retrospect, an escape from danger should it happen again. Social motivations induce one to describe the event repeatedly, to gain support and to warn others of possible danger. Because a high state of arousal suffused the event, recollection of the event even in retrospect tends to induce some degree of arousal; hence the arousal induced by recall of the event reinforces the encoded memory. Under normal circumstances the memory of the traumatic event loses its emotional salience the longer it is relived without the reinforcing presence of actual danger (Maren 2005). But for some individuals the memory never loses its salience, hence any reminder of the traumatic event continues to evoke a full state of fearful arousal. The dread-inducing aspects of traumatic memories will be discussed in the section on alarm.

Flashbacks are a core feature of post-traumatic stress disorder.

### Pseudomemory/Pseudoamnesia

Experiential knowledge is notoriously prone to suggestion and invention. One can vividly imagine having experienced something, perhaps from hearing a story about it or having it suggested by a therapist while under hypnosis (Loftus and Davis 2006). Convinced of the truth of the story, one can reinforce it as one repeatedly stages and restages the imaginary experience in working memory. It is a real, reinforced neuronal network but a false memory. Individuals who describe false memories tend to do so with an air of dreamlike passivity. Under hypnotic suggestion, some individuals have been led to believe wholeheartedly in incredible and demonstrably false tales of having been abducted by aliens or exposed in childhood over many years to satanic rituals of human sacrifice (Ofshe and Watters 1998). In these accounts, there is often, incredibly, no hint of remembered efforts to escape the horror or even to report it to friends, teachers, police, or other relatives. Despite the apparently flimsy basis for such memories, they can feel like fully embodied sensory experiences and thus seem real to the person who experiences them (Kihlstrom 1997), in particular when another person, such as a credulous therapist, shares the belief in their reality and encourages the patient to tell and retell the narrative.

The flip side of false memory is false amnesia. Individuals who had no awareness of having been victims of childhood trauma and were induced by therapists to "remember" what turned out to be fantasies often had been taught early in treatment that they had "repressed" the horrific events (McNally 2005). The more the patient insisted she or he had no memory of a horrific event, the more horrific the event was assumed to have been, to have induced such a severe blockade of memory. There is a kernel of truth in the idea that a horrific event can block memory formation, but such events almost always involve brain trauma, which, like ECT and memory-blocking drugs, can transiently disrupt the hippocampus-dependent process of potentiation. One can never recover such memories, because no organized memory was ever formed.

One other form of pseudoamnesia concerns the claim to have forgotten events from the remote past. One expects some recent memories to fade, because of their relative insignificance. Altered states of mind, from depression or misuse of alcohol or drugs, for example, accelerate the process of forgetting.

Even permanent memories can *seem* to be lost if they fail to resonate with any ongoing experience or feeling, thought, or intention. Memories grow more difficult to retrieve if they are not continuously updated to link them to present experience. It can be disconcerting to try to recall something that was once important—such as the name of one's fourth-grade teacher—and be unable to recall it for several minutes, if at all. But this may be expected to occur the longer one lives without giving a thought to fourth grade.

In the occasional circumstance when someone does recollect after many years a verifiable experience that had apparently been forgotten, almost invariably the event was isolated, confusing, and disturbing enough to the person that it was misplaced, not lost, through a combination of neglect, irrelevance to other experience, and perhaps an aversion to reflection on the event from the time it occurred. An event fades if it is too bizarre or disturbing to gain frequent access to working memory. The fading of even happy memories inspires flights of nostalgia and high school reunions. Re-exposure to old, familiar perceptions reliably accesses those "lost" memories formed from the same perceptions.

A good grasp of the mechanisms of memory and forgetting should give the reader a clue as to the true nature of "fugue" states in which a person claims to have no recollection of identity, personal history, skills, or other events from the remote past (Kopelman 1987). Based on knowledge about the mechanisms of memory, one may conclude that it is physiologically impossible to lose this information without also having a massive disruption of other brain processes. These states of "amnesia" can best be understood the way other pseudoneurological deficits are understood. Like the hysterical person who behaves as if blind or paralyzed, the person in a fugue behaves *as if* memory were lost (Parfitt 1944). One may understand fugue states perhaps as the result of an intense aversion to the introduction of old memories into working memory, if conscious awareness of the facts of one's existence has somehow become sufficiently agonizing.

Fugue states are diagnosed as one of the dissociative disorders. False memories have become associated with dissociative identity disorder historically.

## 3.3. Stark, Craving Mad: Bad Habits

Insanity, in colloquial terms, describes the act of doing the same thing over and over and getting the same bad result. The fact that people repeatedly behave in maladaptive ways demonstrates the power of habit, or conditioned behavior.

The formation of a *classically conditioned* association requires two things: first, an autonomic response to an environmental cue; second, the repeated co-occurrence of that cue with a specific sensory stimulus (Escobar and Miller 2004). Pavlov's hungry dogs salivated without prior training when presented with food, but could be trained to salivate on hearing a bell, when Pavlov fed them consistently every time he rang the bell.

Cues akin to Pavlov's bell pervade our everyday life. When we have an active drive and encounter a stimulus that we have come to associate with its satisfaction, the encounter either expands, maintains, strengthens, weakens, or extinguishes the association (Domjan 2005). Suppose Pat likes the coffee at Ahab's Café. Whenever she sees the Ahab's logo, it reminds her of the satisfaction of drinking Ahab's coffee, and if she is not already feeling peppy, it induces her to think about having some right now. Every time Pat has a satisfying cup of coffee at any Ahab's, the association of the Ahab's logo and desire for coffee grows stronger.

Now imagine that Ahab's suddenly and secretly replaced all its caffeinated coffee with decaf. The effect this would have on Pat's conditioned craving for Ahab's coffee depends on what aspect of the coffee reinforced her desire. If the next visit to Ahab's resulted in a caffeine-withdrawal headache, she might develop a new conditioned *aversion* to the Ahab's logo. If she had a neutral response to the decaf—no withdrawal, but no satisfying caffeine lift either—she might continue to visit Ahab's but the conditioned response to the logo would ultimately weaken and become extinguished, especially if she found a new favorite place to get her caffeine. If she had enjoyed Ahab's coffee for its taste and not its caffeine content, experienced no caffeine withdrawal, and the coffee tasted the same, then the conditioned association of Ahab's logo to the anticipation of satisfaction would continue to be reinforced.

*Operant* conditioning (associated with the psychologist B. F. Skinner) expands on Edward Thorndyke's insight that the likelihood of behavior increases when it leads to a desirable consequence and decreases when the consequence is undesirable (Donahoe 1999). Thus, specific patterns of behavior can be altered when the behavior brings something desired (such as a food pellet for a lab animal or a paycheck to a human) or defers something undesired (such as an electric shock to the floor of the cage or a parking ticket) (Staddon and Cerutti 2003).

Complex behavior thus evolves through a series of steps. In the training phase, each individual step garners reinforcement, as in classical conditioning. So if a person wanted to train a monkey to play the piano, he or she could start by rewarding the monkey for merely banging on the keys. This not only encourages the monkey to make more noise with the piano, but also classically conditions the monkey to become excited in the presence of the piano. If one then rewarded the monkey only when it played certain combinations of keys, this would classically condition the monkey to find the corresponding tones exciting. The end result is operant, but the stages along the way are classically conditioned (Rescorla and Solomon 1967). Humans can replace such step-wise reinforcement with symbolic cues; that is, they are able to read the instructions.

### Addiction

Addictive behavior, whether related to alcohol or a drug, to the avoidance or forced regurgitation of food, or to the habitual pursuit of intense stimulation through gambling, sex, or self-injury, constrains one to a narrow set of actions that transiently resolve a conditioned craving at the expense of other, healthier motives.

Addictions bypass the natural mechanisms of drive and satiety (Goodman 2008). Normally, satisfying a biologically motivated drive results in a brief period of aversion, a refractory period in which one is more motivated to avoid than pursue the thing that one desired a short time ago. Wait a while—a few hours for appetite and thirst, the better part of a day for sleep—and the drive returns. In this way drives regulate themselves. Addictive behaviors, being unlinked to a natural drive, engage only part of the brain's motivational mechanism. They fail to resolve a physiologic state of need, and thus they tend to have an abbreviated refractory period. An addictive behavior may be satisfying, but it does not induce satiety; it generally inspires more, not less, of the behavior. In time, the addictive behavior itself may lose its ability to satisfy, but the craving acts like hunger and thus makes the behavior seem absolutely necessary (Koob and Le Moal 2008).

One can think of the period of craving as like the delay between the bell and the delivery of food for Pavlov's dog. During that time the excited dog drools and expects food. Similarly, outside the lab, a hungry cat rouses from its torpor and sashays to the kitchen when it hears the electric can opener. As a person develops an addiction, the rewarding effects of the behavior become coupled with cues throughout the environment (Hyman et al. 2006). An alcoholic might start to thirst while driving by a local bar; a person who used to snort cocaine might feel the urge again upon opening a packet of white, crystalline sugar; a bulimic might be tempted to binge while passing the cookie aisle in the supermarket. Unlike the hungry pet, an abstinent addict's unfed craving will diminish over time because alcohol, drugs, and binge-eating are not required for survival, but until that occurs an uncomfortable period of arousal draws attention to the object of addiction.

A non-addicted person can indulge in a variety of nonessential but exciting behaviors, such as drinking, sex, gambling, and extreme sports, and will be able to defer the indulgence when it would be inconvenient. What makes some people susceptible to develop an addiction to a narrow range of behaviors? Some factors are probably innate (Comings and Blum 2000). Some people get a more powerful reward from a particular activity or drug than other people; other people may suffer less from the adverse consequences of overindulgence. Either sort of person will be relatively undeterred by the ill effects most people experience from frequent, heavy use. Higher use, under more circumstances, with milder (perceived) consequences, fuels the process of conditioning. Conversely, some people possess innate factors that protect them against addictions; for example, many people, especially ethnic Asians, lack a fully functional enzyme (aldehyde dehydrogenase) necessary for the metabolism of alcohol. When they drink, they get sick, hence they rarely drink often or heavily enough to become alcoholic.

Addictions provide a reliable way to escape, if only for a moment, painful feelings of despair, anxiety, shame, guilt, anger, frustration, boredom, and emptiness. Pervasive dejection and dread, temperamental qualities that make a person vulnerable to intense, negative emotions, and life events that plunge someone into misery become fertile ground for the development of an addiction. Addictions lead to behavior that reinforces the addiction. An addicted person spends time and resources on the addictive behavior, and neglects problem-solving actions that might resolve the emotional turmoil that nurtured the addiction. Most addictions have corrosive effects on interpersonal relationships, finances, and health, and so create more fodder for misery that only the addictive behavior can reliably, albeit transiently, squelch (Sinha 2008).

At the extreme of chemical addiction, the drug alters neurotransmitter function, and craving evolves to physiologic need. As a result abstinence from the drug produces an abnormal brain state (withdrawal), and arouses behavior aimed to resolve the neurotransmitter deficit. At that point chemical dependence entails both unconditioned appetite and conditioned behavior, that is, the need for a substance truly becomes a driving physical requirement like hunger and thirst.

Addiction also encompasses habits carried on despite bad consequences, whether or not they induce a chemical dependency. The motivation may be for pleasure, in the sense that intoxication provides pleasurable diversion, excitement, social bonding, or other secondary kinds of reward. The behavior shades over to addiction when it achieves the status of habit, so that a person cannot plan diverting, exciting, or social activities without the addictive behavior, despite the costs of the addictive behavior in terms of health, finances, relationships, or social status. Thus many chemical addictions thrive not because of the development of a physical dependency, but because they are strengthened by other factors that reinforce their use and diminish the significance of negative consequences.

The diagnoses associated with addiction include dependence and abuse of alcohol and specific classes of drugs (opiates, stimulants, sedatives, cannabis, hallucinogens, cocaine), as well as intoxication and withdrawal from these substances. Addiction is generally a prerequisite for dependence and withdrawal syndromes. Other disorders of addictive behavior include pathological gambling and some sexual and eating disorders (see the following section). Mood, anxiety, and personality disorders contribute to the risk of addiction.

## Restricting/Bingeing/Purging

Anorexia nervosa and bulimia are addictive behaviors, not derangements of appetite (Davis and Claridge 1998). Anorexia is an unusual sort of addiction in that it involves not the ingestion of a biologically unnecessary substance, but the refusal to ingest biologically necessary substances. Although many people attribute the behavior to the cultural veneration of slender attractiveness, this does not explain the persistence of the behavior in some patients, long after they have wasted to an extremely unappealing state of emaciation. Nor does it make sense to see it, as some do, as an exaggerated pursuit of "control"—starving oneself to death can just as easily be seen as the result of a *lack* of control over one's behavior, not of excessive control. Anorexia can best be understood as an addiction to hunger and its physiologic correlates.

What could be motivating about being hungry? Extreme hunger has potent arousing effects (Sodersten et al. 2006). A hungry person may feel more animated and driven; the hunger-induced preoccupation with food may free the mind from worries about other painful problems, like family conflicts. As the anorexic person deprives the brain of nutrients, however, the brain acquires a diminished capacity for plasticity and learning, hence the anorexic person acquires an increasingly rigid behavioral posture with regard to feeding and other behavior. As starvation persists, it becomes physiologically more difficult to adopt alternative ways to behave and cope.

Bulimia does not produce starvation, but similarly can be understood as an addiction to the manipulation of the physiologic power of appetite and satiety. In place of starvation, patients who have bulimia crave the physiologically influenced psychological effects of gorging into a state of dullness and then forcing the body into states of arousal by vomiting or otherwise attempting to manipulate weight (Cooper et al. 1988). Bulimic behavior runs counter to healthy nutrition, disgusts others, and places the bulimic person at risk for serious medical repercussions from metabolic abnormalities and the exposure of the esophagus, mouth, and potentially the lungs to damage from stomach acid. As with other addictions, when used to combat unpleasant emotional states, bulimia does nothing to address the cause of the unpleasantness and generally makes it worse.

Restricting, bingeing, and purging are core phenomena in the diagnosis of anorexia and bulimia nervosa. Many patients manifest elements of both at some point, but tend to be drawn to one or the other by the aspects of behavioral reinforcement they find most salient. In terms purely of the diagnostic criteria, they are differentiated primarily by the factor of weight: anorexia nervosa implies a patient who is dangerously underweight.

### Sexual Deviance

Sexual disorders tend to combine high libido, or sexual drive, with objects of desire that are socially unacceptable and/or interfere with healthy attachment (Bradford 2001). High libido makes the desire more difficult to control. Interference with healthy attachment deprives a person of love; in terms of natural selection and reproductive advantage, it runs counter to rearing well-adjusted children. The question of social acceptance warrants more careful discussion. How do social norms define a medical problem?

The topic of sexual "deviance" as a concern of psychiatry has a controversial history (Spitzer 1981). Most if not all societies, or cultures, deem some sexual practices morally acceptable and some unacceptable. But medicine is a practical art, not a moral platform. Patients need treatment for the problems they have. One's personal aversion to certain practices can cloud clinical judgment, given the opportunity. Sexual acts done for pleasure and in moderation between one or more consenting adults are clinically "normal" regardless of cultural norms because people rarely consult clinicians about "abnormal" desire unless it produces a problem in some other area of life.

The key words in the previous paragraph are *consenting adults*. Our society grudgingly tolerates consensual sex between minors, but otherwise takes the firm view that sexual acts are allowable only between adults who engage in it of their own free will. Sex between adults and minors, or sex in the context of force or coercion exploits the younger or weaker party and is therefore considered a moral wrong. The moral condemnation and legal repercussions for a person who violates this imperative create a de facto medical problem when the person seeks therapeutic counseling or biological intervention to avoid harsh consequences. As a point of contrast, hiring an adult prostitute for sexual intercourse violates the law in most states, but garners far less moral condemnation, so being caught with a prostitute is less likely to induce someone to seek clinical help.

Many individuals who have pedophilic (sexual desire for children) or violent sexual desires find their desires horrifying but also find a life spent in constant, unfulfilled desire to be intolerable (Fagan et al. 2002). Rather than

exploit a child and suffer the consequences, some pedophiles and sexual pred-
ators agree to treatment to lower their libido—a "chemical castration" with
an implantable, testosterone-suppressing hormone. Individuals whose actions
sexually compromise but fall short of sexual contact with children, such as
exhibitionists ("schoolyard flashers") and consumers of child pornography,
risk punishment and condemnation as well. Society also abhors voyeurism
(spying on unsuspecting others while they are in compromising positions),
bestiality (sex with nonhuman animals), and frotteurism (attaining an orgasm
by contact with unsuspecting strangers, as on a crowded subway), though
these practices tend to generate more disgust than horror.

Even when all parties consent, sexual behavior can still be maladaptive if
it is practiced immoderately. Sexual activity that puts survival at risk clearly
poses a problem. Autoerotic asphyxiation—the occasionally lethal practice
in which a person attempts to enhance sexual response by constriction of the
air supply—excites some people but strikes no one as a healthy expression of
sensuality. The risk of death would seem to far outweigh the fleeting benefit
of an enhanced orgasm. Unprotected sex with relative strangers likewise risks
sickness and early death in exchange for transient pleasure. In addition to the
risk to health from sexually transmitted disease, it diverts a person from the
rewards of intimacy and affiliation. Though the term *sexual addiction* has more
popular than professional salience, an addictive pattern to sexual behavior
drives individuals who feel compelled to spend hours surfing for porn on the
Internet, or who masturbate multiple times every day, or who destroy stable
family life in the pursuit of a harem of mistresses, or "nymphomaniacs" who
pursue sexual activity with others on a frequent, regular basis, despite health
and social risks (Rinehart and McCabe 1997). Individuals who engage in these
practices and fail to find happiness or who come to recognize the potential for
harm may feel motivated to seek counseling.

The same potential obstacles to attachment apply to individuals driven to
practices psychiatry and society once saw (and in some cases continue to see)
as "deviant," such as homosexuality, sadomasochism, cross-dressing, and fetishism. But this concern also applies to practices never considered as psychiatric problems, such as adultery, polygamy, and group sex between consenting adult heterosexuals. Whatever legal, non-coercive, and safe thing a person
enjoys, if the single-minded pursuit of sex precludes investment in emotionally intimate relationships, then it is a potential problem for the person. It is
not, however, the case for those in an erotic minority that merely having and

acting on desires precludes a person from having loving, long-term relationships. Many of these practices, along with pedophilia and those that otherwise cause problems socially, share the common feature that the desire to practice them has been imposed on a person, not chosen (Munroe and Gauvain 2001).

Sexual disorder diagnoses are applied to behavior that is patently exploitive of others, such as pedophilia, exhibitionism, and frotteurism, and to alternative sexual behaviors that are purely consensual, when they interfere with healthy relationships. Homosexuality was removed as a diagnosis from an earlier version of the DSM.

### Self-Injurious Behavior

Causing harm to one's body by cutting, burning, pinching, head banging, and so on elicits psychiatric concern (Klonsky 2007). This kind of behavior in a psychiatric setting tends to be driven by one of two motives (Feldman 1988). Some patients derive an emotional reward, either via the sympathy or attention of others, or to experience a transient endorphin-mediated relief of acute angst (Sandman and Hetrick 1995). Others do so out of bizarre motives, fueled by psychotic ideas.

Some other patterns of deliberate self-injury occasionally draw psychiatric concern (Winchel and Stanley 1991). Patients who have some forms of congenital intellectual disability—Lesch-Nyhan syndrome, most notably—have an irresistible urge to gnaw at their extremities. Because of profound cognitive limitations, the interventions required to prevent this often involve simple but severe restraint, though behavioral conditioning methods can at times be effective. Some patients who have severe autism engage in head banging and other self-injurious action, for similarly unfathomable reasons.

Diagnostically, self-injurious behavior is listed in the DSM only as a feature of borderline personality disorder, but in practice is associated with mood disorders, psychotic states, eating disorders, and other addictive disorders.

## 3.4. Executive Bummery: Value Misjudgment

At any given moment, we may entertain dozens of competing drives, at varying levels of urgency. Our appetites, our states of arousal, our habits all connect to programs of action and salient sensory cues that guide action. These components of drive vie for priority in working memory and, ultimately, direct the execution of a course of action (Alvarez and Emory 2006). Executive function refers to this deliberative process that weighs the values of competing drives. Problems develop when we lose the capacity to assign appropriate value to competing drives, and when the power of one destructive drive negates all others and leads to suicide or violence.

Whether to act or not to act hinges on the strength of the drive, the value of available options to satisfy it, and the nearness of an opportunity to do so. A stinging, distracting pelvic pressure might be sufficient motivation to pull over at the nearest, filthy gas station, but a slight tingling in the bladder can wait for a cleaner rest stop down the road. Or, a far milder pelvic tingling that could be ignored for a half hour may prompt an immediate exit, if the next facilities are an hour away. These vignettes suggest that even within the simple act of micturition, there may be complex drives at work: to steer clear of grime and bad smells, to be able to get in and out and back on the road quickly, and to avoid or relieve painful bladder distension.

Other, separate drives may also sway a person to act or defer action. A dwindling fuel level may provoke a full pit stop at the next gas station, filthy or not. Overpriced fuel might push one away from a particular station. Caffeine craving and a sign for Ahab's coffee at one of the competing gas stations might become the deciding factor. To calculate the best outcome for even this apparently simple decision, an algorithm might be helpful.

But does the mind use algorithms to decide (Fellows 2007)? Economists model decisions in terms of the relative utilities or value a person holds for each good, and one could conceivably develop an equation to calculate the best option to maximize value with respect to cheap gas, strong coffee, and a clean place to void, and to minimize the time, effort, and cash expended. But the economists' equations assume a fixed set of variables. A new variable (a sudden yen for a Stuckey's pecan log roll), or a change in utility (a fear that coffee will interfere with sleep later), or a hidden variable (a preference for Exxon because of a love of tigers)—all upset the algorithm.

Prior sections of this book described only relatively simple actions, guided by perception and the prospects of immediate satisfaction. We are normally motivated by goals far more powerful and overarching than immediate needs and wants. Some behavior unfolds over time, with satisfaction measured over hours or years, or anticipated after death, if at all. The driver in the example wants to get to the destination quickly. The driver has a purpose; he or she could pull over and sunbathe along the median strip, stop in a seedy bar in a strange town, or drive off a bridge, but does none of those things because they disrupt the motivation to follow through with the travel plan. The driver also obeys rules; he or she could stop the car in the middle of the road and take care of bodily needs whenever the urge hits, or drive at twice the speed limit to get to the destination faster, or force another driver off the road and siphon off the gas, or worse, but does none of those things because of learned inhibitions against behavior that runs counter to moral sensibility, social mores, and legal prohibitions.

## Disinhibition

Lesions of the orbitofrontal cortex—the region of the VMPFC that overhangs the optic tracts—can produce profound effects on the capacity to make complex decisions. The famous case that illustrates the resulting functional deficit is that of Phineas Gage (Damasio et al. 1994). Mr. Gage in 1848 was a 25-year-old railroad worker who, as the result of an explosion, was pierced through the skull with an iron rod and survived. The rod entered just behind his left cheekbone, traveled behind his left eye, and exited the skull near the midline. Aside from losing a wide swath of the left frontal lobe, he sustained no other known brain damage. Although Mr. Gage survived, he was an irreversibly different man. According to his physician, he changed from being a stable, upright citizen to become "fitful, irreverent, indulging at times in the grossest profanity . . . impatient of restraint or advice when it conflicts with his desires, at times pertinaciously obstinate, yet capricious and vacillating, devising many plans of future operations, which are no sooner arranged than they are abandoned." In short, Mr. Gage could no longer adequately weigh the relative values of possible actions. His character after the injury suggests that he tended always to pursue the behavior that most strongly moved him at the moment.

Common closed-head injuries that cause sufficient shearing force on brain tissue to damage frontal lobes, and degenerative diseases like frontotemporal dementia (formerly known as Pick disease) manifest with similar coarsening of personality. A person who has a "frontal lobe syndrome" of this sort makes decisions apparently without the benefit of algorithmic calculations that weigh the value of present action against all other possible actions, but at a more primal level by urge and opportunity. When a sufficiently interesting cue presents itself, the person who has frontal lobe impairment may drop everything and pursue it, as there exist no competing intentions lurking in working memory with which to inhibit immediate, stimulus-driven action (Hinson et al. 2003).

The cortical code for long-term, overarching motives remains mysterious. Regions of the frontal cortex can be differentiated by their connections; anatomically there are distinct circuits that link specific frontal regions to specific subcortical structures, and ultimately to the thalamus, before the circuit loops back to the cortex (Alexander et al. 1986). However, the cortical geography may tell us as much as the subcortical connections can about the organic basis of executive function. Presumably, from what Phineas Gage and other people who have suffered frontal lobe injuries have taught us, the capacity to plan ahead and to weigh abstract priorities in decision making resides somewhere on the DLPFC (Cummings 1993). In contrast, focal injuries to the VMPFC tend to produce syndromes suggestive of a deficit in motivational and emotional functions.

To extrapolate from our model of the hierarchical organization of coordinated action, one might conjecture that the codes embedded in the outer limits of the DLPFC control not just one twitch or motion, as do the neurons on the motor strip, or one sensory-guided action that requires integration of the frontal cortex with other cortical regions. As one moves out from the motor strip, the codes become increasingly generalized, more engaged with neighboring circuits within the frontal cortex than with sensory association cortex. A neuron on the outer reaches of the DLPFC might encode some program as broad as "keep clean," or "make money," or "be kind," and thus feed innumerable smaller commands encoded in the cortex, like "leave time for a shower," "sell some junk on eBay," or "sign up to give blood tomorrow," increasingly narrow in scope and specific in the timing and circumstances of execution as they radiate back to the motor strip.

The salience of these generalized programs arises from crosstalk between DLPFC and circuits linked back to the motivation/emotion-oriented circuits in the VMPFC. Thus, a general concept—hygiene, avarice, or altruism, for example—originates in the primal sources of motivation, and informs the broadest strategies of behavior more directly than it does the detailed tactics that carry it out. Where the circuits between sensory and motor cortex control a simple stimulus-bound action like picking up a cup of coffee, the action generated by the instruction to "be kind" receives its controlling input from the network in the VMPFC that registers reward from the perception that one has contributed to society. When these circuits go missing from mental life, behavior becomes determined by narrower concepts of appetite and sensory-stimulated impulse, by default.

Disinhibition is a diagnostic feature of brain injury and some dementias and theoretically associated with schizophrenia. A relative inability to suppress impulsive responses is also a common symptom of attention-deficit/hyperactivity disorder.

## Suicidality

Suicide may be the ultimate philosophical question, according to Albert Camus (Camus 1955), but hard to reconcile with behavioral principles. What could motivate a choice to end one's life, when a world of other options is available? If it were a cost-benefit analysis, nothing could justify suicide, as there is no possibility for benefit after the fact. If suicide were simply the logical consequence of low expectations for pleasure, it would be far more common. Suicide tends to be something other than a default option when life loses value. To engage in a suicidal act generally implies an active drive to escape pain. One cannot gain by it, but one can cut one's losses. Not everyone in pain desires death, of course, but the loss of the capacity to anticipate both pleasure and relief from active pain seems to be the necessary combination of elements (Joiner et al. 2005)

Complex, disabling, chronic, and painful psychiatric disorders such as major depression and schizophrenia lead many people to suicide (Harris and Barraclough 1997). A person who has one of these illnesses may lose the capacity for pleasure (anhedonia), even in the fulfillment of basic bodily needs, and for hope, leaving the tormenting experience of a mind that sees only emptiness, threat, and darkness. Other life factors that contribute to the risk of suicide jibe with this model, in that they diminish hope in tangible ways. Older age, isolation, progressive physical illness, and alcoholism all contribute to suicide risk (Moscicki 1997). A host of biological and psychometric factors also contributes, in theory, to the risk for suicidal behavior (Fawcett et al. 1997).

Many individuals, who have committed themselves to a highly lethal course of self-destruction and lived, never choose to repeat (Seiden 1978). Suicidal intentions thus can lead to regrettable single acts, but can also become a persistent part of a person's mental life. People in perpetual pain may come to see the concept of suicide as one of the set of motivating forces that give meaning to their decisions. One can understand the drive to prepare for suicide by fantasizing about methods, by accumulating pills with which to overdose, or by adhering to subcultures that venerate death, as a potential "escape hatch" in case the pain worsens or the pleasure dries up.

The risk of suicide is elevated in most psychiatric disorders and is particularly high in major depression and schizophrenia.

## Demoralization

Demoralization denotes the emotional pain and behavioral inhibition associated with adversity (Clarke and Kissane 2002). In contrast to grief (discussed later in the section on affiliation) events that leave one demoralized tend to lack the finality of death: loss of love, loss of a job or purpose, loss of health, loss of security. When someone has reached a state of demoralization, he or she has lost hope of pleasure and relief from pain, in general. In contrast to anhedonia and dejected mood, however, the capacity to experience pleasure, satisfaction, or relief remains; only the hopeful expectation has been lost. Hopelessness, and the helpless behavior that follows, illustrate a failure of executive functions to permit the pursuit of one's interests to enter into decision making.

The learned helplessness paradigm in behavioral research models demoralization. When one places a rat in a vat of water it will struggle mightily for a time. If one keeps it in the water until it ceases to struggle to swim, the next time in the water it will spend less effort trying to swim. Challenge the same rat in another way—dangle it by its tail, for example—and it will show a blunted tendency to struggle. The rat has evidently been conditioned to view escape efforts as futile in general. It has learned to be helpless (Seligman 1972).

Of course, no one can know whether the rat *feels* miserable at this point (Anisman and Matheson 2005). But people often reach similar points in life, where adversity in one area generalizes to the prediction that there is no escape from adversity in any area of life. It may seem that the struggle to manage one problem makes other problems worse. The biological basis of the painful aspect of learned helplessness involves the glucocorticoid stress response, described in the section on the brain (Shumake and Gonzalez-Lima 2003). Glucocorticoid release after prolonged sympathetic arousal (as would accompany a prolonged exposure to threat) induces the body to stand down from a heightened arousal state to conserve resources, while at the same time mobilizing for a prolonged struggle. The psychological effects of glucocorticoids are complex; cortisol can be activating, but persistent elevation washes away arousal, leaving a person depleted.

To understand demoralization and its relief is also to understand the placebo response and psychological healing. How, for example, can a person recover when given an inactive pill? The answer of course is that the inactive pill does not cure the disease directly, but it does reverse the painful aspects of the demoralization and stress that accompany the disease (Benedetti et al. 2005). The placebo-induced resolution of acute traumatic pain, for example, does not heal the wound, but it does permit the release of endorphins that allow the patient to rest. In therapeutic trials of antidepressants, one often sees the active and placebo groups improve for the first week; subsequently the active group continues to improve and the placebo group worsens. This phenomenon seems particularly remarkable when the depression is the illness in question, because depression tends to be defined by its unredeemable hopelessness. It suggests that even people in the grip of a major depressive illness can be demoralized on top of it. When demoralization occurs without the loss of the capacity for pleasure, that is, without the depressive syndrome, the individual may fail to pursue pleasure actively, but experiences pleasure adequately when it is brought to him or her.

Psychotherapy is not placebo; whereas a placebo can diminish demoralization temporarily, psychotherapy can resolve it (Frank 1974). Following the work of Jerome Frank, the term *psychotherapy* in the broadest sense includes any form of healing in which the elements of an emotionally charged healing ritual is performed in a therapeutic context. We return to this idea in the final chapter on therapeutic principles.

The diagnosis most like demoralization is adjustment disorder. The phenomenon of demoralization, however, is of universal significance in chronic disease, psychiatric and otherwise, and magnifies the suffering experienced by patients.

## 3.5. You Can't Always Want What You Get: Emotional Miscue

Motivation and emotion both derive from the Latin root *motus*, meaning movement. They correspond to the subjective experiences of intention and feeling. One may be moved to intend to do something, or moved to a state of feeling.

Motive goes two ways and variations abound: pleasure and pain, desire and fear, reward and punishment, behavioral activation and inhibition, approach and avoidance, appetitive and aversive, positive and negative valence. In essence, some motivated behavior aims to acquire an object, and the other to be rid of it; some emotion reflects a yearning to embrace an object and some a wish to shun it (Lang and Davis 2006).

These counterbalancing modes of emotion and motivation apply to both classical and operant models of conditioning. A lab animal can be classically conditioned to salivate on cue for food or to freeze on cue before a shock. The animal can also be trained to work to receive food or to avoid a shock. In either case, if a lab animal could report an emotional state, it might describe the anticipation of food as a pleasant feeling of excitement and the anticipation of a shock as an unpleasant feeling of dread. When the animal has eaten the food or survived the shock, excited or fearful arousal dissipates.

Classically conditioned anticipation and learned actions correspond to the same qualities of experience. One might be just as excited by a visit with an old friend whether the anticipation quickens one's step en route to the rendezvous, or merely fills one's head with fantasies about the fun times ahead, while at home awaiting the friend's arrival. The difference lies not in the quality of the arousal but in how one uses the arousal. One might feel a similar sense of apprehension awaiting the arrival of the police to place one under arrest or when making the trek to the station to surrender. And one would be just as relieved to learn that the charges had been dropped whether one had stood before the judge or had heard the happy news over the phone from one's attorney.

Emotion and motivation differ mainly in their proximity to action. Motivation implies an intention to act to alter a state of arousal. With emotion, the plan to act to change the state of arousal has not been fully formed. However, the boundary between emotion and motivation is fluid in both concept and functional neuroimaging (Cardinal et al. 2002). A mere thought separates having a feeling and feeling like doing something, or having a vague yearning and wanting something specific.

In the prescientific or commonsense view of emotional function, a person feels angry and scowls to intimidate a foe and clenches fists to prepare to strike, or feels sad and cries to signal a need for comfort, or feels joyful and communicates it by smiling, to share with others. Early psychologists like William James challenged common sense with the contrary view that one feels angry *because* one clenches one's fists, sad *because* of crying, happy *because* of a smile (James 1884). While appealingly modern, this idea too had flaws; for example, electrical stimulation of nerves to specific facial muscles could induce a grin, but with no subjective sense of pleasure. To account for the concordance of feeling and expression in emotion, the feeling state must be integral to the behavioral response (Cannon 1927).

The modern idea has emerged that emotions combine arousal with context. A person will feel angry when physiologically stimulated and exposed to irritating circumstances, sad when arousal is dampened and something valuable has been lost, joyful when high arousal accompanies a rewarding event. Schachter and Singer's classic experiment demonstrated this point elegantly (Schachter and Singer 1962). Subjects were either knowingly or unknowingly given a stimulant drug and exposed to either an actor who behaved angrily or one who cracked jokes and behaved merrily. Subjects who knew about the stimulant reacted little to either actor, but subjects who did not know tended to report feelings congruent with those of the actor. This experiment showed that, in addition to physiologic arousal and the social context, the final ingredient in emotion is the sense that it is a genuine response to circumstances.

If equivalent physiological arousal can provoke pleasant amusement in some people and irritation in others, depending on their circumstances, it begs the question of how we come to view experiences as positive or negative in the first place. Emotional experience, like organized perception, develops through a long process of conditioning. How do we learn to anticipate pleasure before we experience it? How do we learn to recognize and respond to life-threatening danger without getting ourselves killed? These questions will be addressed in subsequent sections.

Mental problems that illuminate the nature of motivation and emotion include the amotivational states—apathy and anhedonia—as well as the exaggerated defensive drive that accompanies territoriality. Note that a person who has anhedonia or apathy lacks the drive to act, whereas a lazy person finds inactivity rewarding.

## Anhedonia

Anhedonia (from the same root as "hedonism") denotes the inability to experience pleasure. Over time, the person who has anhedonia not only fails to experience pleasure here and now, but also loses the capacity to anticipate pleasure (Pizzagalli et al. 2005). The motivational cycle of drive, satiety, and reward includes several break points, where anhedonia can arise (Wise 2008). For example, under conditions where reward is blocked (that is, where sub-cortical signals of satisfaction and satiety fail to reinforce cortical activity), repeated exposure to any previously pleasurable stimulus will extinguish its association with pleasure. Although satiety functions as expected to abate the biological impetus for a behavior, the absence of hedonic function under-mines the drive to act the next time an appetite pops up. Like the coffee-drinker who missed the caffeine-buzz when Ahab's secretly switched to decaf, an anhedonic person eats to quell hunger pangs, but ultimately will lose the reinforcing properties of food, and thus have no interest in eating.

Anhedonia is a core symptom of major depression. It is present to a less complete degree in some personality disorders, in particular, schizoid and obsessive-compulsive personalities.

## Apathy

Apathy often suggests an attitude of willful indifference (Levy and Dubois 2006), but can also denote a relative inability to care. Whereas an anhedonic person is unmoved by the prospect of pleasure, an apathetic person is un-moved by the opportunity to avoid pain or loss. Anhedonia can lead one to waste away because food seems unappetizing; apathy undermines any sense of concern over this problem. An apathetic person may have no lack of fear, but fails to find safety sufficiently motivating to expend much energy to re-lieve or avoid it. When an apathetic person says, "I don't care what happens to me," it is not an expression or bravery or selflessness; it means "My life has no value, so there is nothing to be lost."

Neither anhedonia nor apathy necessarily implies a pathological inter-ruption of brain functioning, though often apathy accompanies brain disease (Marin 1991). People learn to be apathetic politically, for example, by the ex-perience of disillusionment with public affairs, and they develop diminished anticipation of sexual pleasure if their attachment to a partner is severely strained. Gross disturbances of brain function in which apathy is a character-istic symptom tend to be those that affect subcortical structures, hence the central apparatus of behavior arousal (Cummings 1986).

Apathy is characteristic of major depression, schizophrenia, and subcorti-cal dementias; it may also be an aspect of an adjustment disorder diagnosis.

## Territoriality

Territorial hostility arises from the perception of a threat either to oneself or to the people and things one values (Wilson 1970). Territoriality assembles both motivational forces into one potent, combustible compound; to keep what one values, one must repel anyone who might tear it from one's grasp. One may think of it as the motivational correlate of the "fight" part of the fear-driven "fight or flight" response, which will be described in more detail in the section on alarm. Like any imperiled creature, physically cornered by danger, a human under threat may see no choice but to fight (Blanchard and Blanchard 2003). A threat to one's interests may also compel hostile action, because one cannot abandon one's interests without surrendering some extension of oneself. Thus hostile action serves to defend not only territory or family, but also abstract concepts, such as honor or country or freedom—the kinds of ideas that people fight for in wartime. One cannot flee from a threat to territory or family group or abstract beliefs without losing some essential aspect of the self; therefore one must attack.

Spousal abuse and other forms of domestic violence vividly illustrate this dynamic of hostility. Although much domestic violence can be related to individuals who are aggressive or volatile to everyone, others limit their violence to their families (Holtzworth-Munroe and Stuart 1994). The spouse and children comprise the domain of such individuals—their personal territory. Expressions of dissent seem like treason; a threat to secede from the union becomes a declaration of war.

In many cases, these hostile individuals have witnessed or been the victims of violence in their own upbringing (Feldman 1997). The violent response may thus be partly modeled and partly a conditioned response to any threat to the integrity of the relationship. As a consequence of abuse, the abused partner may reasonably seek escape. The desire to escape abuse truly threatens the relationship, so the cycle repeats and escalates.

One can also understand in this territorial context the hostility that motivates bigotry. Bigoted people despise those of a different race or culture or socioeconomic status or intellectual capacity or sexual orientation. "Those people" are different—unfamiliar—hence the bigoted person perceives a disadvantage when he or she must deal with them, if only from ignorance of their strange ways. Whether or not the despised group poses any material threat, the mere fact of its existence impinges on the domain in which the bigoted person feels comfortably knowledgeable and in control. Hostile aggressors thus tend to see the alienness of members of the despised group as the only salient thing about them (Haslam 2006). At a societal level, the symbolic dehumanization of foreign enemies through caricature and propaganda motivates political violence and warfare. Apparently unprovoked hostility can accompany states of paranoia and other delusions. In these cases the hostile person acts from a perceived threat to his or her interests, for idiosyncratic, possibly psychotic, reasons hidden to everyone else.

Hostility can be seen in some states of depression and mania, especially mixed mania. Patients who have paranoid delusions as part of schizophrenia, or nondelusional paranoia in paranoid personality disorder, frequently live in a state of hostility.

## 3.6. Displeasure Principle: Displaced Desire

We have thus far regarded behavioral motivation generically, equating reward with relief and deprivation with pain. But these distinctions between attractive and aversive motivations matter in mental life. To plan, we must represent in working memory some concept of our aims. Appetitive need, and conditioned environmental cues that promise reward, drive behavior aimed to acquire the needed or rewarding objects (Berridge 2004). We tend to think of these as pleasurable. But why is pleasure pleasant? In other words, what attracts us to pleasure? We are not simple organisms that move always toward the resources we need to survive. We can want what we do not need and cannot have.

Pleasure is currency in the mental economy; it is the basis for comparing the relative value of competing drives. Disturbance in the capacity to arouse or control pleasurable motivation in mental illness causes unfathomable suffering. The inability to be motivated to pursue pleasure, as we have seen, constitutes anhedonia, and is the source of despair in depressive illness. The insatiable pursuit of pleasure—a greed for pleasure—defines the core phenomenon of depression's counterpart, mania.

Pleasure resembles the relief from pain, qualitatively. Strong desires often have a painful quality, such as intense hunger or the pressing urge to empty the bladder. The yearning for companionship and sex is an aching feeling; Cupid shoots arrows, not marshmallows. Whatever the need, the pleasure in relief is generally proportional to the intensity of the ache. Physiological states like dehydration, breathlessness, and hot or cold body temperature have qualities as urgent motivators, and similar mechanisms of reward when they are relieved (Seymour et al. 2005). The mechanisms that mediate the satisfaction of appetite and the relief from pain overlap. Communication between subcortical nuclei and prefrontal cortex ensures that we retain, within our repertoire of encoded action programs, whatever we did to achieve satisfaction or relief (Everitt et al. 1999).

But the reward system seems inadequate to explain the mutability and power of pleasure (Berridge and Kringelbach 2008). If the satisfaction of a specific appetite or drive, or relief from a specific source of pain, yields simply the reinforcement of a learned response, we might have a myriad of specific satisfactions, but not a unified currency of pleasure. The general attraction to pleasure, or the pleasure response, derives from our earliest experiences of satisfaction and from its physiologic correlates. We become conditioned to expect pleasure not only in the objects or activities that satisfy or relieve specific drives, but also in the other objects, activities, people, and circumstances that accompany satisfaction.

Newborns seem unable to anticipate reward and certainly lack the power to seek it. A newborn's first lesson in operant reward conditioning begins the first time he or she cries from hunger. The newborn does not know that crying will trigger events that will relieve hunger; any intense, uncomfortable state of arousal leads to crying. The sound of crying moves the mother (or other caretaker) to provide comfort and milk. Milk produces taste and visceral stimulation and yields nutrients that reverse the hormonal signals of hunger and induce hormonal signals of satiety (Cota et al. 2006). Satiety inhibits sympathetic activation, raises parasympathetic tone, and thus quells motor activity. The baby settles. The baby has now begun to learn that crying initiates a process that provides relief.

How did the baby learn this? Satiety signals initiate activity in subcortical dopaminergic neurons that project to the prefrontal cortex and associated basal ganglia structures (Schultz et al. 1998). There, they facilitate the retention of prefrontal cortical networks that encoded the sequence of actions that produced the satiety response. Whatever the baby did at the time the satiety-producing event occurred, she or he will now more likely do again, the next time the same feelings and perceptions emerge (Schultz 2006).

Over time and with repetition, the cortical networks associated with hunger, crying, mother's face, milk, the warmth of being held, reliably come together whenever hunger is superseded by satiety. These experiences classically condition a hungry infant to *anticipate* pleasure when the mother approaches, well before food is ingested, before the infant is even painfully aware of hunger, and without the great effort involved in crying. Some of the factors that at first induced pleasurable relaxation only after feeding now produce the anticipation of pleasure before feeding. Hunger becomes an excited feeling of anticipation—perhaps even pleasant—rather than a desperate sense of emptiness.

As a baby becomes mobile, the sight, sound, taste, touch, and smell of desirable things and people excite not only yearning, but active exploration. Thus, we humans learn to gauge how close we are to encountering in the environment perceptions that match our internal representations of pleasure. If what we have been conditioned to want grows larger, louder, or more fragrant in our perceptions, our excitement increases; if it fades, excitement wanes. As excitement wanes, the prefrontal cortex receives signals to inhibit, not activate, behavior (Matsumoto and Hikosaka 2009). Trudging through the desert, the sight of an oasis quickens the traveler's step; but when it turns out to be a mirage, that sinking feeling is the dissipation of anticipatory excitement.

Babies reared without warmth and affection often fail to thrive, even when they are given food, shelter, and safety (Ainsworth 1962). If there is a failure to associate feeding and the relief of hunger with a variety of other cues (warmth, attentive mother's gaze), then the capacity to anticipate pleasure based on these or any other cues grows impoverished. If an infant reared in a reward-impoverished environment does survive, there may be persistent problems with feelings, affiliative, and cooperative behavior.

## Dejection

Mood can be defined as a persistent, pervasive, and free-running state of emotion, unmoored from the normal influences of the environment and physiology. The feeling stays, even when context shifts. A person in a truly happy mood may exclaim, "Nothing can bring me down!" Dejection, with its scatological undertones (in medical jargon), suggests the opposite: a mood that nothing can elevate. Dejection is one of many ways one can describe the mood of one in a depressed, or melancholic state. The term *depression*, however, sows much confusion because it can refer both to a common symptom of low mood, and to a diagnostic entity related to a crippling mental illness, so in this book the term *depression* refers only to the illness.

A dejected mood implies anhedonia (Naranjo et al. 2001). If a dejected person could experience and anticipate pleasure, then the emotional state would no longer be immune to environmental influence and therefore could not be considered a true mood. Thus the key difference between a dejected person and a demoralized person is this: a demoralized person lacks any opportunity to feel better because of adverse circumstances or because she or he has become too discouraged to seek pleasure; a dejected person feels bad despite having opportunities for pleasure.

In a dejected mood state, a person's self-attitude suffers. Self-attitude can be understood as the quality of pleasure or satisfaction a person may enjoy in reflecting on his or her own past accomplishments, present mental and life activities, and future prospects. A dejected person takes no pleasure in the contents of his or her own mind, and may even have a painful reaction to the recollection of personal history, reflection on the contents of working memory, or anticipation of future actions. A person who lacks the capacity to find reward through any form of self-reflection becomes conditioned to seeing the self in a negative light. A person who has a low self-attitude thus may consider himself or herself a failure in past deeds, ineffectual in the present, and worthless with respect to future value.

Dejected mood characterizes the major depressive syndrome, where it may manifest as pervasive sadness, angst, irascibility, or numbness. In milder degree it is the core feature of dysthymia. Dejection may also accompany psychotic disorders, borderline personality disorder, and other disorders in the mood spectrum.

## Excitement

Excited emotions are normal in the context of eager anticipation and active enjoyment. A high or elated mood state describes persistently excited emotions in the absence of appropriate stimulation. For a person in an excited mood state, the exaggerated motivation for and emotional response to the prospect of pleasurable reward persists beyond the point of satisfaction (Johnson 2005). The potential to become aroused to action attaches itself to whatever drive seems most salient moment to moment. Whether this manifests as action or merely fantasy, the excited person may feel literally as if she or he can do no wrong.

When all actions promise equally exciting rewards, behavior hinges on opportunity, not the rational calculation of costs, risks, and benefits. This loss of rational processing leads to uninhibited excesses of spending, speeding, sexual adventuring, and other forms of impulsive, high-risk activity that can derail the life of a person with an intensely excited mood. In contrast to the self-attitude of a person in a dejected state, a person who has an elevated or grandiose self-attitude finds rewarding aspects to all internal experience and mental content, so the person logically concludes that the high value attached to all thoughts and actions proves superiority as a person.

Excited mood typically accompanies heightened energy. As described in the section on arousal, the feeling of having or not having energy, of feeling anergic or vital, demonstrates how motivated a person feels toward action. In contrast to the anhedonic, anergic, dejected person, who must laboriously find a motive to undertake every step in a mundane task, the excited person is driven forward by the ultimate reward of actions today, compounded into a future, glorious destiny. Thus, it is no trouble to find the energy to work tirelessly, around the clock, and then to abandon one task for another that seems even more promising.

Excitement primarily characterizes mania, which is the core feature of the diagnosis of bipolar disorder. The virtually universal occurrence of depressive states in people prone to manic states suggests a pathology of motivation as the common cause of the wayward moods in bipolar disorder (Depue and Iacono 1989).

## Irascibility

An irascible person expresses florid hostility, triggered by minor provocations. Excited moods often give way to irascible states. Irascibility and excitement together can be understood functionally as related by the dynamics of motivation, hostility, and territoriality. A person in an excited state sees treasure all around, and figuratively, if not literally, assumes ownership. But if everything one surveys comprises one's personal fortune, then the territory one might feel the need to defend is also virtually limitless. An irascible person may thus perceive an innocent statement about the weather as a threat if it contradicts that person's own, absolutely definitive opinion about it. When one feels a personal stake in everything, opposition makes one fight because one cannot flee.

How does a delightfully excited mood give way to a mean, irritable mood? Initially in an excited mood it may seem that nothing could threaten well-being, as everything seems part of one's personal territory and all is well. But the world inevitably offers resistance to this expansive viewpoint. Territoriality, hostility, and an irascible mood follow. Moreover, the heightened state of autonomic activity in a state of elated excitement cannot be maintained indefinitely, and so the stress response may at some point undermine the normal process of emotional adaptation (Zalcman and Siegel 2006). By contrast, when irascibility occurs in the context of a dejected mood, it can be understood as the exaggerated perception of loss predicated not on the illusion of overinvestment in objects, but on the illusion that one is losing what little of value remains.

Aggression and irascibility are common to manic and mixed mood states, and may arise in people who have schizophrenia. Individuals who have paranoid personality disorder may appear irascible to others who are not aware of their secret resentments, and those who have borderline personality tend to manifest rageful reactions to the threat of losing a relationship.

## 3.7. Fear Factory: Hyperactive Alarm

Things we desire pull us forward until they fill our senses; they cease to move us when we lose desire. What force motivates us to steer clear of danger? First is painful experience. Having burned one's hand once on a hot stove, one learns not to touch it again. But how does one learn to fear deadly things like rattlesnakes and speeding cars? Not from experience. We rely on the startle reflex (Grillon 2008). The startle reflex halts us in our tracks and jolts the sympathetic nervous system to prepare to overcome or escape an imminent threat. Analogous to the pleasure response, which emerges as one learns to anticipate reward, we learn to anticipate being alarmed—startled and aroused by fear—under certain general conditions, and we are motivated to avoid this unnerving experience. The motivation behind much defensive behavior is largely the drive to reduce the possibility of an unpleasant surprise. We can either steer clear of things that have startled us, or we can pre-empt startle by becoming pre-aroused to the prospect of danger.

Alarm begins with the startle reflex, and then progresses to a sympathetic surge to mobilize the body for "fight or flight." The startle reflex freezes us in our tracks and focuses all attention on incoming perceptions. Startle involves a relatively simple neuronal relay: sensory organ to thalamus to amygdala to subcortical structures to motor inhibition and autonomic output (Davis 1998). Note that the neuronal pathway of the startle reflex bypasses sensory cortex.

We startle before we have time to process the perception. Specific, scary things like sharks, earthquakes, or muggers do not startle us because we know them to be dangerous, though they may frighten us once we recognize the danger. They startle us because they share the one unifying aspect of startling stimuli: they are strong stimuli that occur abruptly. Startle can follow any significant, abrupt change in sensory stimulus detected in the thalamus as an unanticipated shift in activation of a population of sensory neurons. These neurons register sudden, strong sensory stimuli, for example, a bright flash, loud bang, sudden force on a limb, noxious smell, or rancid taste. When these qualities of a stimulus are detected in the thalamus, they relay a signal to the amygdala to initiate startle.

Startle arrests all other goal-directed action. This serves two purposes: it denies a predator the sight and sound of our motion, and flushes all but immediate perceptions from our working memory. To freeze when chased by a wild animal may expose one to the risk of being pounced on, but may be adaptive when the nature and location of the possible threat is unknown. When a person routinely encounters strong, sudden sensations, startle may be maladaptive. We do not startle every time we turn on a bright light or hear a car horn on a busy street. Nor does a seasoned deep-sea fisherman startle upon seeing a fin, or a senior seismologist when the earth shakes, or a veteran tight end as he is blindsided by a linebacker. In spite of its intensity, the stimulus in each of these examples lacks the element of surprise. How does one learn not to be surprised?

Newborns have a sensitive startle reflex. A face thrust into view, a mild shake, or a sharp clap often produces a characteristic momentary inhibition of motor activity. Every sensation is surprising when it is unpredictable. Infants have the capacity to learn to inhibit the startle response through experience (Bridger 1961). The newborn's hypersensitive startle fades early in life, at around the time the capacity for pattern detection has begun to gel in the cortex.

With the development of neural pathways involved in sensory processing, information begins to feed forward to the thalamus. That is, based on what the cortex detects at this moment, it primes the thalamus to expect to receive certain kinds of sensory signal in certain locations of the visual field (or tones in the auditory field, or points on the skin surface, and so on) (Yarrow et al. 2001).

Thus, the major inhibitor of startle is simply the present content of perception. The moment-to-moment persistence of the objects already in our perceptual world dampens our surprise if we look away or close our eyes for a moment, and then return to the same scene. However, the sudden *disappearance* of something we saw a moment ago would almost certainly seem startling. Nor does predictable change startle us. The cortex devotes much of its acreage to the analysis of patterns in the size, location, tone, intensity, clarity, and motion of objects in perception; all of this feeds forward to the thalamus and other regions projections of where and at what size and quality we can expect to perceive objects in the next moment (Simo et al. 2005). Thus, we would be more startled if a ball sailing through the air were suddenly to freeze in midair than by its continued travel, because we anticipate its location to change continuously. This inhibitory aspect of sensory processing suggests there must be an automatic mechanism to inhibit startle. In laboratory settings, it has been established that the reflexive response to a startling stimulus weakens with repetition, when the stimuli are presented close together in time. This phenomenon is known as pre-pulse inhibition, and is a putative psychophysiologic marker of schizophrenia (Braff et al. 2001).

Fortunately, most of the things that startle us are benign. We hear a door slam and we freeze. A split second later, before sympathetic arousal can begin in earnest, before we begin to truly feel fear, we have realized there is no threat, the startled arousal dissipates, and we get on with our day. In the rare situation when startle does produce a full-bore sympathetic response that arouses and fuels defensive action, the experience conditions future behavior (Delgado et al. 2006). Jolted by the sudden jiggling of the ladder one has climbed, one takes pains to plant the ladder more firmly next time, to avoid that terrifying lurch. Conversely, if threat proves illusory or exaggerated, the cues we encounter in those circumstances may become the cues that condition us to suppress startle in future, similar circumstances.

When danger seems present, we respond first with heightened vigilance. Monoaminergic activation arouses both motor and sensory systems (Lang et al. 2000). Stronger arousal of sensory cortex means enhancement of the signals traveling through it, which in turn means more information to the thalamus. The more information flows through the cortex and back to the thalamus, the less likely one will encounter an abrupt, unexpected change in sensory input to the thalamus, and the less likely one will be startled. This may explain the preternatural calm that overtakes some individuals when they find themselves in danger. The brain, primed to anticipate dramatic changes in sensory stimuli, loses its sensitivity to be startled by anything.

Alert to danger, we can go into either active or passive defense. Active defense is the familiar, energetic flight or fight. With an active defensive strategy, an organism requires accurate and dynamic sensory information about the external environment, where the threat lies. Passive defense, in contrast, reflects an apparent dulling of sensitivity toward the environment, and weakening of the connection between threat-driven arousal and execution of a plan of action (Bracha et al. 2005). A threatening stimulus, coupled with the deprival of the means of defensive action, provokes a state of inattention to perceptual cues and to plans of motor action. In this state, surprising stimuli apparently meet with a dampened subcortical response. If, for example, one has been conditioned to helplessness as an adverse response to many commonly encountered visual cues, all vision may seem to lack salience. "Blind" to the significance of visual information, nothing visual can be surprising. This mechanism has been proposed in the section on perception as the basis of conversion, or hysterical pseudosensory symptoms.

Fear denotes anticipatory arousal of sensory, motor, and autonomic systems that sharpen our perceptions and move us to action as they also reduce the chance of our being surprised and possibly harmed. Fear motivates us to remove the signs of danger from our presence, or remove ourselves from the signs of danger, so danger may not surprise and alarm us. The arousal gets us to run or struggle; the removal of the dangerous cue from our perceptions reduces arousal and allows us, eventually, to stop running. Surprise also diminishes when we confront the source of danger; direct engagement provides us with more information about the severity and nature of the threat and, if we prevail in the ensuing struggle, eliminates it.

## Dread

The alarm response normally mobilizes attention and metabolic resources to generate defensive action when it is necessary to escape or overcome danger. Fearful feelings accompany defensive action when danger is imminent, and reflect hyperarousal of attention and autonomic function (Sullivan et al. 1999). Fear and anxiety can be separated by their neurobiology (Davis 1998) and by their motivational functions. Like the term *depression*, however, the term *anxiety* alludes to both symptoms and diagnoses, and so may not be useful as a means to clarify concepts. *Dread* constrains the concept of anxiety to its anticipatory aspects.

The anticipation of an unpleasant emotional response to danger, not danger itself, generates anxiety, or for our purposes, dread (Reiss 1987). Interviewed on a battlefield, the soldier under fire feels fear; the soldier back home, awaiting orders, feels dread. Fear motivates cautious behavior, to minimize the possibility of being startled by danger; cautious behavior has little effect against dread, as long as the threat remains abstract. Safety from danger relieves fear but not dread. One can eliminate from one's perceptual world the cues that signal danger, but one cannot eliminate the cues for dread, because they are internal cues about possible future threats, not avoidable threats in the immediate environment. One can run away from something that inspires fear, but not from the possibility that something dangerous might happen.

Dread emerges from situations in which threat is symbolic, or implied, or anticipated. Fearful arousal stimulates attentiveness and worried rumination. Rumination—"chewing over" worrisome thoughts—reflects heightened attention to one's own thought contents. Thoughts become an acute focus of attention because they are the only salient input available as one attempts to formulate a plan of defense against anticipated threat. Relief from dread thus requires new knowledge or a belief that changes the prediction that danger might happen. However, new information might also provide more fodder for rumination and dread, if it happens to be ambiguous or, worse, frankly discouraging. Thus, some people who suffer from dread actively avoid any additional knowledge about the thing they dread.

The fearful arousal associated with a specific state of dread can also be overcome via a reduction in the state of general arousal, as might occur from a strong satiety response. This creates an incentive to overeat, engage in compulsive sexual activity, or seek chemical sedation with alcohol or a drug (Kelley and Berridge 2002). For some individuals, dread may lead to an *increase* in risk-taking behavior, as the feeling of relief that follows will also wash away the original fearful arousal state.

Fear may begin naturally and later convert to a maladaptive state of dread. A traumatic event can induce a classically conditioned fear response to cues that remind the person about the event (Fendt and Fanselow 1999). Normally this fear response subsides over time, if the cue is no longer reinforced by an actual threat. For example, the recent victim of a mugging in Miami might experience a touch of fearful arousal whenever the news reported the score of a Dolphins football game. After sufficient exposure to "Miami" without further harm or threat, the name of the city would evoke only a neutral recollection, if anything (Hermans et al. 2006). But some people never quite extinguish the conditioned fear response to cues of a past traumatic event. Pictures of palm trees and pastel stucco might continue to bring to mind vivid memories and feelings of terror. More accurately, perhaps, the fearful response to cues about the traumatic event persists because it is reinforced by the alarming experience of fear itself, and the unpleasant physiologic arousal that accompanies it. Hence any subsequent experience of fearful arousal prompts intrusive memories (flashbacks) of the traumatic event, which further inflame the state of arousal, which in turn stimulates more intrusive recall (Brewin 2001). It is not so much that the person dreads Miami because she expects to be mugged again in Miami; she dreads and avoids Miami because she feels horrible whenever she is reminded of Miami. She becomes afraid not of again being the victim of a crime, but of being reminded of a crime that already happened.

Remember the stressed-out rat, never knowing when its tail would get a shock? The situation is similar here. A person could return to Miami, enter into a state of high alert at the scene of the crime, and then later feel safe, secure, and relaxed back at the hotel. But a person who lives in fear of even being reminded of the mugging never knows when someone will mention the Dolphins, so maintains a prolonged state of defensive alert, which can lead to the stress response, high cortisol, and the gradual depletion of resources (Korte 2001). Lacking a way to cope with an amorphous threat, the person in a state of dread may cling to any excuse to stay home or may seek sedation in order to get through the day.

Anxious feelings associated with dread are a characteristic symptom of the diagnosis generalized anxiety disorder, a common mood state in depression and bipolar disorder. Dread of a hypothetical harm is a direct motivating force in the avoidance associated with phobic disorders, obsessive-compulsive disorder, and post-traumatic stress disorder, and often an indirectly motivating force in substance use disorders.

## Paroxysms

A terrifying encounter causes sudden hyperalertness, pounding heart, breathlessness, cold sweat, fluttery stomach, tingling extremities, lightheadedness, a sense of unreality, senses primed to scan the environment for danger and take defensive action. Paroxysms of abject fear that arise for no apparent reason define the common experience of panic attacks. In a panic attack no threatening stimuli exist to fight or escape, not even an imaginary or hypothetical threat. The only unusual phenomena in the perceptual world of someone in the midst of a panic attack are the signals from the body, especially the pounding heart. The suddenness with which the terrified feeling overwhelms a person—the paroxysmal fear or feeling of panic—compounds the sense of alarm; hence many individuals in a panic state assume they must be in the midst of a myocardial infarction, and feel certain death is imminent (Austin and Richards 2001).

Panic attacks aversively condition people to avoid stimuli they associate with panic attacks, whether or not the stimuli had anything to do with inciting the attack (Bouton et al. 2001). Panic often leads to agoraphobia—literally, fear of the marketplace, but understood as fear of being in any public space. Vulnerability to an agoraphobic response hinges on the aversive power of the panic attacks, and also on the incentive to function despite the risk of a public paroxysm. Some particularly avoidant individuals whittle away their world to a safe, small scope. To avoid being surprised again by a panic attack, they stay away from the mall, the grocery store, the local convenience store, until ultimately, the only safe place may seem to be at home.

Paroxysmal attacks of panic often occur to people who experience other abnormal mood states, which also suggests a possibility of a deficit in the mechanism by which emotional responses in general are tied to environmental stimuli. Repeated, acute, intense states of fear and dread accompanied by the physiologic symptoms of sympathetic arousal are the core symptoms of panic attack.

## Guilt

A guilty feeling can be understood as the dread of punishment; in mental illness this occurs most often when no punishment is forthcoming. To feel guilty, a person must be aware or believe he or she has done something criminal or sinful or immoral or unethical, or something sloppy or negligent or halfhearted, or have failed to act when action is called for. Generally, he or she must also have been conditioned to expect to be punished for such misbehavior. These two conditions are not entirely independent. What a person is conditioned to think of as misbehavior has much to do with what the person was punished for during the formative years.

Pathological guilt accompanies dejected states, sometimes as an understandable reaction to the distorted observation that one has let other people down, for example, by being unmotivated to continue to love and support them. Guilt in dejected states also may accompany a depressive delusion in which one is falsely convinced one has committed some loathsome act. In this case, the guilt might be the primary abnormal emotion that drives the delusional belief, and not simply the consequence of having the belief. Only the horrifying conviction, perhaps that one has been the source of a deadly influenza epidemic, can adequately account for the intensity of one's feelings of dread and self-loathing.

Guilt is a characteristic symptom in the diagnosis of major depression and may occur frequently in diagnoses of adjustment disorders and obsessive-compulsive personality. Obsessive phenomena of obsessive-compulsive disorder often develop around themes of guilt.

## Paranoia

A person who is in the grip of paranoia sees cues of danger everywhere; however, the cues are all false. Paranoia may begin with an unexpected, neutral event that aberrantly stimulates an alarm response (Freeman 2007). Most people would be surprised to see a quarter on the sidewalk, but not startled or aroused to alarm, because the intensity of the stimulus is too weak. A person who is prone to paranoia has a lowered threshold to perceive the quarter as an alarming sign, and the hyperaroused mind scans the memory and immediate environment for clues about its salience as a threat. Perhaps someone has left that quarter there deliberately as a trap, as a test of honesty. A paranoid person feels surprised and alarmed almost constantly, hence strongly motivated to adhere to a theory about the nature of the threat (Garety et al. 1991). Convinced that others are trying to lay a trap, such a person will cease to find it alarming to see a quarter on the sidewalk. Now, she or he expects the unexpected and finds that to possess a ready explanation for uncanny events may prevent an unexpected encounter from flowering into an uncomfortable state of fearful arousal. A conspiracy theory provides some comfort because it encompasses all possible surprises. A world full of surprises frequently elicits the paranoid theory and thus reinforces the comfort it provides; hence such theories may be hard to eliminate.

Paranoia, described further in the section on delusions, is a core symptom in schizophrenia and delusional disorder and is often seen in mood disorders. Paranoid personality disorder involves a similar approach to life; however, the theories fall short of being accepted as certain facts, compared to someone who has frank delusions.

## 3.8. Summary: Integral Mind

The brain systematically integrates the elements of mental life into the familiar subjective phenomena of thoughts, feelings, and intentions. These, in turn, form the basis of the uniquely human capacity to translate the mind's own workings into useful information.

*Attention* denotes a state of readiness for action, contingent on new information. New information and context flow through working memory, where they mingle with the residue of past experience and the sketches of future plans. Inattentiveness may follow from a problem with arousal. Too little arousal leaves one adrift in sensation and reverie; too much arousal leads one to become easily distracted. Apparent inattentiveness among schoolchildren often reflects lagging cortical development, and a tendency to allow extraneous stimuli to distract them from the task at hand. Pathological mental phenomena may affect the flow and content of attention. The sense among some patients who have psychosis that the contents of working memory have either been removed from access to attention, or that some alien thought has been forced into attention, comprise the characteristic symptoms of avulsion (thought withdrawal) and intrusion (thought insertion).

*Memory* refers to the active retention of information salient to desire or survival. The most useful memories persist, permanently enshrined in cortical networks. Memory is selective, not complete. In general, the more a memory (and its associated cortical network) is accessed, the easier it is to find and activate it the next time it is needed. Raw episodic memories retain the flavor of events, but when only certain specific elements of an event in memory are accessed many times in many contexts, the unique elements of the event may be stripped away, and yield freestanding knowledge, that is, factual or semantic memory. Loss of hippocampus function produces primarily anterograde amnesia, or the inability to form and retain new memories. Common progressive dementias impede memory formation as they interrupt a variety of other mental processes that require widespread brain connectivity. On the other hand, some people can be said to have too much memory. When full-bodied recollection of a past painful event intrudes as a flashback into working memory, it may induce a painful emotional response in the present. Even in the absence of brain pathology, memory is not infallible. Complete retrograde amnesia in the absence of gross brain pathology may affect certain emotionally troubled people, who feel as if they have lost themselves. And some individuals have the traumatic experience of recovering memory for horrific events that never happened.

*Habits* can be adaptive or maladaptive. To retain in memory a close linkage between sensory cue and an appetitive drive, or between a cue and a learned course of action, saves one the trouble of having to find what one needs through trial and error. The capacity to link sensory and internal cues to the mechanisms that drive behavior also contributes to maladaptive, addictive behaviors. Addictive behaviors co-opt normal drive mechanisms. Drug and alcohol addictions lead the addict to satisfy a craving that fills no biological need, but induces the brain to falsely ascribe salience to the addictive agent, that is, to find it rewarding. Eating disorders illustrate the point that addictions require no actual substance, only a physiologically provocative behavior that produces a desired internal state. Self-injurious behavior, like cutting or burning oneself, similarly accesses the reward system and conditions behavior, thus constituting a form of non-chemical addiction. Sexual behaviors considered deviant are culture-specific to some degree. However, in the context of medicine, the relevant issue is whether the consummation of one's sexual desire is likely to prove harmful to oneself or disturbing to the other person.

Adaptive behavior requires one to juggle competing drives. To choose adaptively entails executive function: comparison of the *values* of different courses of action. Frequently, one ascribes the highest values to actions motivated by abstract or future rewards. Individuals who have frontal lobe damage tend to lose the ability to forgo immediate rewards in favor of richer rewards that unfold over the long term. Failure of executive function leads primarily to stimulus-driven, disinhibited behavior because the diffuse cortical representations of these deferred goals fail to entrain plans of action that might lead to attaining them. By default, the attraction of the immediate object wins out, because only immediate objects can be "seen" and selected by the frontal cortex. One can understand suicidal behavior as a kind of failure of executive function in which the salience of pursuing even the normal appetitive satisfactions of life loses value relative to the salience of escaping from pain, when there is a loss of hope that life will regain value. When a person has suffered adversity to the point that he or she can no longer see the point of putting out the effort to struggle for gain and against pain, the person has fallen into a demoralized state.

*Motive* refers to motivation, or the value of a drive one aims to satisfy, as well as to emotion, or the value of a drive one cannot, will not, or does not know how to satisfy. Drives come in two major varieties: some drives move one to approach or acquire an object, perhaps to consume it, and some move one to escape from or avoid an object. The failure to be moved to approach, acquire, or consume objects of positive value describes the common symptom of anhedonia, the inability to experience pleasure, or more accurately, to be motivated to pursue pleasure. Apathy, in contrast, describes the inability to be moved to avoid pain or loss. The hostility inherent in territoriality mixes the drive to embrace and the drive to repel, tragically when the objects one wishes to embrace and repel are one and the same.

One learns to *desire* pleasurable people, places, and things by developing an extensive array of conditioned cues to the satiety response. One can thus take pleasure in many things beyond those that satisfy a particular appetite. Dejection, a painful mood state that persists despite the absence of immediate painful stimuli, stems from severe anhedonia. To be in a state of emotional pain and to be incapable of being moved by pleasure is to be dejected, and probably in the grip of a major depression. By contrast, an excited mood implies excess capacity to anticipate pleasure. Satisfaction of an excitement-driven desire does not quell the drive but enhances the motivation to pursue more pleasure. Excitement tends to confer a feeling of ownership over everything in one's world. Excitement can, and often does give way to irascibility, a state of ready emergence of hostility, when the pleasurable emotion fades but the investment in many things remains, hence there is more territory to be defended, and more potential for an angry, defensive, hostile response.

How does one learn to become *alarmed* by threatening things, if they have caused one no harm? States of alarm, or fearful arousal, occur when one either has already been startled by an unexpected, sudden, powerful stimulus, or has entered an environment in which one has been conditioned to anticipate a startling stimulus. Startle is a reflex; strong sensory stimuli may trigger an amygdala-mediated relay and initiate a freezing response before the stimuli have reached the cortex to be processed into an organized perception. The result of startle is to cease all motion and attend to the environment for sensory cues to the nature of the threat. A state of alarm, in essence, is one in which senses have been aroused and defensive responses primed, in anticipation of being startled. Under many conditions, such as crossing a busy street, this is a highly adaptive state. Problems occur when the focus of alarm has turned inward, to autonomic cues rather than environmental ones. To become hypervigilant to internal cues of defensive arousal is to experience dread: a state of fearfulness over the possibility of being afraid. Guilt represents a special case of dread: fear of the painful effects of being punished for some transgression, real or imagined. A paroxysm of panic, complete with physical symptoms of sympathetic arousal, occurs pathologically in the absence of any relevant threat. Paranoia may be the end result of an overactive state of alarm that leads one to see threat in all unexpected stimuli; paranoid ideas survive because they make one less surprised by unexpected occurrences.

# CHAPTER FOUR

# Synthetic Mind

Now the story advances from the elemental and integrative mental processes found in many animal species to the uniquely human processes that permit us to weigh options when motives clash and to act intelligently in uncertain circumstances. These synthetic processes create mental models of reality that we employ to navigate successfully in a complex world.

The forces that drive behavior do not always compel it. A person who is in good mental health may choose to seek evidence or accept things on faith; choose to challenge authority or heed conscience; choose to defer reward indefinitely or cash in; choose to hold, fold, or double down. Mind provides the means to escape the bonds of determinism, to imagine, hope, and plan. Or so it seems.

Is free will an illusion? If one believes that all mental life derives from brain activity, where can one place the power to choose one's actions amid the axons, dendrites, synapses, neurotransmitters, receptors, action potentials, and other workings of neurons? The embodiments of our free will are neurobiological phenomena that arise from chemical phenomena that arise from physical forces set into motion, ultimately, by the Big Bang. If one takes the material world seriously, mental phenomena arise from the brain, not from some *deus ex machina*, and consciousness is merely along for the ride (Mc-Ginn 1989). But belief in free will unites worshippers of omnipotent gods who see it as a tenet of faith, with atheistic existentialists who regard it as a human responsibility. The logic of neurobiology leaves no room for it, but in an individual human being failure to experience a power to choose to act or not to act is distinctly odd. Indeed, the sense that one is unable to think or choose freely defines many states of mental illness, from obsessions to catatonia to addiction and demoralization.

The concept of free will poses a paradox (Feigl and Meehl 1974). It may defy neurobiology, but it defines mental health. Fortunately, there is no need to resolve the paradox. It is not important to the question of freedom whether one's mental life up to this moment has been fully determined by physical forces. Freedom concerns the future. If the concept of freedom implies a lack of *any* external constraint or influence, then it is nonsensical to apply it to past actions. One can always find a constraint or influence to explain any past action as a rational choice, or else it would be irrational by definition—done for no reason at all. To act freely in the future, however, means to allow factors other than the expedient execution of present demands to impel one's actions. To have free will is to have the power to act against expediency. Whenever we defer immediate gain in favor of some other long-term project, such as building character, making a fortune in stocks, getting to heaven, fighting the enemy, winning an election, running a marathon, raising children, or attending medical school, we assert our freedom from the tyrannies of reflex, appetite, and conditioned responses.

Note that many of these long-term purposes live far from the forefront of our motives. When we become aware of them, their satisfaction may become expedient. The motive to attend medical school, for example, moves to the fore during the application process, and the act of filling out the forms becomes expedient. However, once one has gotten into medical school, on a day-to-day basis the motive to become a doctor recedes, unquestioned, into the background, while more immediate concerns, like memorizing the Krebs cycle, or tracking down labs, or finding a set of well-fitting scrubs, predominate. The background motives tend to remain hidden, until circumstances flush them out. When one can trace a motivation readily to its source, the source determines the course of action, and the action no longer seems to have been freely chosen. When motivation has complex and ultimately irreducible sources it seems free because in fact it is free from expedient motivations.

If we could predict all our actions, we would not feel free. As a thought experiment, imagine that a psychomathematician has collected all relevant data about your mind right now and claims to be able to predict what you will do five days from now in response to an event only she knows will happen. To be sure, she puts the prediction in writing and seals it in an envelope. Five days hence you face an unexpected decision. You deliberate carefully, make a choice, and only later learn that this was the event in question. You tear open the envelope to learn that you did exactly as predicted. Stunned, you consult with the psychomathematician. She shows you the models and equations that calculated with airtight certainty that you would act as you did. Would you still feel you had made a truly free choice? Or that what you perceived as a freely made decision was the end result of forces set in motion in the past, acting as an impersonal algorithm within your brain, knowable to anyone with the data, the psychomathematical software, and unlimited RAM?

If the idea that your actions might conceivably be predictable undermines your confidence in the concept of free will, then you may agree that our experience of freedom rests on our being *unable* to know everything about our own minds. The mental systems described thus far provide the veil between our thoughts and motives necessary to account for free will.

Mind flows from two complementary systems, one concerned with information and the other with arousal. The information system uses a combination of excitatory and inhibitory connections to construct a perceptual representation of the world and a set of instructions to organize bodily movement. The connections are largely forged by neurons that employ the neurotransmitter glutamate and are modulated by GABA. Alterations in glutamate receptor composition determine the ease with which certain of these representational/ instructional networks can be activated. They encode information and store it not in the roadmap of the brain's circuitry, but in the pattern of differences in the readiness of certain circuits to become activated by other cortical associations and by arousal signals.

The phasic arousal system uses monoaminergic neurotransmission. Neurons that secrete dopamine, norepinephrine, and serotonin radiate from subcortical structures to points throughout the cortex. In this way signals of autonomic and physiological state affect the likelihood and degree of activation of specific circuits encoding information and action programs. Arousal signals alter neither the content of the mental representation of the environment nor the instructions for bodily movement. They simply reinforce whatever circuits were active when these monoaminergic neurons were active, and restimulate these circuits when a need arises. In essence, the monoaminergic signal adds an additional spur to the informational system either to induce an association between neurons in a circuit or to awaken dormant circuits (Gu 2002).

To review how this might work, imagine a hungry person with nearly empty pockets, walking the backstreets of a city in search of a cheap meal. Arousal is high because the hunger is intense, and no fast food is in sight. Each of the three monoaminergic systems has a role to play. The division of labor among them is a subject of speculation, but roughly speaking, norepinephrine sharpens the senses and quickens the step, dopamine drives the search procedure, and serotonin guides the search toward the needed object: food.

The hungry person takes a detour down an unfamiliar side street and luckily encounters a souvlaki vendor. The detection and consumption of souvlaki satisfies the state of arousal, producing pleasurable satiety. Satiety signals have stimulated the cortex to retain as favored circuits the sensory and spatial representations of the stand and the sequence of actions that led to it. The next time hunger strikes and funds are low, the heightened monoaminergic activity will illuminate these cortical representations of souvlaki and map how to find it. Conversely, an incidental reminder of the souvlaki experience—the act of walking down the same side street for some other purpose—may trigger not only a recognition of having been there before, but also a classically conditioned recollection of the feeling of enjoying a souvlaki there while in a state of dire hunger.

When arousal signals selectively reactivate information-enriched cortical circuits, the result is a thought or an intention. When the cortical circuits that store perceptual representations and action programs become engaged in working memory, they may activate a classically conditioned drive, as the sight of the Ahab's logo made Pat want coffee, in a previous section. The complementary systems that store information and induce arousal thus communicate with one another, but remain separate domains. Their functional asymmetry is reflected in their anatomic distribution. Informational circuitry occupies the vast cortical expanse of the frontal, parietal, temporal, and occipital cortex (Constantinidis and Procyk 2004). Arousal systems use a few small, remote areas of cortex, and emanate mainly from a diverse collection of subcortical nuclear centers.

Incidentally, this asymmetry of influence and structure suggests a biological basis for the Freudian unconscious. In Freud's view, the unconscious mind consists of the primal drives that civilization trains a person to suppress (Freud 1961). To a Freudian, the unconscious is impenetrable to self-reflection; it emerges only indirectly through unintentional thoughts, feelings, and actions. To Freud the unconscious has much more to say about the nature of a person's mental suffering than do the more accessible conscious contents of mind. Freud argued that mental suffering follows from inadequacies in mental efforts to suppress unconscious urges. But it may be more consistent with biology to say that the unconscious remains poorly accessible not because it is suppressed, but because it is inarticulate. The forces of arousal that comprise the unconscious mind contribute no direct information to cortical processes. They do, however, maintain a rich and nuanced influence over which mental representations and action programs will be retained and will gain access to working memory and behavior.

To recap: conscious information and unconscious arousal systems communicate asymmetrically. Paths between cortex and subcortical structures mediate the interaction between them. A primary state of arousal induces cortical activity in certain encoded representational and instructional circuits by monoaminergic stimulation. Cortically encoded thoughts can, in turn, revive dormant states of arousal.

The mind seems free because one cannot trace this process of cortical to subcortical communication the same way one follows a moving tennis ball or the plot of a book or the logic of a mathematical equation, where all of the variables are in view, or on the page, or explicitly rational. When competing motives arouse competing visions of what would be the outcome of a choice, the decision to do this and not that is influenced by forces deprived of direct access to working memory (Kihlstrom 1987). One can own one's decisions as the product of free will because one cannot trace them to some immediately identifiable motive, or to some impersonal algorithm. Therefore, they seem free and undetermined by any influence but one's own character.

To illustrate, suppose a hungry person was presented with a rotisserie chicken a friend had stolen from a grocery. Appetite might compel the person to eat it without hesitation, but in the brief time it takes to reach for a drumstick, the incidental information that it was stolen awakens other cortical circuits invested with significance by past conditioning—perhaps the person had been punished severely for receiving stolen goods in the past, or has worked in a grocery, so feels empathy for the store owner. A moment before the friend appeared, honor may have been the last thing in the person's mind, but now it emerges as a dominant motivator. The temptation to engage in dishonorable behavior has activated a classically conditioned response, mediated by some of the same subcortical structures that were aroused in past experience.

In an honorable person, the conditioned response is likely to arouse a set of thoughts, feelings, and intentions that would lead the person to refuse the stolen food. The person must choose to eat or be honest. This seems like a free choice because some of the roots of these aims cannot be traced back to a logical point of origin; a moment ago the person was painfully aware of being hungry, but may have had minimal awareness, if any, of honorable intentions. Whatever makes the person go one way or the other seems like an essentially free, unforced reflection of the person's character, even though at some level the process is rooted in biological activities of the brain. By contrast, a hungry person who refuses a meal because of a (paranoid) conviction that the food has been poisoned can say exactly why consuming it is not an option; the thought was never out of mind. The choice to abstain is not free; the paranoid person feels compelled to refuse the chicken upon pain of death.

The point of this philosophical digression has been to provide a plausible basis for the aspect of mental life that seems most inexplicable and human. It would be implausible to build a model of mental life in which behavior follows logically from explicit perceptions, drives, and memories. We simply do not experience life that way. Uncertainty, therefore, is not only an unavoidable fact of life, but also the heart of our indispensable concept of free will. However, up to this point in the book, the discussion has always been predicated on the assumption of certainty: that the healthy mind processes true information derived from actual experience.

How do we cope when we need useful information about things that are intrinsically uncertain or unknowable? It is relatively easy to predict the outcome of decisions when they involve knowable, static objects, like lamps and biscuits, and changeable but natural law-abiding objects like gladiolas and riptides. We use experience to predict complex natural phenomena on the scale of weather and ecosystems, but with the caveat that our predictions are probabilistic, not certain. Social interaction requires information beyond what

*Table 6.* Synthetic Mind: Employment of Secondary Mental Functions of Memory, Drive, and Emotion under Conditions of Complexity and Uncertainty

| Function | Description | Disruptions |
|---|---|---|
| Bias | Reflexive predisposition to value one anticipated outcome over another | Ambivalence, avoidance, impulsiveness, inertia |
| Personality | Patterns of habitual behavior associated with bias | Anankastic, histrionic, labile personalities |
| Belief | Prediction of the long-term consequences of anticipated action | Delusions, overvalued ideas, doubt |
| Identity | Beliefs about one's values | Gender disorientation, projection, dissolution |
| Cooperation | Strategy to reduce uncertainty about the actions of other people by engaging them in mutually beneficial actions | Asociality, sociopathy, shame |
| Communication | Strategy to reduce uncertainty by exchange of symbols that represent one's mental state | Dysfluency/hyperfluency, derailment, telemission, misrepresentation |
| Affiliation | A cooperative relationship in which benefit to one party is shared with another | Grief, overdependency, egotism, eccentricity |
| Help-seeking | Cooperative behavior aimed to relieve a state of distress, dysfunction, or danger | Psychosomatic complaints, denial, parasuicide |

can be learned through or extrapolated from personal experience. People are neither constant nor predictable; therefore a large part of our mental focus must be devoted to the effort to estimate, or model, how other people will respond to our actions.

We routinely face uncertainty when we anticipate how we will feel about today's actions tomorrow and when we try to predict what other people may do. We often rely on intuition and hearsay to fill the gaps in our observations. If we are alert to our biases and the tentative nature of our beliefs, we have more freedom to act rationally in our own future interest. And, to the extent that we communicate with other people about our own and their experiences, and live with other people and share common ends, we become much better at predicting what they will do. Thus, we limit uncertainty about other people through cultivating ongoing relationships with them.

Mental symptoms and deficits of the kinds described up to this point profoundly affect our capacity to manage uncertainty and maintain relationships. When our biases are poorly modulated, or our beliefs fall into error and doubt, or we fail to make our thoughts known to others, our choices may be led astray. Deficiencies in the capacity to cooperate, or to heed other people's intentions, or to feel their pain, or to enlist others to assist when one is in need, all contribute significantly to mental suffering and impairment. Table 6 summarizes the components of the synthetic mind.

## 4.1. Leaning Disability: Unbalanced Bias

With sufficient information and time to weigh options, a person employs information from past experience to guide future actions in the context of present arousal and appetite. Knowing the rewarding or painful outcome of past behavior, one sets one's sails for the port one desires, steering clear of rough seas.

Once the goal is fixed, however, there may be different paths to attain it. How do we choose which way to go? For example, imagine driving up behind a slower car in the middle of three lanes of an otherwise empty highway, as sketched in Figure 4. We can pass the car on its left or its right. We might, without hesitation, stomp on the gas and swerve out and around the car ahead, going right or left depending on which hand happens not to be holding our beer. Or timidly hit the brakes on the assumption that we must have been speeding. Or ponder whether it is proper road etiquette to pass on the left or right. Whatever we choose to do, chances are we would make the same choice most of the time, under similar circumstances.

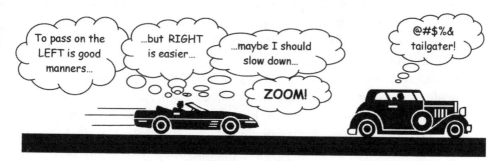

*Figure 4.* Bias in decision making arises from temperamental traits.

The biases toward reckless, or timid, or rational kinds of action—temperamental *traits*—reflect enduring qualities of a person's individual emotional tone, specifically, the tensions between attraction and aversion; fear and comfort (Whittle et al. 2006). Traits are a product largely of innate sensitivity to the motivating forces of alarm and desire (Kagan and Snidman 1991). Thus a particularly hedonistic person might demonstrate a consistent bias to take the more immediately pleasurable of two options, but another person who has an equally strong hedonic drive but greater sensitivity to aversive consequences would consider strongly hedonistic urges a warning to proceed with caution.

To know someone well is to know the person's traits, that is, to be able to predict with some accuracy how the person is likely to respond when faced with a choice or challenge. We know something may be seriously amiss with the individual when his or her behavior deviates from predictions. When a normally hesitant person makes reckless choices, or an exuberant person withdraws, friends and family report that he is "not himself." Whatever his traits, we say that the person is not in his normal *state* when actions deviate from expectations. As discussed earlier, our decisions and state of mind reflect the strength of arousal for pleasure and relief from distress, and the ease with which we can satisfy desire and forestall alarm.

The concept of temperamental traits permeates medical history. For the ancient Greeks and Romans and generations of Western physicians who followed, temperamental qualities were believed to be a function of humors, or bodily fluids (Howarth 1988). A person was thought literally to possess greater or lesser quantities of some bodily substance that made his or her character sanguine (blood), phlegmatic (phlegm), melancholic ("black bile"), or choleric ("yellow bile"). The sanguine person tended to be affable and buoyant and not easily bothered. The phlegmatic person tended to be pensive and serene. The melancholic person tended to be passive and pessimistic, depressive (if not clinically depressed). A person who had a choleric temperament tended to be angry and hostile, "hot-headed."

Although the ancient linkage of bodily fluids with temperaments seems fanciful today, the model's grasp of temperamental types has remained sufficiently valid to endure for ages. The widely used schema of Hans Eysenck updates the ancient model, replacing humors with traits along two main axes: introversion/extraversion and stability/instability (Ruch 1992). All else being equal, an *introverted* person trades some opportunities for pleasure in order to achieve freedom from the fear of a painful experience, and finds the resulting inner harmony to be more salient than the drive for pleasure and stimulation. An *extraverted* person prefers the latter, hence tends to find shared experiences with other people the most salient motivators, because other people heighten the potential for both pleasure and stimulation. Stability/instability refers to the rapidity and intensity with which the emotions may shift. The choleric person in the ancient humoral schema would most resemble an unstable extravert, the sanguine person a stable extravert, the phlegmatic person a stable introvert, and the melancholic person an unstable introvert. Clinicians frequently describe people in Eysenckian terms, based on impressionistic assessments. However, the terminology has been adopted and altered in the hands of different theorists, so upon hearing a person described as an introvert or extravert, it is wise to ask the speaker to define his or her terms.

Is there an objective basis for temperamental assessment, or is it all in the eye of the beholder? How useful is it to estimate a person's behavioral biases? Two modern approaches illustrate some of the strengths and weaknesses of the clinical concept of temperament. The five-factor model of Paul Costa and Robert McRae grew from empirical research into the terms and concepts people use to define their own inclinations (Costa 1991). People rated how much they thought each of a large series of adjectives applied to them (for example, lonely, gregarious, stoical, fearful, skeptical, belligerent, and so on). From factor analyses of these data emerged five cardinal traits, which have since been assessed for their reliability and predictive validity (Saulsman and Page 2004). Two of the five traits overlap, roughly, with Eysenck's two axes: Neuroticism (similar to stability/instability) is defined as the propensity to experience strong negative emotions and Extraversion is the capacity to experience positive emotions. The three other factors of this NEO-AC model (Neuroticism, Extraversion, Openness, Agreeableness, and Conscientiousness) split off other qualities that vary independently of one another.

An alternative model developed by C. Robert Cloninger and colleagues maps traits according to the monoaminergic arousal systems that are hypothesized to account for them (Cloninger et al. 1993). The three traits are reward dependence (dopamine), harm avoidance (norepinephrine), and novelty seeking (serotonin). Thus, the advantage of the five-factor model is its basis in empirical research, whereas the advantage of Cloninger's is its theoretical appeal to students of the brain and human nature.

Although bias does not set our goals, the choice to follow or not follow one's inclinations may have a significant impact on success. If the driver in Figure 4 swerves recklessly around the car in front and veers into the median strip or attracts the notice of a highway patrolman, then the bias is maladaptive. Similarly, if the driver too timid to pass becomes angry and frustrated and blames the slowpoke in front for making him or her late, the consequence of heeding his or her overcautious tendency is needless distress.

## Ambivalence

Ambivalence manifests as indecisiveness, of a particular sort (Sincoff 1990). An ambivalent person avoids making mistakes by opting to do nothing. There is not necessarily a general preference for safety over reward, but rather a specific fear of choosing the less valuable among competing opportunities. Relative to a more decisive person, an ambivalent person may overvalue the difference in expected value between two options, while undervaluing the risk of losing the opportunity due to hesitation. More information might resolve the impasse for some ambivalent people, but not always. In contrast to avoidance, which is a bias toward the less risky of two paths, the ambivalent person does not necessarily prefer the safest course, but does fear making the wrong decision and so avoids taking any path.

Ambivalence in the context of psychosis arises from problems more profound than temperamental bias. A person who has psychosis may appear ambivalent because additional meaning has been attached to the options. The question how to maneuver around a slow car is no longer a matter of style; it may seem to be a matter of profound existential or historical significance because one is convinced that the driver ahead has nuclear waste hidden in the trunk of his car and is it better to avoid him, or try to force him off the road before he can use it to build a dirty bomb? Thus, the person hesitates, perhaps indefinitely, fearful of making the wrong move. A person with a subcortical dementia, on the other hand, may appear ambivalent because the push and pull of bias is weakened to the point of paralysis, and the person is left at the crossroads of a decision, unable to imagine or feel any difference one way or the other.

An ambivalent attitude is characteristic of obsessive-compulsive personality disorder, and may explain some of the asocial aspects of schizoid personality disorder. Ambivalence may occur as well as a psychotic or cognitive symptom.

## Avoidance

An avoidant attitude is driven by the overvaluation of imminent risk. It biases a person to focus excessively on possible harm in the short term, at the potential sacrifice of greater pleasure and reward (Heinrichs and Hofmann 2001). The main consequence of avoidant bias is "phobic" behavior. The person who has an avoidant attitude must act, as any other person must act, on essential desires and appetites, but does so in the way that arouses the least potential for alarm. If a person fears shopping at the supermarket to the point of refusing to try, then the options to obtain food are limited by the availability of friends, carryout, and grocery stores that deliver. If a person fears new people, then the desire for social engagement must be met by the same set of people he or she already knows, even if they are unpleasant to be around.

Avoidance is central to the construct of so-called avoidant personality disorder which, in turn, has been associated with phobic disorders in which an exaggerated fear combined with avoidant behavior together impel a withdrawal from normal life functioning. Avoidance may be linked as well to major depression, where it characterizes a state rather than a trait.

## Impulsiveness

Confronted with a decision about how to attain a goal, a person might opt to act now on what is known, or await further information. As with any decision, the choice depends on factual knowledge ("I will wait until I see the quarterly report before I buy stock in that company"), belief ("The early bird gets the worm"), or impulse (a bias toward a rapid decision versus deliberation) (Hinson et al. 2003). It takes less time for the brain to arouse action toward a goal than it does to process information, so an impulsive tendency toward quick decisions is generally a decision to go for it and damn the consequences. Impetuousness is a common quality of youthful inexperience; when there have been fewer adverse experiences from which to learn, there are fewer experiential brakes against hasty action.

The impulsive attitude is thus the polar opposite of the ambivalent attitude. When a person has been around long enough to be able to anticipate a wider range of consequences, impulsiveness tends to be viewed as evidence of emotional immaturity. Immaturity may result from exposure to an environment in which one has been shielded from consequences, or it may reflect an innate, relative inability to learn from consequences. Impulsive decisions are not always wrong or harmful, but they may bias toward undesired outcomes, because they produce action that fails to take into account information that might rationally cause a more careful person to defer action (Ainslie 1975).

Impulsiveness is characteristic of several of the cluster B personality disorders, including antisocial, borderline, and histrionic personality. In mania, impulsiveness is a state rather than a trait. The impulsive bias may contribute as well to substance abuse, bulimia nervosa, kleptomania, and pathological gambling. Intoxication on alcohol or drugs may further weaken inhibitions and thus facilitate impulsive acts.

### Inertia

A body at rest tends to stay at rest. A person who has an attitude of inertia has a bias away from change, even when change promises a high likelihood of substantial reward (Baumeister and Scher 1988). Inertia causes poor recovery from illness and rigidity when confronted with challenges to habits of living. Inertia may be a residual effect of a mental illness that impedes motivation. To resume goal-driven life functioning, it may be necessary to overcome inertia by structured rehabilitation, as a person would overcome muscle wasting after a limb injury by engaging in physical therapy.

Inertia, as a learned attitude rather than a trait of temperament, is found primarily as a characteristic of residual and partially treated phases of psychotic and mood disorders. Trait inertia is not a feature of any particular diagnosis, but may pose a significant hindrance to successful maturation in a society that values individual achievement and the pursuit of independence.

## 4.2. Veer Goggles: Personality Non Grata

Personality is part temperamental bias, part habit, part style (Rutter 1987). The interaction of these factors over decades of our lives can define us as it steers us toward certain kinds of actions, but still allow us freedom to adapt our responses to a given environment. Or, the combination of a strong temperament, adverse circumstances, and maladaptive actions can leave us with a stereotypic set of responses that constrain freedom (Svrakic et al. 2009). Personality affects not only how we react, but also how we see the world.

In the discussion of temperament as a form of bias, the critical factor differentiating temperaments was the individual's attitude towards value—to what extent does pleasure trump the risk of pain or loss or uncertainty? Where temperamental bias is not overly strong, a person may learn what choice works best in a given situation. Such a person is defined not by personality, but by his or her powers of critical judgment.

The effect over time of a strong bias, however, is a skewed reality. A person with extreme temperamental bias does not learn to bend judgment to circumstances, but rather to read the circumstances to fit the biased choice she or he is strongly inclined to make. If the outcome of a decision cannot shape the future choices of a strongly biased person, it also teaches nothing useful about the world. To cope with a world in which many decisions seem to have poor outcomes (at least in the eyes of others), the person tends to focus only on a small part of the outcome.

Thus, a person's strong temperament may make one source of information seem more salient than all others (Shapiro 1965). Someone who has a bias toward caution attends more closely to signs of danger in the environment than to his or her own appetites and desires. Someone who has a strong bias toward feeling may neglect vigilance about the environment while savoring the nuances of pain and pleasure. To further complicate matters, strong temperament biases one to avoid or embrace certain kinds of environment, and these environmental exposures in turn bring out the best or worst in a temperament (Kendler et al. 2003). A careful person prefers to avoid volatile situations like bar fights and ménages à trois; an emotive person might yawn at analytic pursuits like chess and estate planning.

Bias in perceiving the salience of one aspect of experience versus the other, repeated daily over many years, under many circumstances, lies at the heart of personality development. When a person has spent years attending more closely to the minutiae of perception to the neglect of the emotional consequences of actions, the person comes to be an expert at detail while remaining a novice at emotions. Conversely, the person who is biased to attend to the subjective nuances of experience becomes a virtuoso of feelings and may inhabit a world of fantasy and wishful thinking, while remaining myopic about the real-world signs of danger.

## Anankastic Personality

Emotionally rigid, habitually stubborn perfectionists preoccupied with minutiae over the "big picture" are often called *obsessive-compulsive personalities* (Pollak 1979). This is a confusing term, because it sounds like *obsessive-compulsive disorder*, to which it is only tangentially related. It is also inaccurate;

such individuals do not necessarily have obsessions or compulsions. As defined in the section on action regulation, obsessions and compulsions are abnormal mental phenomena that arise from a failure to detect the satisfactory completion of simple intentions or actions, and manifest as thoughts or actions that arc unnecessary or absurd, and resisted by the patient. Another oft-used term, *anal-retentive,* reflects an old Freudian theory of the developmental origins of this personality type, said to emerge from conflicts over toilet training in toddlerhood. *Anankastic* is an old clinical descriptive of this type of person, and lacks the linguistic baggage of these other common terms. In other contexts, the term implies compulsory action. In grammar, an anankastic conditional construction takes the form: in order to X, you must Y.

Anankastic people follow rules. People who have anankastic personalities do not always suffer from their traits. Emotional stoicism, steadfast reliability, and careful attention to detail can be adaptive virtues. The problem for the anankastic person is the excessively and inflexibly unemotional, rote, and particular approach to complex situations and especially to other people. In the face of uncertainty, an overly anankastic personality may cause a person to delay rather than risk a bad outcome predicated on incomplete information. Anankastic traits tend to interfere with relationships as well; many qualities of the personality can make it hard for such a person to cope with the apparent irrational unpredictability of other more emotionally demonstrative people.

Strongly anankastic traits primarily characterize obsessive-compulsive personality disorder, and some mild diagnoses in the autism spectrum. Milder, more adaptive anankastic tendencies are prevalent among professionals.

## Histrionic Personality

Anankastic people are the engineers; histrionic people are the actors and actresses. The world as seen by someone who has the emotionally expansive, serendipitous, sweeping approach to life differs radically from that of the anankastic person. Reality to the histrionic person is more firmly rooted in feeling and belief than fact and knowledge. The thread that links experiences together as coherent elements of knowledge is the flavor of the feelings associated with them. For the histrionic person, feelings are essential bits of information (Clore and Huntsinger 2007).

There are significant implications for behavior when knowledge from personal experience and from others is based more on feeling than perceptual nuance. First, to get a predictable outcome from behavior with respect to others, the histrionic person is less apt to be concerned about objective markers than about the interpersonal consequences. To the outsider it may seem that life for the histrionic person is one sudden drama after another, a source of stress best avoided, but in fact the histrionic person anticipates a volatile emotional landscape. The stormy outcome only confirms the histrionic person's point of view, because a storm was anticipated, perhaps intended. The fact that the emotion seemed painful is of lesser consequence, because the second significant implication of a histrionic outlook is that emotional valence swings quickly with a change in circumstances. Because present and past experiences are linked by their emotional and not their sensorimotor content, all the histrionic person has to do to change bad feelings is to change the present experience. Thus, from the outsider's perspective the drama swings, maddeningly, chaotically, from tragedy to comedy, and from the histrionic person's perspective what matters most is that he or she feels better, for now.

Histrionic traits are at the core of histrionic personality disorder, are common in borderline personality disorder, and are written about extensively in the Hollywood tabloids.

## Labile Personality

One personality subtype of clinical significance stands apart from rigid anankastic personality, and reliably overreactive histrionic personality: the type of personality forged by chronic emotional instability. People with labile personalities create turbulence around them as they move rapidly through phases of excitement, dejection, and irascibility for no apparent reason.

 Our model can account for the core phenomenon of labile personality—emotional instability—as a failure to integrate environmental cues efficiently and appropriately with the apparatus of phasic arousal. We have seen several ways that context normally guides arousal. Strong appetitive or defensive motives prime us to attend to the environment for the cues that would resolve the state of arousal. When we encounter someone or something salient to our fears and desires, a well-tuned arousal system fixes attention and drives action, and winds down when our senses register that we won the prize, smashed the mosquito, or fled the Rottweiler. In an emotionally unstable person, despair can arise without disappointment, anger without threat, and elation without victory. The arousal mechanisms that drive emotion percolate on their own.

Whatever the cause of unstable emotions, the labile personality emerges through years of chaotic encounters with the world. One day the labile person hears an off-hand comment about her hair and interprets it as a compliment, the next day the same comment plunges her into suicidal despair. Or one day is pulled over for speeding, cheerfully accepts the ticket, and motors off, too elated to care. The next day when the same thing happens, he erupts with rage and nearly gets hauled off to jail. In either case, the labile person is unable to learn from experience, as the same experience has led to vastly different outcomes; the salience of consequences has become warped by the individual's wildly variable emotional states.

If the same stimuli meet with widely disparate affective responses over the course of years, the expected result is a person who finds love perilous, work fleeting, and the future bleak. The labile person's relationships with family, friends, and physicians range from adoration to loathing, rarely settling in the middle. Labile people seek out intoxicants as a way to force some measure of chemical predictability upon the mess within. Because labile people often inspire angst, hostility, and mistrust in those around them, the transition from moody kid to mercurial adult may be compounded when chronically unpredictable emotional responses must cope with a world devoid of the stabilizing influence of people who have been driven away by the turmoil.

Labile personality is the core problem for many individuals diagnosed with borderline personality disorder. Rapidly changing moods also occur in a subset of individuals considered to have cyclothymia, rapid cycling or mixed forms of bipolar disorder.

## 4.3. Cardinal Knowledge: Beyond Belief

Information guides all goal-directed behavior, from scratching an itch to running a country. But people take many actions in the absence of direct experience. Where do they acquire the information needed to act intelligently? Belief serves as a proxy form of information, to guide behavior when direct experience is lacking, either because of naïveté, or because the necessary information concerns events that have not happened yet or occur, if at all, beyond human experience.

Information can be acquired directly from personal experience and indirectly from the words of other people. When we rely on information from others, we accept it on faith until we have had a chance to test it in our own experience. Stable knowledge that cannot be tested remains as belief. A body of belief therefore consists largely of the information we borrow from others to guide our behavior when we lack direct experience (Lund 1925).

Some information simply has not yet been tested in experience, though conceivably it could be tested. One might know the next date of Halley's comet, and if one lives long enough, test that knowledge personally. Such knowledge is more stable than mere belief because it came from many other trustworthy people who have personally charted Halley's appearances. Or one may *know*, rather than merely believe, that variation across species demonstrates natural selection. No one has observed it directly, but the theory has been tested in many indirect ways and thus need not be taken solely on faith. But some knowledge predicts things that are unverifiable—this is the domain of pure belief.

Statements that adherence to a religious faith will bring eternal happiness, or that honesty is the best policy, or that science is a force for good, are pure belief. No individual experience can prove any of these ideas true or false. There exists no objective test for the truth of predictions across infinite time, or of sweeping generalizations, or of judgments of the value of abstract entities.

We acquire belief in much the same way we acquire many other verifiable forms of information, from the minds of other people. Despite its lack of objective proof, we may accept and use it because other people we trust also accept it and base their actions on it. The social reinforcement of this faith-based knowledge overcomes its lack of verifiability. If you and those around you believe honesty is the best policy, you gain social rewards when you find examples from your life to support it. You can try to verify it objectively, but be forewarned that game theory models suggest honesty may be the *worst* policy if you find yourself among dishonest people (Pruitt and Kimmel 1977). This information is unlikely to change a belief if the belief is based on socially reinforced moral precepts.

To deal with other people requires belief. One can never know exactly what is on another person's mind nor, if asked, offer a complete account of what is on one's own mind. There is a Heisenberg's Uncertainty Principle of mental life—when we examine it, we change it. Thus, any behavior that involves other people must be based on an assumption—that is, an implicit belief—that other people will behave predictably. To know another person's character is to extrapolate a belief about that person from prior experience with that person, and from experiences with people in general.

Self-knowledge is just as belief-based as knowledge of other people. One may assume, for example, that an eagerness today to be married is adequate to make an accurate prediction of one's feelings in the far-off future. But if this were a reliable indicator, then there would be much less divorce. Socrates' advice to "know thyself" does not implore one to navel-gaze, but to see one-self as a human being moved by forces both familiar and unfamiliar. We return to this topic, of self-knowledge as a form of belief, in the following section on identity.

The impossibility of testing some beliefs does not necessarily make them untrue. A moral precept or an axiom about human nature or an attitude about society may be an accurate enough prediction about human behavior to make it useful information. Those who wish to understand human nature do well to observe when certain moral precepts apply and when they do not. The end point of the quest to know human nature is wisdom. A wise person not only has acquired information about the world, but also has tested his or her be-liefs about human nature, transforming belief into reliable knowledge.

Belief is judged to be true if it reliably predicts contentment when it is ac-cepted and discontent when it is not. With a false belief, the consequences are unpredictable. False beliefs that are shared with others are especially perni-cious if the people who share and socially reinforce the belief trust it despite its false predictions. Thus, if one devotes one's life to high finance in the belief that vast wealth ensures contentment, one may find plenty of encouragement from colleagues and the *Wall Street Journal*, but little solace when the bubble pops. False but firmly held beliefs that are shared with no one—delusions—characterize severe mental illness.

### Delusions

A delusion is an impossible and unshakeable belief unique to one person (Ghaemi 2004). The person who has a delusion fails to amend beliefs when the evidence contradicts them and no one else shares them. The nature of delusion has long baffled philosophers (Rhodes and Gipps 2008) and inspired numerous explanatory models (Roberts 1992). For the purposes of this book, and the functional view of mental life, a behavioral model to explain the power of delusional beliefs may prove useful. In such a model, delusions start with a fixed state of arousal that becomes a lens between new experience and its perceived salience. The thoughts and actions of a person who has a delusion can best be understood as motivated by aberrantly aroused thoughts, feelings, and intentions, rather than by verifiable facts. Delusions thus often lead to erratic and incomprehensible behavior, incongruous and intense states of distress, and alienation from the shared beliefs of others.

Delusions tend to emerge when the unexpected happens. Normally, an odd encounter would lead a person to acquire more information. If a man unexpectedly runs into a casual female acquaintance in two different stores on the same day, he may be moved to wonder if she shares his tastes. But a man who has a paranoid delusion may find the unexpected meeting ominous confirmation of a conspiracy. A man who has a grandiose delusion may find the woman's presence to be proof of her desperate sexual attraction to him. A man who has a depressive delusion may be convinced that the woman is a stalker out to punish and humiliate him. In each case the false belief explains a puzzling experience in terms of something other than evidence, and may motivate markedly different behaviors.

Delusions tend to be reinforced by mood; when delusions lack consistency with a state of dejection or excitement or alarm they generally reflect some other kind of pathological arousal. Thus, a manic person who has an excited mood, faced with uncertainty, predicts certain reward. As the mood state precludes the experience of any other outcome from her or his actions, the manic person may begin to understand her or his gift for always being right and fabulous as the correlate of some power or ability or religious significance beyond mundane human experience. As long as the manic mood state and grandiose delusions persist, it is difficult to realign these predictions with actual experience. Thus, even as the consequences of a manic jag begin to hit home—encounters with police, friction with the boss or spouse—the threat-inspired emotions are rationalized grandiosely as a plot to impede the manic person's upward thrust.

A dejected person anticipates no benefit from any course of action, only loss and pain. If a belief forms around an idea that could explain the painful mood, then the persistence of the dejected mood will reinforce it. These delusions tend to revolve around themes of disease, punishment, bankruptcy, humiliation, or other forms of loss and torment. A person who has a delusion of criminal guilt may regard hospitalization as part of the punishment and may even expect that electroconvulsive therapy has been proposed not as a means of relief, but as a death sentence for the person's imagined crimes.

The emotional substrate of paranoid delusions is a fearful mood, a state of unremitting anticipation of menace, foreboding, or dread. Ambiguous statements or looks or behavior or headlines or spam email messages are be-lieved to be the warning signs of some horrific event. When the anticipation of menace persists over a long period of time, a person comes to incorporate the world in detail into the delusional system. At first the belief may be sim-ple, but over time it can become more elaborate as the attempt to figure out a way to cope with the threat becomes integrated into all experience. In time, the paranoid person may learn to hide the belief from others, as a further act of self-defense.

When the person who has a paranoid delusion first "identifies" its source, there may be a sense of satisfaction in knowing the enemy. The predictable fear that arises in the face of the unexpected, and the satisfying feeling of relief that the threat can be identified together reinforce the delusion. The false belief seems true because its predictions always ring true in one's al-tered emotional state. After the paranoid person is conditioned to expect threat from specific people, the maleficent intentions of these people may then become a fixed idea. The paranoid delusion becomes self-perpetuating. Reinforcement of the belief comes from the predictable feeling of threat whenever those people bring the delusion to mind, and the feeling of relief that ensues when one can plot defensive action (whether or not one chooses to act on it). The paranoid delusion cannot be extinguished by objective evi-dence, because the aspect of the belief that makes it seem most true is not its consistency with reality or its logical coherence, but the predictable feeling it inspires.

Other common delusions can also be understood as erroneous predictions based on aberrant states of emotional arousal, whether the arousal accompa-nies a mood disorder, psychosis, or a toxic insult to the brain (Kunert et al. 2007). People who have jealous and erotomanic delusions begin with the pervasive, unmovable feeling of lost or found love, respectively, and interpret their faithless or unwitting lover's every move accordingly. Those who have delusions of reference detect evidence in things they read or encounter to explain their overwhelming feeling of strangeness and foreboding. Religious delusions of ecstasy and damnation tend to occur with manic and depressive states, congruent with the high or low mood. A paranoid patient who alter-nates between manic and depressive episodes might be convinced she was the object of surveillance and sabotage in either mood state, but for different reasons. In the manic state, the strange things that befall her are seen as en-coded messages from the government to keep quiet about the conspiracy that only she comprehends. In the depressed state, the same odd occurrences are meant to punish her because of a minor error on her 1997 tax return.

A delusional belief held for weeks, months, or years becomes an anchor for all experience in the meantime. Once a person's mood has returned to normal, she or he must still unlearn the connections that had become forged between day-to-day events and the overarching explanatory idea, that in essence burned the association into permanent memory. Delusional patients in recovery tend to develop parallel ways of thinking about the delusion, or compartmentalization. He or she may begin to doubt the beliefs, but often the beliefs remain tucked away somewhere in reserve.

Delusions occur in schizophrenia, delusional disorder, mood disorders, delirium, and dementia.

## Overvalued Ideas

To overvalue an idea is essentially to continue to believe something false, because the belief holds some value beyond its value as an agent of accurate prediction (McKenna 1984). Overvalued ideas often subvert the adaptive function of belief, which is to serve as a placeholder for experiential knowledge in the informed conduct of complex behavior. Behavior conducted under the influence of overvalued ideas lacks even the rudimentary rationalization that drives delusions. Overvalued ideas are held not because of their applicability to reality, but because holding them provides other rewards. For example, rigid adherence to a belief shared by other people confers membership in a group. Most overvalued ideas, like those shared within subcultures or religious sects or political parties, are of no clinical significance and are considered to be pernicious mainly by those who do not share them.

But if the group is a religious cult bent on mass suicide, their beliefs are obviously dangerously maladaptive. While such groups have a short existence, their beliefs may outlive them. The group to which a person may wish to belong may be a group in concept only. A man who castrates himself to adhere to the tenets of an ancient sect acts from shared beliefs and an overvalued idea (that he may someday regret) of the rightness of his path to salvation. In contrast, a man who castrates himself because voices told him to, or because he believed the devil literally intended to use him to father the antichrist, is psychotic.

Whether the belief is held by a select group or society at large, overvalued ideas become clinically significant to the degree that they spawn maladaptive behavior. The physiological arousal that accompanies starvation makes food restriction a rewarding act in patients who have anorexia nervosa. Belief in the absolute goodness of being thin and badness of being fat support the addictive aspect of the behavior with a worldview that sustains it even when the craving is absent. Similarly, a manic patient may stop medication and smoke more marijuana in the false (and unfortunately, far from unique) belief that mental illness is a social invention and pharmaceuticals are unnatural (whereas cannabis is not).

Overvalued ideas that move patients to behavior contrary to their interests and to good medical advice contribute significantly to therapeutic resistance. Thus, the clinician often must not only perform an accurate assessment and choose an effective treatment, but also persuade the patient to adopt a new belief about the nature of mental illness and the need to follow psychiatric advice.

Overvalued ideas are apt to occur in paranoid personality disorder and schizotypal personality disorder. In cases of so-called shared delusions ("folie à deux"), where one party is frankly delusional and persuades another party of the delusional idea, the quality of the second party's belief is that of an overvalued idea, motivated by the need or wish to appease the delusional person.

### Doubt

Beliefs change. When one's beliefs consistently fail as predictions, then it is rational and in most cases adaptive to upgrade them. The abandonment of even an old, faulty belief can be a painful process if there are strong interpersonal or social attachments to the person or community that reinforced those beliefs. The process of readjustment to a different perspective motivates many patients to seek psychotherapy, to allow them to fully reap the benefits of a changed belief consistent with new knowledge.

Doubt is a common phenomenon, contributing to existential dilemmas that motivate or arise in the course of psychotherapy. One might argue that they emerge inevitably in psychotherapy as part of the process of transforming one's attitudes.

## 4.4. No Thyself: Misshapen Identity

The concept of personality captures the patterns of behavior that develop over time out of one's volatility and temperamental biases. Identity, in contrast, refers to a set of beliefs one maintains about one's own experiences, feelings, and actions. Thus a person's identity is comprised not so much of the bare facts of his or her life, but of the way these facts may be applied as a narrative to comprehend memories and guide future actions (Eakin 2004).

Belief functions as a proxy in decision making when experiential knowledge is lacking. Because people are complex and free to act as they will we can have no firm a priori knowledge of what they will do when we involve them in our plans. With time and much patience, one may begin to know someone well enough to predict that person's behavior with reasonable accuracy. This applies to one's own behavior, as well. To plan one's actions, one must rely on a belief about the likely satisfaction to be experienced in the future from actions today. The set of beliefs about the likely actions of another person concern the person's *character*. The beliefs one holds about oneself concern *identity*. The stronger the sense of a person's character, the better able one will be to predict the person's future actions. The stronger one's own sense of identity, the better one can apply good judgment to decisions that affect one's future.

A person's sense of identity typically develops over years. In earliest childhood, at the dawn of self-consciousness, one tends to draw no distinction between self and world. Children grow to lose this mindset as they develop a sense of empathy for others. If another person can experience something in a different way, then the world one sees is not identical to the world the other person sees.

In the process of forming concepts of the worlds of others, one's own individual identity emerges. As one begins to define other people by their membership in a family or gender or religion, it becomes evident that these same kinds of distinctions can be made about oneself. As concepts of the character qualities of other people grow more nuanced, so do concepts of identity. Thus, in early childhood, the salient aspects of identification with one's brother may be simply that he's different because he's younger and messier, but the same because of shared home, parents, and surname. As one matures and comes to appreciate the nuances of character, one may appreciate that one is like one's brother in many obvious qualities, but different in ways that only someone with intimate knowledge might appreciate. For example, one's brother's taste in expensive wine informs one's knowledge of his character and in a way adds one more facet to one's own identity, as something that defines what one is not.

Identities, like beliefs, vary across many dimensions. Some identities are grand and ambitious, some modest and circumscribed, some scrawny and warped. Some identities are oceanic in fellow feeling; others hold other people in contempt. Identities evolve throughout life; many readers of this book may now be in transition from unfettered student to responsible professional. In other words, the reader has begun to assimilate by teaching and example a new set of predictions about how he or she will act over a range of circumstances.

Identity goes awry when it conflicts sharply with social expectations, when it remains underdeveloped and immature, or when it lacks shape and form.

## Gender Disorientation

Gender is one of the first aspects of identity most people claim. Usually it is overdetermined, so no cause of conflict. If one's first name jibes with one's genitalia, and these match the tastes and aspirations typical of one's gender, one can quickly declare oneself a girl or a boy. When these fail to mesh, the results can be awkward, painful, or even tragic, depending on the circumstances (Zucker 2005).

The causes of gender disorientation are clear in some cases, murky in others. Children born with ambiguous genitalia, whose obstetricians could not declare them boys or girls at birth, were in past eras assigned to a sex (Wisniewski and Migeon 2002). If the assignment consisted merely of giving the child a gender-specific name and raising the child as if the child belonged to one or another gender, the error might emerge a few years hence when the child began to show gender-contrary preferences for clothing and play, and the opportunity would exist to simply change the name, buy a new wardrobe, and otherwise follow the child's lead.

However, some infants have undergone sexual assignment surgery, based on the discredited theory that gender is almost entirely a result of postnatal hormonal influence and social conditioning, so one could simply remove the underdeveloped testicles and penis, surgically build a vagina and vulva, and teach the child to be a girl. The tragic consequence of this occurred when some of these children began to mature and declare themselves boys. It turns out that one's sex is written into the brain (specifically, the hypothalamus) prior to birth, so postnatal removal of testosterone by castration does not make an infant a sexual *tabula rasa*. This mechanism of sexual determination in the brain may account for young children who have otherwise unambiguous genitalia but express from an early age a preference for clothing, toys, and friends consistent with the opposite sex.

Many cases of gender identity disorder in people who have normally developed genitalia present in adulthood, and almost all such cases report that they always "knew" they were really of the opposite sex. Surgical transformation is still possible, though it is probably more rarely done now than it was in decades past. One caveat offered to potential candidates for surgical gender transformation is that in many past cases life became no more satisfying after surgery (Lothstein 1982). In these cases the notion of being the wrong sex may have served as an overvalued idea, essentially a motivated distraction from other more salient life problems. Another reason surgery may be more rare is that increasingly among substantial segments of many societies a "transgendered" identity is perfectly acceptable, so there is little motivation to undergo the trauma of surgery.

Gender identity disorder is diagnosed when a person complains of feeling uneasy in his or her public gender, and more comfortable with the idea of being the opposite gender.

## Projection

Identity formation hinges on recognizing the fundamental difference between the perspectives of the self and other people. Failure to observe this difference gives rise to interpersonal behavior predicated on projection: the assumption that another person feels and will act as one would feel or act in the other person's position (Murstein and Pryer 1959). Projection is a common expression of immature or regressed psychological development with or without other psychopathology. It is not specific to a subset of psychiatric diagnoses.

Projection is not an inherently maladaptive or pathological phenomenon. Frequent projection occurs normally in childhood social development. Accurate projection with respect to others may simply reflect that one has chosen to associate with people who share one's temperament and outlook on life. When projection frequently goes awry and occurs to excess in adults it tends to signify immaturity and to lead to maladaptive behavior.

As a familiar clinical example, patients often project onto clinicians the expectation, perhaps reflecting experience forged in the parent-child relationship, that the clinician will be personally affronted and inclined to act punitively if the patient questions the treatment plan. This may lead to an assortment of maladaptive help-seeking behaviors. A patient may resent the punitive intentions the patient imagines the clinician to harbor, and so sabotage the treatment plan in retaliation. Conversely, a patient from an abusive background may crave punishment paradoxically—in childhood experience punishment grew to be a familiar mode of parental engagement—and so may sabotage treatment in order to provoke punishment. Or, to pre-empt the anticipated punishment, the patient may attempt to engage the clinician in flirtatious banter, or to plead for forgiveness over a minor lapse in healthy habits, or to complain bitterly about being made to wait for five minutes. In cases like this, it may seem to the clinician that he or she has become a character in the patient's own personal drama. That is close to the truth. Patients who behave badly in the clinical setting often have developed assumptions about the treatment they wish or fear to receive from the clinician. The clinician, meanwhile, has been cast unwittingly in the role of authority figure along with all that entails for an individual patient, derived from the patient's lifelong attitudes about other authority figures.

## *Dissolution*

Dissolution applies to the failure of some individuals to establish a coherent identity. Such individuals may struggle with gender identity, or at least with sexual orientation; they may commonly practice projection in personal interactions. Most significant, they seem to lack a concept of self-integrity that would normally facilitate making wise and adaptive life choices.

Identity dissolution suggests fundamental problems in development. Failure to form a coherent identity might be the result of a childhood-onset mental illness that diverts the child from normal developmental learning. Or, in someone who has lifelong, severe temperamental vulnerabilities that impair interpersonal relationships or, worse, a labile personality, it might be difficult if not impossible for the person to define his or her own identity compared to others, because there is so little opportunity to acquire useful information about the rational mental processes of others. Early and severe traumatic experiences that impede trust and undermine developmental tasks contribute to dissolution for similar reasons.

Though the term is not part of any diagnostic criteria, the phenomenon of dissolution is a common denominator in conversion symptoms and dissociative disorders. Dissolute patients are prone to pseudoneurologic, or hysterical symptoms (Kihlstrom 2005). The reader may recall from the discussion earlier that hysterical symptoms arise from the individual's dread of the contents of his or her own mind, which leads to the avoidance of certain modes of mental activity. Dissolution is the overarching phenomenon behind such splintered consciousness. Similarly, a dissolute identity is likely a prerequisite for dissociative disorders, such as the so-called multiple personality disorder, in which the integrity of individual identity is so weak that the person is easily led to create many elaborate "alters," which may or may not be in communication with one another (Spanos 1994).

## 4.5. Quid Pro Woe: Cooperative Contretemps

Human infants are among the most helpless creatures in the animal kingdom. Infants, and children in general, need more than material support and nurturing. Children model the skills they will need for self-sustenance and self-defense through interactions with other people. In the process, children learn to express their own wants and needs, and to understand the wants and needs of other people. These comprise the essential skills of cooperative behavior.

Not all species live cooperatively, and the value placed on cooperation varies across individuals and cultures, but some degree of cooperation appears to be essential to human survival (Fehr and Fischbacher 2003). Cooperation among mating partners ensures that genes are passed on to a new generation. Cooperation among larger groups ensures that those to whom genes have been passed thrive long enough so that they, and their children, and their grandchildren, all survive to propagate. Social cooperation thus serves as a hedge against natural selection. Humans live longer and propagate more efficiently than many other species thanks to the social protections that permit pair-bonding for the protection and nurture of offspring, the care of elders to foster social continuity and cohesion, and the capacity to sacrifice some individual pleasure and safety to benefit the group as a whole.

Cooperative behavior works on the same principles as any goal-directed, adaptive behavior, but with added complexity because other people are involved. Motivated behavior that involves other people must account for the freedom of people to behave in ways other than hoped-for, planned, or predicted. One can reduce the degree of uncertainty if one can motivate another person to act in a particular way. The socially acceptable way to motivate another person is to offer something in return: to cooperate (Axelrod and Hamilton 1981).

One can also minimize uncertainty in dealing with other people by acting like them. Every human passes through phases of life when access to the basic needs of life, pleasure, and safety from harm depends on the protective care of parents and other caregivers. It becomes clear to most people from an early age that one can earn the favor of these caregiving figures by mimicking their behavior. Indeed, the ability to imitate others predates the ability to formulate behavioral plans and rules based on verbal instruction, so for a time it may be the only coherent way for a young child to act (Lakin et al. 2008).

The drive to conform can be so potent that it motivates people to deny their own senses, as demonstrated in a famous experiment (Bond and Smith 1996). An unwitting subject, surrounded by a group of actors, can be induced to agree that two line segments are the same length, when they are obviously different, after seeing that every one of the actors makes the same wrong judgment. In another famous series of experiments, led by Albert Bandura, not only the judgment but also the apparent emotional state of others proved transmissible by imitation (Bandura and Ross 1961). Children were induced to play violently with toys when they were both aroused by frustration (in one phase of the experiment, they were denied access to available toys), *and* when they had been exposed to adults who played violently with toys. Without the modeled violent behavior, the children behaved less angrily. Under normal circumstances, the drive to conform to the behavior of others, whatever the behavior may be, facilitates cooperation.

Cooperative behavior can be classed according to how the mutual benefit is managed. The simplest method is reciprocation. In its basic societal form, reciprocal cooperation includes barter, a cash purchase, or a contract, in which the terms of exchange and the end point are specified in advance. As parties learn to trust one another, some credit may be extended, and the end point may be waived so that one party may help another with the expectation that at some unspecified time, the favor will be returned.

In a long-term cooperative relationship, there may be instances of explicit, contractual cooperation ("If you wash the dishes, I'll put the kids to bed"), but there will also be times when the effort is one-sided, as when a parent is raising children or a child cares for an ailing parent. Taken at face value, this may be explained partly by the belief that it all evens out in the end; parents care

*Table 7.*    Modes of Cooperative Engagement

| Type | Description | Mental Faculties/Dysfunctions |
|---|---|---|
| Isolation | Refusal or denial of cooperation with others | May imply asociality, eccentricity, if the task would be more readily accomplished with others |
| Coercion | Enlistment of others in one's interests by threat or force | Implies sociopathy or hostility when imposed by another individual or group in a free society |
| Servitude | Service of other's interests out of fear or coercion | In a free society, suggests overdependency, inertia |
| Manipulation | Enlistment of others in one's interests by misrepresentation of mutual benefit | A favored, nonviolent approach by individuals with sociopathy, egotism, overdependency |
| Mutuality | Service of common interests simultaneously | Implies recognition of common cause with another |
| Exchange | Direct and explicit, *quid pro quo* arrangement | Requires one to negotiate one's own and the other party's values simultaneously |
| Contract | Explicit but perhaps indirect exchange | May involve abstract calculation of benefits and commitment to a plan |
| Relationship | Implicit expectation of exchanges over a prolonged or indefinite period | Involves significant degree of mutual trust that both parties value parity |
| Attachment | Assumption of the interests of another as one's own | Motivated by pleasure rather than fear |
| Altruism | Sacrifice of one's personal interest for the benefit of others in general | Implies a strong, unbreakable attachment to an abstract entity |

for children so they will be cared for in old age. But in the long run, *quid pro quo* is too simple to explain such altruistic acts. People often devote enormous effort to others they know are unlikely to be able to reciprocate. We understand this kind of expenditure of effort as a derivative of affiliative behavior, driven by the embrace of someone else's welfare as influential to one's own welfare. Affiliation is discussed in a later section. Table 7 contrasts the common modes of cooperative and non-cooperative engagement.

## Asociality

Asociality describes a global impairment in the capacity to work or play effectively with others. Cooperative social behavior builds on two premises:

one, that other people can help one to achieve one's ends; two, that one can get other people to be helpful by being helpful to them. Asociality hinders a person from being able to competently engage other people in the process of reciprocal cooperation.

Social reciprocity takes complex calculations. In the development of cooperative relationships both parties form highly sophisticated models of what to expect in the course of a cooperative venture. In solo behavior, the actor has only to model her or his own variables. To engage in cooperative behavior, the actor has to first form a mental representation of the goal of her or his own behavior, as well as the anticipated steps to completion. If any of the steps require another person, she or he must include a subroutine to effectively enlist another person's aid. To succeed at this, a likely partner must be identified (and some assessment made about the partner's character) before negotiation can begin. To negotiate, the request for cooperation must anticipate the goals the other person may have, and construct a feasible set of actions that could be taken to serve the other person's interests. In other words, one must possess a "theory of mind" in order to see the world from the mind of another person and thus predict what he or she might want and might be willing to do to obtain it (Baron-Cohen et al. 1985).

For example, Jack plans to move and rehearsing the task in his mind realizes there is no way he can get his couch out of the house on his own. Two people, he calculates, could do it. None of his good friends are free (that is no open-ended cooperative relationships to draw on). He runs into Jane, an acquaintance. He wants to ask Jane to help, but in the absence of an ongoing cooperative relationship with Jane, knows he will have better luck if he can offer something in return. He thinks of offering money, but projects she will find it a crude gesture. He thinks of offering to help her move, but knows her circumstances well enough to know she has no plans to move in the foreseeable future. Finally, he proposes to treat her to pizza and beer, and she accepts.

Although this seems a mundane and simple interaction, the capacity to incorporate not only one's own plans but also to model the character and desires of another person into the cooperative proposal requires complex computations. The mental construction of models within models is so highly demanding of swift, integrated calculation across the entire cortex that a brain malfunction that merely slowed down intercortical communication over a prolonged period of development might permanently damage the cognitive capacity for cooperative behavior (Ciaranello and Ciaranello 1995).

When the capacity to calculate a reciprocal course of action is impeded early in life, before someone has developed cooperative skills, it can produce profound lifelong impairment, as seen in patients who have autism disorder. Like many neurodevelopmental processes, there is likely a critical period during which these skills must be mastered if they are ever to be fully acquired. The risk for new onset of autism likely diminishes with age because by the end of childhood the skills needed to engage others in cooperative action have already been learned and cemented in permanent, procedural (skill) memory. Once learned, the skill becomes second nature, like walking or talking, practiced without fail long after the brain begins to deteriorate. This is illustrated in progressive cortical dementias, such as Alzheimer disease, in which a person may lose all capacity to learn or plan or even to speak coherently, but retain social skills almost to the end.

Asociality can be acquired later in life, in the context of chronic mental illness (Lee et al. 2004). Individuals who have chronic hallucinations and delusions often undergo a devastating deterioration in social skills. This may result from a deficit in cognition or it may develop as the psychotic contents of mind render social interactions less predictable and meaningful over the course of years. The psychotic experience of reality may in effect provide pathological feedback that conditions behavior away from effective interpersonal interactions and toward an idiosyncratic, untrusting, asocial approach to other people. It is hard to enter into a trusting, cooperative relationship with someone if voices are saying, daily, that the person wants to kill you.

Diagnostically, asociality is the hallmark of autism, childhood attachment disorders, schizophrenia, and schizoid personality.

### Sociopathy

Certain individuals in society find ways to motivate other people to serve their interests and offer nothing substantive in return. The threat or infliction of harm to another person is a crude and socially unacceptable example, but manipulative behavior provides a less dangerous method that flies under the radar of social disapproval. Manipulation of others superficially resembles cooperation, but the mutuality of the benefit is illusory. A practitioner of manipulative behavior does offer something in return for someone's attention, effort, and resources, but the offer is false in some way.

Most well-socialized people abhor the thought of threatening or cheating others. The principle of the "Golden Rule," to do unto others as you would have done to you, works best if one person can model in his or her own mind how it will in fact feel to be in the other person's position. That is, most people employ empathy both to guide successful cooperative interactions and also to avoid actions that harm or use others. Sociopathy, or antisocial behavior, involves the failure of this latter aspect of empathic understanding (Moll and Schulkin 2009).

Success at manipulation suggests a sociopathic person is unimpaired in the cognitive capacity to model the perspective of other people, or else it would be difficult for such a person to gauge what to (misleadingly) offer the other party as a cooperative gesture. But a sociopathic person may be unable to find adverse consequences salient. If the sociopathic person underestimates the severity of bad consequences for himself or herself, why not for others as well? In some cases the capacity for empathic understanding may exist, but the sociopathic individual may have been conditioned in an environment where the long-term adverse consequences of selfish behavior—or the benefits of cooperation—were never experienced. A sociopathic person regards other people as a means to an end, and so learns crude means to make use of people, but lacks the wherewithal to engage people in relationships that will ensure cooperation in the long run.

Some individuals seem to acquire sociopathic behavior from impoverished environments, in which they were rarely treated with compassion and empathy, and then grow out of it once they reach adulthood. Many others, however, develop sociopathic behaviors despite being raised with adequate nurturing, and go on to maintain sociopathic patterns throughout life (Loeber 1982). This was demonstrated in adoption studies, in which having a biological parent with sociopathy predicted lifelong patterns of sociopathy, whereas bad conduct in adopted children of nonsociopathic biological parents tended to wane over time (Crowe 1974). Thus, some who have sociopathy may have a true biological deficit in the capacity to model the emotional states of others and rarely grow past it (Kiehl 2006), whereas others may have acquired sociopathic behaviors as means of survival. On reaching adulthood and perceiving the limitations to the manipulative approach, the person who has learned sociopathy has less difficulty acquiring the necessary social skills.

Some people who have mania develop a sociopathic attitude toward others, at least while manic. Narcissistic and borderline personality disorders often incorporate some sociopathy. Active substance abuse often fosters sociopathic behavior in the pursuit of the drug. The diagnoses most characteristic of sociopathy are conduct disorder and antisocial personality.

## Shame

Shame is a potent motivator and a key civilizing influence, especially in childhood. Its power stems at least in part from the associated fear of the withdrawal of cooperation. Shame is not itself a sign of mental illness, but it often worsens the suffering that follows from illness, mental and physical.

Shame can be either real or misplaced. When a person has broken the social contract, and the misbehavior is common knowledge, it changes the structure of that individual's relationships, and alters the ability to negotiate cooperative agreements in the future (Gilbert 2000). The people with whom the person might wish to cooperate may refuse in the future to extend trust. Part of the painful emotional experience of shame is the feeling of loss, because in losing the trust of others the shamed person has lost something of real value.

The painful feeling of shame in some individuals motivates addictive behavior to suppress it. The success of the Alcoholics Anonymous / 12-step approach to the treatment of addiction, in which the addiction is considered a "disease," is understood in this light as a useful fiction to steer the recovering addict around relapse-provoking feelings of shame. An alcoholic may have done some shameful things, but need not be ashamed of having a disease that cannot be controlled (Potter-Efron and Efron 1993). Freed of this seemingly inescapable shame about the weakness to control drinking, the recovering alcoholic is less motivated to seek solace in drink, and can work on redressing the shameful things done in the course of alcohol addiction.

Misplaced shame often occurs in the psychiatric context in the form of stigma (Hinshaw and Stier 2008). Thus, the converse of the alcoholic who feels less ashamed because the addiction is seen as a disease imposed on the mind and body is the person who has depression or chronic psychosis or some other malfunction of brain processes and avoids help because it seems shameful to admit to having a mental illness. This can become a particularly insidious problem with depression, because the dejected state biases a person to the most negative self-assessment. As the idea of mental illness as disease becomes increasingly widespread in our culture the stigma diminishes, albeit at a glacial pace.

Shame is not specific to any diagnosis, but is widespread across many psychiatric disorders, in the form of stigma. Narcissistic personality disorder behaviors can be seen as intended to ward off feelings of shame. Shame can compound role dysfunction particularly when it occurs with social phobias and depression.

## 4.6. Piece of Mind: Communication Breakdown

Communication is both a tool and a rewarding, motivated behavior. A typical baby just learning to speak develops speech not from having anything specific to say, but from a drive for social engagement with parents. Early in life, infants begin to utter modulated sounds when others around them are in conversation. The infant's random efforts at vocalization produce the desirable consequence that they gain attention from parents and other cooing adults. By this time in the infant's development the experience of a familiar human face in the infant's field of view has come to be associated with pleasure, because the same face has been seen frequently in the context of other pleasures like feeding. Thus, vocalizing earns the parental gaze, which provokes pleasurable excitement. This makes vocalization a rewarding activity for the infant, and in subsequent interactions between child and parents repeated over years the child's random vocal output is molded into meaningful language (Meltzoff et al. 2009).

The cooperative aspects of communication become most apparent in development as a child begins to learn verbs. The first verbs we use tend to be actions that involve other people. When a toddler says "go," it generally means not that the toddler wishes to go somewhere alone, or wants someone else to go somewhere, or has remarked on some third party in the process of going somewhere; it usually indicates a desire for the person being addressed to take him or her someplace. The simple "throw ball" statement entices one to throw the toddler the ball, and when one says the same thing back to the toddler, the ball is returned, and the game is repeated. Over nearly 20 years the child's verbiage increases in complexity and the direct reciprocity of early play is replaced by less immediate motivators. However, the aims of conversation remain the same. We express what is our mind in order to engage another person in our interests, with the expectation that cooperation, affiliation, and mutual benefit in some form will result (Reddy 2003).

## Dysfluency/Hyperfluency

Inhibited and excessive speech are common consequences of severe mental disorders. Asocial individuals communicate little because, in the absence of an organized capacity to engage others in cooperative action, communication has limited salience. In states of dejection, in which motivations and emotions are not sufficiently aroused toward action, a drive to communicate may also be underactivated. There is no point in the effort to engage others in one's plans if there are no plans.

Excessive speech, writing, and other modes of communication, on the other hand, is a hallmark of an excited mood and generated by the same brain processes associated with artistic creativity (Flaherty 2005). In extreme cases, it may be difficult to interrupt a person with excessive speech, or to follow her or his skips in logic. The give-and-take aspect of speech may be lost, as the person's speech becomes what is described as "pressured." The manic person is so motivated to engage others in her or his many and shifting interests and plans that she or he cannot resist the urge to interrupt, change topics without notice, and otherwise dominate the conversation. Excessive speech in the context of anxious hyperarousal, in contrast, seems motivated by the fear of a silent pause in conversation, and what alarming thing might come up if silence is allowed to persist.

Voluntary perturbations of communication are often manipulative. The willful refusal to communicate bypasses expectations of cooperation. Heightened flow of speech (logorrhea), as employed, for example, by a high-pressure salesman or a drug-seeking clinic patient exhausts the listener and leaves little room to escape the conversation, other than to accede to the demand to buy or prescribe.

Quantity of speech is at times a purely dimensional characteristic and not diagnosed. Relatively increased speech may be a feature of histrionic personality while diminished speech a quality of schizoid personality. Elective mutism is a behavioral disorder diagnosis in childhood. Speech may increase or decrease in quantity with mood disorders and in anxious states.

## Derailment

Disorganized cognition manifests as a derailment of logic in the train of spoken thought. In excited mood states, speech may flow copiously but be so full of obscure references and unrelated ideas that it seems clear there are many thoughts competing for expression all at the same time. To the listener, reader, or interpreter, the communication becomes increasingly disjointed. At somewhat lower levels of arousal, whether excited or anxious, the train of thought never comes off the tracks, but it takes excessive time to get to the caboose. Overinclusive speech has logical coherence but contains more detail than is necessary to convey the thought. The difference between circumstantial, digressive speech and tangential speech hinges on whether the speaker remembers to return to the main topic of conversation. True derailment reflects either a pace of thought exceeding the capacity to precipitate it into coherent prose, or idiosyncrasy in the logical world of the speaker (Spitzer 1997).

Significant thought disorder is characteristic of mania, schizophrenia, delirium, and, to a lesser degree, some dementias. Mildly meandering speech ranges from normal personality quirk to generalized anxiety to some personality disorders, including histrionic and narcissistic personalities.

## Telemission

Thought broadcasting—to silently send one's thoughts abroad, involuntarily, to all around—is an experience primarily found in schizophrenia. The term *telemission* is coined here to juxtapose the phenomenon to its better-known opposite, telepathy, in which one claims to receive the thoughts of others from afar. Unlike hallucinations, extravolitional (passivity), intrusive (thought insertion), or avulsive (thought withdrawal) symptoms, the abnormal phenomenon is attributed to other people, whom the person believes are in possession of the person's thoughts. How can one understand this as the disruption of a normal mental function?

The existence of such a symptom suggests there may be a specific mental faculty that detects when we have made successful communication, akin to the faculty that detects when we have satisfied some other motivated behavior. This might work by predicting the sensory cues we expect to see and hear if we have successfully communicated something—the nod, the murmured "uh-hunh." Because the pace and quality of communication is finely tuned to the detection of comprehension in the listener, this capacity must normally be well developed, and have ready access to the cerebral apparatus that generates communicative behavior. Although it may seem odd that such an essential skill might be practiced so frequently and yet be so removed from awareness, it is clear that the time it takes to "read" a face is far shorter than the time it takes to be aware of what we are reading. Thus, experimental studies of emotion recognition demonstrate a normal ability to correctly identify the emotional quality of a facial expression despite having no conscious recollection of having seen it (Dimberg et al. 2000). This suggests simply that one may readily pick up social cues without conscious awareness that one has perceived them.

The psychotic experience of telemission, then, may be seen not as a belief about other people's perceptions or even about the auditory properties of one's thoughts, but rather as the misinterpretation of social cues that normally signal comprehension. The perception of a nod, a grunt, a minute intensification of eye contact, a pursing of the lips, that collectively signal "message received" in a particular part of the cortex somehow has been activated aberrantly, and one experiences this as a feeling that other people know what is on one's mind, without having to say it out loud. The mind may thus be fooled into believing it is in a state of active communication while it continues to process normal, private streams of thought.

## Misrepresentation

When communication is represented as true but is demonstrably false, it is considered confabulation if the speaker is unaware that the words are false, and lying if the speaker is aware of but deliberately misrepresents reality. Confabulation occurs with some dementia syndromes, and seems to reflect an inability to align established knowledge with an accurate grasp of the present context (Schnider 2003). A person confabulates unaware of the falsity of the information he or she provides. A person telling a lie, on the other hand, willfully misrepresents fact. Lying manipulates the listener. Although lying is occasionally benign if it spares the listener needless pain, more often it is selfish if the intention is to profit by moving others to do one's bidding, or exploitative and possibly destructive if done to enjoy the pleasure in the power to move or manipulate others.

In clinical settings, the question whether a patient is lying or not is most significant in decisions about whether to start or stop treatment. Some patients may misrepresent that they have symptoms when they do not, to gain intoxicating drugs or disability compensation, while others may falsely claim significant improvement in symptoms, to be released from unwanted treatment prematurely. This is part of what makes psychiatry so challenging: there are no completely objective gauges of illness. When in doubt, the truth of a patient's report can be validated by records or reports of other people. In the rare case of factitious disorder (Munchausen syndrome) the misrepresentation is nonverbal—these individuals in the patient role actively mislead clinicians by placing a drop of blood in a urine sample, or painting the arm red with makeup to resemble cellulitis, or hyperventilating to induce a period of hypocarbic apnea (Spivak et al. 1994). In contrast to individuals with other somatizing behaviors, who seek the reassurance or caring attention of the clinician, those with factitious presentations seem motivated by the desire for all the trappings of medical care, including invasive procedures, intravenous lines, sponge baths, and rectal temperature measurements.

Demonstrably and deliberately false speech suggests malingering and antisocial personality. Falsifying symptoms in order to receive unnecessary medical care is factitious disorder; malingering is the falsification of symptoms for some material gain.

## 4.7. Social Insecurity: Disaffiliation

Cooperation and communication provide the motivation and tools for reciprocal social behavior. Affiliation with other people provides something more than reciprocal benefit. A partner in an affiliated relationship does not merely help us find rewards in the world; time spent with a partner *is* the reward. Cooperation can occur without affiliation but misses this extra benefit of being able to share pleasure with another person.

The story of the development of affiliation picks up at the point where the infant has begun to anticipate satiety and pleasure in the presence of the mother. Over time the sights, sounds, smiles of approval, and touches of the mother initiate the pleasure response when there is no specific need or desire. The infant can begin to feel warm, safe, and secure just by seeing, and later, thinking about mother (Bowlby 1977). A series of famous experiments with monkeys has shown that baby monkeys become attached to the cozy cloth mother doll and not the wire figure from which they obtain milk (Harlow and Zimmerman 1959). Thus the most essential ingredient of healthy affiliation is not, in fact, the meeting of physical needs, but the emotional response to the physical comfort of a mother.

The process of affiliation might never occur, however, without the physiologic influence of the oxytocin/vasopressin peptide hormone system, mediated via the hypothalamus. In other animals there is clear evidence that these hormones determine the capacity for affiliative behavior. Two subspecies of the vole—a small rodent—that differ only in the presence of these hormones differ markedly in the pair bonding and nurturing behavior they exhibit (Young and Wang 2004). Similarly, a key difference between bonobo apes, who display complex erotic behavior and bonding relationships reminiscent of humans, and chimpanzees who do not, appears to be the presence in bonobos of active oxytocin/vasopressin function (de Waal 1988). In humans, oxytocin/vasopressin function facilitates affiliation from mother to infant, as well as between romantic partners (Insel and Young 2001). Analogous to the bond between child and mother facilitated by the child's satiety response to feeding, the bond between parent and child and between sexual partners becomes cemented when the child or sexual partner is in one's arms at the moment of hormone release. Hence behavior that leads to more encounters of this kind is encouraged by the mechanisms of conditioning.

A stably affiliated person learns to reframe the interests of the other person as his or her own. In an affiliated relationship, it seems that an act done for the benefit of the other person will benefit both people. In a strong and lasting relationship, one may imagine this cycle of shared benefit generates a positive feedback loop of goodwill that keeps it running smoothly in perpetuity.

Pleasure is important but disappointment is also essential in the development of mature relationships. One day the infant awakens from sleep, hungry, while the mother is in another room. The infant scans the room, sees no mother present, and then cries. What had begun as pure pleasure when the mother relieved hunger and pain has become painful, as positive expectations exceed the mother's capacity to satisfy them. The frustrated desire for mother may create conflict in the infant. The mother's presence is no longer a matter of pure pleasure, as experiences of frustration and fear become associated with the desire for her. But these mixed feelings can be the starting point of secure, mutual attachment, as the growing child learns how to manage them, for example, by anticipating that the needs will be met eventually (Ainsworth 1969). The child accustomed to immediate gratification may grow to lack the motivation to learn how to engage in cooperative behavior. A measure of the strength and stability of a relationship is how harmoniously the parties negotiate their expectations of one another.

## Grief

The developmental sketch in this section portrays the dawn of attachment, the formation of a conditioned anticipation of pleasure in the company of the mother. Grief is its end point, the extinction of the conditioned expectation of pleasure in someone with whom one has become affiliated. Normal grief leads to a readjustment to the world, and ideally a set of fresh desires (Maciejewski et al. 2007). Someone may grieve not only for people who have died, but also for other irretrievable losses, such as health, innocence, culture, or the fruits of one's labor. In a sense, the things one can grieve for are all concepts or beliefs or institutions that can be adopted as one's own interests and to which one can therefore become affiliated.

One grieves for people who have given one pleasure, even if these people also caused a lot of pain. To think about the person or look at his or her picture or hear a recording or read a letter associated with the person cues a conditioned expectation of pleasure in the person's company. After the loss of that person, these stimuli arouse happy expectation and an instant later frustration from the reminder that the anticipation is misplaced. Over time, the disconnection of cues from the active reinforcing experience of pleasure weakens the automatic arousal of desire, and emotional life returns to normal.

Grief is a normal human response to loss; if demoralization or functional deterioration follows, it may become the impetus for treatment seeking. Clinicians will encounter it in their patients routinely. Diagnostically, when the major depressive syndrome accompanies an important loss, it may be considered major depression and treated accordingly.

## Overdependency

Affiliation fails if it is inflexible. Mature and adaptive mutual dependency characterizes long partnerships and marriages. Mature affiliation mitigates the pain of separation, and may even enhance the relationship ("absence makes the heart grow fonder"), because the expectation of mutual reward has so often been met. Unstable relationships, in which the expectation of mutual reward has often been raised and frustrated, tend to produce demoralization, anxiety, hostility, and stress with separations. Often the inability to form stable relationships has been conditioned by experience, but other factors such as temperament may exert the greater destabilizing force (Rutter et al. 2009).

Overdependency has less to do with how much one wishes to be with someone, or relies on someone else for help and support, than with the quality of the emotional response to being without that person. A partner in a romantic relationship may grow overdependent through a clash of styles, in which one partner aims for interdependency in all things, while the other behaves inconsistently, gratifying the need one day and pulling away the next. Conflict in an overdependent romantic entanglement manifests in behaviors like clinging and jealousy that tend to undermine the mutuality in a relationship. When the less dependent partner decides to sever the bond, the resulting distress may trigger all manner of misery and maladaptive behavior to quell the pain of loss, up to and including rageful violence and suicidal behavior. The degree of desperation and pain in these situations suggests the feelings one might have if one's spouse or parent or child had died and one believed one could reverse death by screaming, sobbing, and rending one's flesh.

A diagnosis of dependent personality disorder encompasses the concept of overdependency; relationship conflicts are responsible for many episodes of emergency treatment for suicidal ideation in which adjustment disorder is the most appropriate diagnosis.

## Egotism

The term *narcissism* comes from the ancient tale of the young man, Narcissus, who was so besotted with his own reflection in a pool of water that he fell in and drowned. It has a variety of popular connotations, including vanity or excessive self-love. Its usage in psychiatry is somewhat confusing, as in practice the patients who tend to be called "narcissistic," while self-centered, are anything but self-adoring (Bushman and Baumeister 1998).

A more accurate clinical term might be *egotism*, which implies a priority for self-satisfaction, but without the assumption of excessive self-love. There is nothing intrinsically wrong with looking out for one's interests, but it does become a problem when the priority of immediate self-interest impedes the ability to form stable relationships. In general the egotist has, for whatever reason, not come to anticipate pleasure from affiliation with other people. This might reflect a dysfunction in the hormonal reinforcement of attachment, or an attitude learned from hard experience among uncaring caretakers, or a view of other people dimmed by apathy and anhedonia. Or, the egotistical person might possess a temperamental disposition toward impulsivity, hence undervaluing future rewards from long-term relationships (Vazire and Funder 2006).

But people and the world at large can and often do disappoint. Whereas a person with a healthy affiliation has a ready source of comfort in the person of a loved one, the egotistical person has no one from whom he or she expects to find solace when the world fails to gratify. Thus the egotistical person may seem arrogant or vain, because the only reliable sources of satisfaction have become self-satisfaction and self-reflection (Campbell and Foster 2007). Egotistical people engage in relationships, but dismiss the value of affiliation (Bartholomew 1990). Unlike people who have sociopathic tendencies, egotistical people are not looking to exploit others for material gain; they exploit others, intentionally or not, for the emotional reward of being held in high regard by others. Whereas healthy relationships grow from past shared rewards and subsist on the anticipation of future shared rewards, the egotistical person has a low expectation that others will provide future reward, so finds less motivation to act in the direct interest of a partner, and so less opportunity to learn that the benefits will accrue in the end.

In contrast to an overly dependent person, an egotistical person at the end of a relationship does not feel fear but intense frustration. From a behavioral perspective, the egotistical person holds on to a relationship in the anticipation of personal pleasure. To lose a relationship, such as it is, is to lose a source of satisfaction. And, because the egotistical person has not come to associate self-satisfaction with the partner's, the loss of the pleasures of the relationship stimulates rage and despair, at being denied pleasure, rather than sympathy or guilt over the unsatisfying experience the other person has had in the relationship.

Egotism is most characteristic of narcissistic personality disorder, and it contributes to domestic violence.

### Eccentricity

A subset of individuals appears to have little interest in affiliation with other people. Unlike the egotistical person, who desires the benefits of a relationship but may be unable by nature or conditioning to fully embrace one, the eccentric person is either unmotivated by the emotional benefits of a relationship, or impaired in the faculties needed to overcome the uncertainty and friction that must be navigated in forging an interpersonal relationship (Tantam 1988).

The term *eccentric* commonly means unusual or odd or different in tastes and behaviors; for the eccentric person this may be a consequence rather than a cause of the diffident attitude regarding relationships. If a person fails to engage with other people, then it follows that the person may form beliefs that seem odd to other people (Bell et al. 2006). Whether this follows from a constitutional weakness in the appraisal of human behavior, or inexperience with it, the eccentric person may remain naïve to the motives and expectable actions of other people. Thus a person who has vast experience in human affairs doubts conspiracy theories categorically because it is practically impossible to organize large numbers of people in a secret common cause, whereas eccentric people who lack much messy human experience may have less reason to doubt the plausibility of mass conspiracies about the Kennedy assassination, alien abductions, and so on.

Although the causes of these patterns of poor affiliation and odd preoccupations have been linked to schizophrenia and autism in many cases, eccentricity per se is not generally a clinical problem, until it becomes maladaptive (Raine 2006). If an eccentric person fails to anticipate that mutual cooperation is essential to survival under some circumstances, such as dire medical or financial trouble, then the failure to develop relationships may leave the person vulnerable to serious risks to life, health, and well-being. An eccentric person may desire some of the pleasures of a relationship, such as sex, and may become frustrated over the difficulties of finding them.

Eccentricity with respect to interpersonal attachments is a common feature in Cluster A personality disorders: schizoid, schizotypal, and paranoid, as well as pervasive developmental (autism spectrum) disorders such as Asperger syndrome.

## 4.8. Complain Speaking: Help-Seeking Misbehavior

Healers have always been around. Before the modern era, healing flowed from the healer's access to supernatural power or at least from his or her worldly wisdom and spiritual insights, in addition to a specialized knowledge of the body and physical remedies for ailments. The model medical encounter involves a patient with a problem who contracts with a healer to improve health, resolve symptoms, and above all, alleviate distress. Whether the distress is as sharp as the acute abdominal pain signaling appendicitis, or as amorphous as the vague fear of premature death that prompts the generally well person to submit to a full physical exam, the aim is to help the patient feel better and preserve life functions.

Rational pursuit of treatment for medical illness occurs when the consequences of untreated illness are dire and treatment efficacy is predictable. Conversely, when there is low risk of morbidity, and the obstacles to treatment are high, and the effectiveness of treatment is doubtful, then unreasonable forces must explain help-seeking. These forces include fear and dread of illness and belief in the power of the healer.

The term *patient* commonly and imprecisely refers to any person who shows up in a hospital or clinic to see a clinician. But some people seek out clinicians for motives other than the fear of morbidity and faith in the healer. A true patient, in the ideal, has entered into a healing relationship in which all relevant information is revealed unreservedly and the healer's interventions accepted with full and faithful adherence. In return, the healer suspends personal interest in order to attend to the patient's problems. This is not to say an ideal patient should practice blind obedience; quite the contrary. Whether the plan is negotiated or dictated, having agreed on it, the true patient makes no unilateral changes without the healer's agreement that the change is consistent with the healer's plan of therapy.

Some patients do not seek the healer, but are forced into clinical attention. A defiant child coerced into the office by worried parents, or a raging, agitated adult delivered by the police, may have no trust in the clinician's healing power; in fact he or she likely rejects the need for healing. In these cases, the faith in the healer transfers to whatever authority has brought the patient to medical attention. Society invests in clinicians a legal and moral duty to try to protect patients and others from avoidable, harmful consequences of mental illness. Society also invests in families the duty to act in the best interests of a sick relative incapable of rational judgment. Persuasion, cajolery, and frank manipulation are routinely exercised for the good of the ill family member.

In reality, many individuals who seek the attention of healers do not yield full authority to the healer. In these instances, help-seekers are better described as "clients" than as patients. The healer-client relationship rests on the preferences of the client. In the real world, people who consult clinicians often demonstrate a mixture of patient and client characteristics. When a person takes the antibiotics exactly as prescribed, but fails to follow the clinician's advice to lose weight and stop smoking, the person has a mixed patient-client relationship with the clinician.

Certain individuals mimic help-seeking behavior in order to enlist the clinician's assistance for some material end, such as a prescription for narcotic drugs, a disability form, or admission from the cold streets into a warm hospital bed. One might call a person who has these help-seeking motives a "user." A user of medical treatment, unlike a client, has no interest in receiving help for a medical problem. However, many users and clients have serious medical problems, and some can ultimately be converted to patients.

A caveat to the young clinician: it is strongly advised that you should assume any help-seeker is a true patient, unless there is solid evidence to the contrary. The risk that you will offer too much care to someone who does not truly want or need it is benign compared to the risk that you will fail to offer help to a true patient who, for whatever reason, strikes you as false or ambivalent. Incorrigible clients and users declare themselves eventually.

## Psychosomatic Complaints

Patients (as well as clients and users) often present to clinicians with complaints or concerns about physical ailments that turn out to have little or no basis in organic pathology. This kind of behavior can manifest in a variety of ways. Some help-seekers (described earlier) have unexplained pseudoneurological deficits, otherwise known as hysterical, or conversion symptoms, that appear to derive from the powerful, perhaps reflexive avoidance of awareness of frightening feelings, thoughts, and actions. In contrast, people who have *somatizing* behavior present with physical symptoms or complaints that engage the clinician's attention, but are difficult if not impossible to validate physically (Lipowski 1988).

In many such cases, a diagnosis can be assigned from the domain of amorphous diagnostic entities like chronic fatigue syndrome, fibromyalgia, and irritable bowel syndrome (Barsky and Borus 1999). This is not to say that every case of one of these disorders has a psychosomatic cause; the conceptual problem with these diagnoses is similar to the problem with many psychiatric diagnoses; they are defined by symptoms, not function or pathophysiology. By making the leap from symptom to diagnosis to presumptive disease entity, the focus of treatment often remains stuck on biological therapies, and overlooks or devalues approaches that might address the maladaptive patterns of behavior that tend to develop around such symptoms. An otherwise demoralized help-seeker whose vague physical complaints acquire the gravity of a medical diagnosis may come to embrace the diagnosis as a license to be disabled.

Reinforced materially, identification with a symptom-based diagnosis can take on the quality of an overvalued idea via self-help books, support groups, websites, and accommodating clinicians.

*Hypochondriacal* help-seekers fear rather than embrace a diagnosis, and seek frequent reassurance regarding the disease they worry about. At the same time the person fears the diagnosis, the diagnosis serves a function as the one thing that might explain the dreadful aches, pains, gurgles, secretions, and anguish. Thus highly stressed medical students often develop hypochondriacal worries early in medical school, as they begin to learn about disease, but lose the tendency to confuse symptoms with disease once they gain confidence as budding physicians and begin to meet truly ill patients on the wards (Hunter et al. 1964). A hypochondriacal person often grows frustrated when informed there seems to be no evidence of the dread diagnosis, because the angst that the diagnosis would have explained remains.

Although disparate in their motives and methods, individuals who have primarily psychosomatic problems knowingly or unknowingly aim to exploit the healer-patient relationship in order to gratify a desire for a certain kind of interpersonal engagement. Often one can understand this as a replication of patterns of behavior that failed, to varying degrees, to forge attachment between the help-seeker and parental figures in the formative years of life. The search for a rescuer is not confined to medicine. Lawyers, teachers, and clergy no doubt have their fair share of clients, students, and acolytes who are motivated more by the desire for reassurance and comfort than by any specific problem that demands expertise. When clinicians are sought out for this kind of service, the problem takes a psychosomatic form. A psychosomatically motivated medical visit provides an avenue for a person to receive parentlike attention and care, while offering only a token symbolic reciprocation in the form of a fee, which is more often than not covered by insurance.

Psychosomatic help-seekers tend to be incensed at the suggestion "it's all in your head," and with good reason. The symptoms feel real at the time. What is the basis of a psychosomatic symptom? In many cases the symptoms that give rise to complaints, or hypochondriacal worries, are benign physiological processes that have assumed exaggerated importance. If one is primed to fear for one's health, then one tends to feel a powerful sense of dread about symptoms, perhaps accompanied by sympathetic and stress responses that add the physiologic correlates of these states to the list of worrisome symptoms.

If a healer takes the complaints at face value and overlooks the hidden motivations of the consultation, this now shared worry about a phantom disease can escalate to an overvalued idea that draws the help-seeker further into the vortex of physical complaining. The healer may unwittingly exacerbate the behavior by labeling the symptoms with a technical-sounding but merely descriptive diagnosis. It may also be the case that the healer, although paid and duty-bound to do so, is the only kind person willing to listen to the person's troubles. This added emotional reward from a clinical encounter might undermine any countervailing motivation to stoically ignore a passing symptom.

A variety of diagnoses, as described above, are included under the rubric of psychosomatic complaints, including somatization, somatoform disorder, hypochondriasis, and factitious disorder.

## Denial

Denial in psychiatry suggests a lack of insight or self-knowledge. Thus, a person in denial poorly predicts the health consequences likely to result from symptoms and actions. Some forms of denial are obvious. When an addict claims, "I can quit any time," anyone who has been with the person, and anyone who has experience with addicts, knows how little it means. Self-knowledge can be particularly prone to error with mental illness because the illness itself can make a person a poor judge of his or her own mental state. A person who is in a manic state often has great difficulty seeing the abnormality of that state, as the excited mood obscures painful consequences and induces an attitude of arrogance that can make the person impervious to counsel.

Denial can occur with any psychiatric diagnosis.

## Parasuicide

Suicide attempts in which there was the potential for lethal consequences, made by people who clearly wished to avoid being caught in the act and who were convinced that the act would be lethal, are a matter of serious concern and intervention whether the patient agrees to it or not. But the vast majority of suicide attempts are made by people who, if not witnessed in the act, acted in the expectation that other people would discover them and intervene. Often the person was intoxicated or emotionally upset, so rational thought was impaired, and the aims of the suicidal act ambivalent or indistinct even to the patient. Such low-lethality, low-intent suicidal acts are termed by some as "parasuicide."

In contrast to a true suicide attempt, in which the aim is death, or more accurately perhaps, to avoid pain by inducing death, the parasuicidal person aims to intensify the focus of other people on his or her distress or grievance, to relieve pain not by aiming for death, but by changing the terms of a relationship so that the other party must set aside points of contention, or other concerns, to engage in rescue activity (Gunderson and Ridolfi 2001).

Parasuicide may occur with mood and adjustment disorders, and among personality disorders is particularly associated with borderline personality disorder.

## 4.9. Summary: Synthetic Mind

Uniquely human aspects of mental life begin where certainty and simplicity end. To navigate life despite incomplete personal experience, the mind may act on preference rather than information, or may substitute second-hand knowledge for first-hand experience. To navigate a world filled with unpredictable other people, the mind extends itself to model the perspectives of other people, and communicates its own contents symbolically to others. Most minds have the capacity to detect when their functions have gone awry, and this motivates the pursuit of help.

When competing paths yield no useful information to differentiate their values, one's behavior may be *biased* to follow one or another path according to one's motivational propensities, that is, one's temperamental traits. Temperament is an ancient concept, encapsulated in the humoral theories of prescientific medicine. One may understand temperamental bias in physiologic terms as a function of the rapidity and strength of arousal responses to environmental cues. Commonly troublesome biases include ambivalence, avoidance, impulsiveness, and inertia. An ambivalence-prone person suspends decisions because he or she identifies no definitive difference between two options and thus fears regret in choosing the wrong course. An avoidant person consistently values fearful motivations over pleasurable ones, hence misses opportunities for satisfaction. An impulsive person, opposite to an ambivalent one, overvalues the difference between two options and undervalues the risk of regret. A tendency toward inertia tends to reflect an overvaluation of known rewards relative to unknown, potentially greater rewards.

*Personality* can be understood as the end result of behavioral habits predicated on strong temperamental bias. People who have distinct personalities may experience reality in quite different ways, because they have tended over the long run to trust sensory over interoceptive information, or vice versa. Anankastic personality refers to one common type encountered clinically: an emotionally rigid, detail-preoccupied person, who may well have strong emotions, but pays little active attention to them. In contrast, the histrionic personality reflects an emotionally expressive approach to life in which trouble may be encountered because of inadequate attention to the real-world consequences of actions motivated by emotional temperature. Perhaps the most troublesome sort of personality emerges from chaotic mood swings, as these individuals fail to acquire a set of competent responses to life challenges, having never experienced consistent reinforcements to shape adaptive behavior.

When information has been acquired by word-of-mouth, or otherwise in the absence of direct experience (for example, dreaming or imaginary speculation), and is then used to inform behavior, this information takes the form of *belief*. Some beliefs can be converted to experiential knowledge in time, some never can because they concern matters that are abstract, speculative, general, and/or immeasurable, hence beyond an individual's direct experience. A belief is useful, but not necessarily true, if holding it forges bonds with a protective, like-minded social group. A belief can be considered true if it proves both useful and accurate as information. A delusion is a pathological, false belief. Delusions survive and often grow because they help the delusional person make sense of a persistent, pathological mood state. Overvalued ideas, unlike delusions, are reinforced not by the pervasive emotional state of the person, but because they serve another behavioral function for the person who has them, for example, they may cement one's membership in a social group, or justify one's self-destructive but somehow satisfying behavior. Doubt, or the loss of belief, may be adaptive, but can be painful, as the abandonment of belief deprives one of a source of information one has come to rely on in uncertain times.

*Identity* can be understood as the information one uses about oneself to predict how one will experience the outcome of a course of action. It is a form of belief in the sense that it is irreducible to a simple point of fact. The development of a mature identity can be a lifelong task. When one has an accurate belief about one's identity, one has insight. Gender disorientation presents a fundamental problem of identity; a person, often a child, has the body of a boy and the mind of a girl, or vice versa. In many cases, there may be a biological explanation for this: gender-specific preferences (such as what kind of play the child most enjoys) are encoded in the hypothalamus before birth. People who have poorly conceived identities in general are more prone to maladaptive patterns of interaction such as projection, in which the person acts on the assumption that another person thinks, feels, and intends just as the projecting person does. Identity dissolution represents a complete breakdown of belief about identity. Dissolution often follows from disruption in emotional maturation through emotional trauma, neglect, strong temperament, or childhood mental illness, and can become disabling if it leads to a sense that one's mind is occupied by many distinct personalities, for example.

People need other people, hence must contend with the fundamental unknowability of other people's minds. To engage in *cooperative* behavior is to enhance one's ability to predict what another person may do so one may engage the person in mutually beneficial actions. Cooperative behavior entails a set of sophisticated cognitive maneuvers: one must be simultaneously aware of one's own values and accurately predict the values of the other person, in order to negotiate. In addition to its material rewards, cooperation reflects an innate drive to imitate other people, apparent even in young infants. The idea that faulty cortical development produces the tragic inability to engage in cooperative behavior is one way to understand childhood autism as a cognitive deficit. Other socially impaired individuals seem to have the cognitive apparatus to model the desires of other people, but not the capacity to model the emotional responses of other people (or else they undervalue the painful ones); this may lead some people to sociopathy and lives of crime. Shame, in contrast, occurs to individuals who perceive the painful effects of losing the trust of other people, and suffer as a result.

*Communication* serves as both a tool and a rewarding behavior. The translation of one's mental experiences into symbols that can stimulate reflections of these phenomena in the mind of another person is a marvel, and also a necessity for all but the simplest modes of cooperative behavior. Communication failure can occur from an excess or paucity of output, either of which may deprive other people of essential information. Or it may occur because of a fundamental disorganization in expression or comprehension; this may reflect a mind running faster than words can convey, or a loss of congruence between the symbols of one person and another. The phenomenon of telemission, or thought broadcasting, suggests there may be a highly developed cognitive capacity to detect that one's message has reached another person, and that this capacity may be falsely triggered by aberrant brain activity. Misrepresentation is of course a problem in all walks of life. When it is not the result of a pathological process that renders a person unable to know the truth (confabulation), it implies manipulative motives.

Cooperation and communication tend to facilitate the satisfaction of a variety of drives. *Affiliation* between people provides a means to experience satisfaction directly from engagement with another person. Affiliation is catalyzed biologically, by certain hormones secreted during bonding behaviors, like nursing and coitus, and reinforced as one becomes conditioned to find pleasure from the presence and in the well-being of another person. Grief is a normal, painful response to the loss of a relationship. The pain occurs at the moment some stimulus arouses the conditioned anticipation of pleasure, when that anticipation is frustrated by the reality of the other person's absence. An overly dependent approach to relationships implies a failure of reciprocity—one party tends to experience fear at the prospect of absence from the other, but the feeling is not necessarily mutual. The fear of loss differentiates it from healthy bonding, in which loss may arouse sadness, but not much fear. Individuals who engage in relationships without a sense of true reciprocity often can be seen as egotistical. For them, personal satisfaction is primary, the well-being of the other is secondary. Eccentric people who seem unable or unwilling to attach to other people in meaningful ways may be content, more or less, though they may also be vulnerable to social marginalization and to fantastical overvalued ideas about government conspiracies, extraterrestrial visitations, and so on.

A variety of motives impel *help-seeking* behavior. Help-seekers may be roughly classified either as patients, clients, or users. True patients seek help to resolve a problem, and engage in full cooperation with the clinician to resolve the problem. Clients seek out clinicians but may value other things more highly than they value the resolution of the problem, hence they may pick and choose which advice to follow. Users of clinical services see merely the opportunity to have a need met, and are not motivated by a clinical problem, even when they have a clinical problem. Psychosomatic complaints are a ubiquitous issue in clinical care. There may be any of a variety of motivations to present to clinicians in the absence of true pathology. Some people seek the emotional reassurance of a caring professional, some are driven by an overvalued, hypochondriacal idea that they have an illness that explains their troubles, some have misinterpreted a relatively normal physical symptom as a sign of somatic illness when their problem is essentially mental. Patients in denial pose challenges to clinicians, who must often win a patient over to a new set of beliefs about his or her problems before appropriate care can begin. Parasuicide—suicidal behavior in the absence of serious intent—is an extremely common phenomenon in psychiatric settings. This is not always benign or should not be easily dismissed, as the parasuicidal patient may inadvertently place his or her life at risk. But the motivation, if not for death, is likely to be to manipulate other people to engage in rescue activity.

# CHAPTER FIVE

# Psychiatric Mind

We have come to the end of our trek through the mind and mental dysfunction, from norepinephrine to neurons to neuroses. We now can map troublesome mental symptoms, propensities, experiences, and behaviors to specific adaptive functions.

If this were a standard textbook of psychiatry the chapters would have been patterned after the official manual of psychiatric diagnosis, the DSM, which chops psychiatry into a manageable number of classes of disorder (mood disorders, psychotic disorders, personality disorders, and so on), comprised of rule-based diagnoses. Instead, this book has deconstructed these diagnostic entities and distributed their components throughout the entirety of mental life. Has it made psychiatry more complicated?

Indeed it has, but only in the sense that a modern textbook of general medicine complicates the simple and elegant but artificial categorization of disorders developed before the modern medical era. For example, William Cullen's nosological grouping into pyrexic (fever), neurotic (neurological), cachexic (systemic but neither febrile nor neurological), and local (confined to one organ or body part) syndromes had a pragmatic logic, but with respect to the modern classification of diagnosis by function and cause, it often lumped where it should have split, and split where it should have lumped (Cullen 1800). With the sacrifice of simplicity, one gains a logical framework to understand the relationships between brain dysfunctions, behaviors, innate vulnerabilities, and the meaning the patient attaches to his or her experiences.

In this chapter, the various manifestations of mental dysfunction are sorted roughly into groups defined by the nature of the illness. Borrowing (and paraphrasing a bit) from Paul R. McHugh and Phillip R. Slavney (McHugh and Slavney 1998), there are essentially four distinct methodological approaches to mental illness: to see it as a disease, as a dimensional aspect of a person (trait vulnerability), as maladaptive behavior, or as a disrupted life story (adverse experience). Each of these employs a different logic to gauge the identity, significance, and severity of illness. One employs these distinctive modes of clinical reasoning in the typical patient who presents with a complex clinical problem: a disease that incites maladaptive behavior, as obsessive aversion to the touching of different foods on a plate may constrain the food choices of a person with anorexia; or a temperamental vulnerability that exposes one frequently to adverse experience, as histrionic overdependency may strain relationships and bring on the abandonment the person most dreads.

## 5.1. Psychiatry Rebuilt

Each of the mental dysfunctions described in the book falls more or less into one of four types of problem. In this section, we will reorganize them according to the type of dysfunction they represent, and show how the identification of these manifestations of illness leads to a useful formulation of a patient's clinical problem. For simplicity, the mental dysfunctions are assigned to only type of problem, based on clinical relevance, though in some cases (for example, dysregulation of appetite), they could be discussed and employed to understand the patient's problem in several ways (for example, as a deficit in the biological regulation of food consumption, or as a trait of excessive hunger, or as a maladaptive behavior).

### Disease States

Many diverse phenomena are attributable primarily to expressions of abnormal brain activity.

*agitation, delirium, dysregulation of sleep, appetite, or libido; hallucinations, illusions,*
*agnosia, disorganization, catatonia, apraxia, dyskinesias, extravolition, obsessions/*
*compulsions, avulsion/intrusion, amnesia, disinhibition, anhedonia, apathy, dejec-*
*tion, excitement, irascibility, paroxysms, paranoia, delusions, asociality, dysfluency/*
*hyperfluency, derailment, and telemission*

If a person has several of these dysfunctions, or a severe and persistent form of any of them, then he or she almost certainly has a disease: a biological abnormality in brain activity. A patient who has pathological symptoms is likely to have other problems as well. Each of these pathological symptoms can and does contribute to other kinds of problems, and each may arise as a complication from other kinds of problems.

If one does not know the pathological cause of a symptom, how does one know it is pathological? One can infer this when the same symptom can occur from a *known* biological malfunction. For example, steroid and stimu-lant medications each can induce states of excitement alternating with irrita-bility, agitation, and paranoia (Hall et al. 1979; Snyder 1973). This does not tell us the cause of these symptoms when they occur without drugs, but it strongly suggests that the symptoms arise de novo as a result of some similar alteration of brain activity. The second key to a pathological symptom is that it occurs in essentially the same form in different individuals, across different cultures, and cannot be stopped—only tolerated—by an effort of will or change of attitude.

In combination with one another and with other kinds of mental dysfunc-tion, these symptoms add up to a handful of common syndromes. The com-mon syndromes or disease entities in psychiatry and their typical pathological symptoms are listed below. Note that the list is organized so that the symp-toms of a syndrome lower in the list may occur as an element of one or more syndromes from higher in the list.

The common disease syndromes (and common symptoms) in psychiatry include

- delirium (agitation, delirium, illusions)
- Alzheimer disease and other progressive dementias (agnosia, apraxia, amnesia, disinhibition)
- intoxication (agitation, lethargy, delirium, irascibility, excitement— depending on the drug) and withdrawal from alcohol, amphetamines,

opiates, sedatives/hypnotics, and cocaine (delirium, agitation, or lethargy)
- major depression (anhedonia, apathy, dejection, dysfluency) and mania (excitement, irascibility, hyperfluency)
- schizophrenia (hallucinations, disorganization, catatonia, extravolition, avulsion/intrusion, disinhibition, paranoia, delusions, asociality, derailment, telemission)
- autism (asociality)
- obsessive-compulsive disorder (obsessions/compulsions)
- panic attacks (paroxysms)

If a patient has a pathological symptom, then it is incumbent on the clinician either to diagnose a disease syndrome or to explain why the symptom is not truly pathological. If the symptoms do not add up to a specific syndrome, more information from the patient or from others should resolve the issue. Whether or not there is a pathological symptom, the next step in the application of the organic model of mind is to assess the significance of any vulnerability the patient may have.

### Trait Vulnerability

Some dysfunctions of mental life involve predispositions within the wide range of normal performance that manifest as problems when patients are tested or under stress. But predispositions are abstract. As constructs they predict and explain rather than exist as tangible entities. We cannot grasp them directly. We can measure them quantitatively on standardized tests, or we can observe their likely influence across a variety of aspects of mental life, where they trigger symptoms and promote behavior. The reader has encountered a variety of patterns of dysfunction that arise as the result of strong predispositions.

> low intelligence, distraction, ambivalence, avoidance, impulsiveness, inertia, anankastic, histrionic, and labile personalities, sociopathy, overdependency, egotism, eccentricity

A few of these expressions of trait vulnerability may actually have a pathological cause. Sociopathy, for example, might ultimately turn out to be caused by a biological deficit in the neurohormonal mechanisms of attachment (Kiehl 2006). Conversely, some pathological symptoms might be the end result of trait vulnerabilities. Thus, one might have panic disorder the way one has asthma, in which paroxysmal attacks are often precipitated by environmental allergens. Under sufficiently adverse circumstances, such as inhaling carbon dioxide-enriched air, almost anyone might have a panic attack (Bailey et al. 2005), but some people have such a low threshold that it becomes a clinical problem for them (Rassovsky et al. 2000). When it is difficult to say in an individual case whether the problem is a disease or vulnerability, then one may look at the problem both ways at once until more information becomes available.

Temperamental vulnerabilities map roughly to the personality disorders categorized in the DSM. Low intelligence maps to the diagnosis of intellectual disability (mental retardation). These specific vulnerabilities tend to be associated with maladaptive behavioral responses to adversity, and to adversely affect a person's overall experience of life.

One may uncover trait vulnerability through formal testing, but most of the time a clinician will offer an educated guess, while trying to make sense of a patient's persistent tendency to respond badly to certain situations. Because they are tendencies and not symptoms they manifest differently among individuals who have different backgrounds and cultures. Moreover, a person can suppress the effects of trait vulnerability if not the trait itself through effort of will and change of attitude.

Traits can therefore be tricky for the beginner to discern with confidence. If one listens carefully to a person's story and begins to see patterns in the way the person approaches things like relationships, major decisions, conflicts, social engagements, and changes of fortune, then the data are there to make a conjecture about a possible trait vulnerability, to be tested as one gets to know the person better over time.

Disease states and trait vulnerabilities oftentimes are not a person's primary concern when the person seeks help. The need for intervention in many cases is triggered by the maladaptive or dangerous behavior driven by the symptom or by the trait-skewed response to adversity.

## Maladaptive Behavior

When change in a person's voluntary actions could alleviate the harmful, costly, or painful aspects of a problem, the problem is behavioral. The motivation for the behavior may be pathological, or may reflect trait vulnerability, and these must be addressed from the appropriate perspective. Reduction of the troublesome motivation will make it far easier for a person to change behavior, but if the person fails to change behavior, the problem remains.

Many problems in mental life are essentially the products of maladaptive behavior.

*maladaptive choices regarding sleep, feeding, and sexual behavior; hysterical (pseudoneurological) symptoms, pseudohallucinations, addiction, restricting/bingeing/purging; self-injurious behavior, suicidality, territoriality, misrepresentation, psychosomatic complaints, parasuicide*

The person often rejects the idea that changing the behavior would fix the problem, or even that he or she has the power to change the behavior. It seems that the urge must weaken its hold first. But behavior problems feed themselves. They narrow options and nourish the adverse circumstances that fuel the urge behind the behavior. In other words, a person drinks to ease the pain caused by the terrible things that happened the last time the person drank.

Persistent maladaptive behaviors challenge the assumption that people always seek pleasure. Where is the payoff from self-induced starvation or vomiting, or selling one's body for drugs, or waking up shaking and desperate for drink, or slicing one's forearm with a razor, or submitting to an unnecessary medical procedure? The motivation is not for pleasure, but for relief from the craving. We can understand craving as the state of arousal spanning the time between conditioned cue and consummation of the drive it induces. Craving resembles pain more than desire—an urgent need, not just a want. The craving is born at the moment when the behavior first quelled some other psychic pain or distress. It grows as the relief of psychic pain becomes far more salient than the physical pain (for example, from an intravenous needle or razor self-mutilation) or loss (of job, family, money, health, self-respect) that follows from the behavior.

Pain of all kinds motivates maladaptive behavior because the satisfaction of the conditioned craving eases, for a while, all pain. To alter such behavior may require one to address the pain at its source. Disease-related pain may require a biological intervention, trait-related pain may call for personal guidance, the pain of a hopeless outlook on life may respond to engagement with an empathic healer. None of these methods works if the maladaptive behavior continues. As long as a person invests in the pursuit of maladaptive rewards, the more elusive but stable rewards that follow eventually from pain-relieving, restorative, and adaptive behavior remain neglected.

## Adverse Experience

Adverse experience pervades the lives of psychiatric patients, often as the direct result of a disease state, or as the response to a vulnerability stressed to the limit, or as the consequence of maladaptive behavior. Some adverse experiences occur to intact, well-adjusted but unlucky people. This book has touched on a few painful or maladaptive responses to adversity.

*flashbacks, demoralization, dread, guilt, overvalued ideas, doubt, gender disorientation, dissolution, grief, denial*

These examples of responses to adversity relate to a person's life story. A person plots his or her life course through challenges large and small, and by having some clear sense of identity and purpose. If one sees oneself as an active protagonist, with the wherewithal to learn and grow and overcome adversity, then one tends to be happy. If one has a poor sense of identity and feels buffeted by life's turmoil, one tends to be unhappy. A person may be quietly unhappy in this sense for years and never come to clinical attention, but an adverse experience, or crisis, can convert a previously happy or quietly unhappy person into a patient.

Problems related to adverse experience may result from a fundamental weakness or confusion in the definition of character, for example, dissolution of identity or gender misidentification. Or one may have been overwhelmed by trauma, loss, or stress, manifest as dread, guilt, flashbacks, demoralization, and grief. Or, one may be hampered by poor choices made in the effort to interpret and cope with adversity. Overvalued ideas, projection, and denial patch over a faltering life story, but fail to engage reality constructively; doubt may occur to those who have a more mature perspective but have nevertheless lost hope.

## Complex Problems, Complex Patients

Psychiatric patients rarely have only one problem. Pathological symptoms cluster together to form disease syndromes. Trait vulnerabilities remain latent until awakened by adverse experience. Psychiatric disease is itself an adverse experience that upsets a person's life story. The distress aroused by disease, triggered by stress, imposed by adverse experiences, may motivate self-destructive behavior to assuage the pain and anguish. Certain trait vulnerabilities predispose a person to undervalue risk and thus engage in addictive or self-destructive behaviors. As a consequence of maladaptive behavior, a person may fall into a disease state, encounter stress, and throw his or her life story completely off track.

The model of mind as an organic function described in this book, applied to the complex problems of real patients, provides a path from one kind of mental problem to another.

For example, consider the syndrome of schizophrenia. Pathological symptoms of schizophrenia arise throughout the levels of mental function. The hypothetical mechanism for several of these symptoms—aberrant arousal of sensory pathways, both primary and integrative—suggests a common pathophysiology, and an explanation why dopamine-blocking drugs may help quell a wide variety of symptoms (Kapur et al. 2006). Dopaminergic pathways throughout the brain normally enhance cortical function in the service of executing goal-directed behavior; misfiring dopamine-mediated connections may stimulate a variety of abnormal expressions of cortical activity disconnected from the active contents of thought, such as hallucinations, telemission (thought broadcasting), intrusion (thought insertion), and so on. Blunting of the dopaminergic neurotransmitter system will not only inhibit this aberrant arousal, hence the symptom, but it will also inhibit spontaneous activity in general, hence the blunting of will and expressiveness as side effects of many drugs in this class.

From another angle, the experience of hallucinations, a low-level phenomenon in the perceptual organization of mental activity, potentially affects all higher cognitive functions. The information one can use is only as good as the information one gathers. If false signals taint one's perceptual experiences over years, then the effects may be felt in a variety of behaviors and experiences: bizarre ideas and memories, idiosyncratic modes of speech, asociality as it becomes increasingly difficult to mesh one's own mental world with that of other people. A person may embrace eccentricity, or become demoralized by the loss of social engagement and the shame of being ill.

Consider as another example a patient who makes a host of psychosomatic complaints and other hysterical symptoms, like pseudoneurological deficits and pseudoamnesia. One may understand complaints about these symptoms as behavioral manifestations of fearful arousal. A person beset by persistent dread must be on alert full-time; perhaps this follows from traumatic experience and a reflexive need to anticipate intrusive, frightening memories. Or, perhaps the dread arises from a weak sense of identity, or dissolution. A person who has identity dissolution, who lacks a strong self-concept, may be unable to predict his or her likely response to upcoming events. Hence the person remains on perpetual high alert against a bewildering and possibly ominous future. Under some circumstances the belief that one has a somatic or cognitive illness may grow to become an overvalued idea because it confers a sense of relief to be absolutely certain about the nature of one's distress—even if one is completely wrong about it.

Or, one more example: picture a young, anankastic individual who has become overstressed by a major life transition and expanded responsibilities, say, to college or a new job; marriage, or a new baby. The transition fosters stress, as the individual's heightened alert to the details of a novel situation finds no solace in routine, predictable behavioral responses. A pervasive inability to anticipate reward (anhedonia) has taken over. The mood has consequently become dejected, as there is no expectation of pleasure. The dejection blossoms into a hopeless sense of demoralization, as none of the lifelong methods of self-soothing seem to work; there seems to be no way out of misery. Even the taste for food has been lost; the awareness of hunger is there, but it does not arouse an appetitive drive. Cognition slows; it is increasingly difficult to register any salience to the words on a page. Work performance suffers, and the person may drop out, resign, or hole up in his or her room. Secondarily, the person feels guilty for the inability to fulfill life roles and satisfy the expectations of others. Daily experiences of pain only reinforce the social and functional withdrawal. In short, the person now has a full disease syndrome of major depression.

Eventually, perhaps with medication that enhances synaptic serotonin and thus heals the deficit in reward motivation, the appetites return, lethargy fades, but the person remains withdrawn. In this anankastic person, the painful experience of falling into a depressive state at the moment of an increase in responsibility has conditioned the person to fear responsibility. The person has acquired an aversion to life. Disability seems an adaptive response. Perhaps at some point in the illness cannabis relieved the pain and restored the appetites temporarily, and so even after recovery, the person feels reluctant to give it up. While all other rewards of life faded, cannabis remained a source of pleasure, and so it continues despite the growing costs to relationships (intoxication hinders true empathy) and cooperation (nothing is more motivating than the drug).

To assign an orthodox multiaxial diagnosis to any of these patients, or to explain away the problems as expressions of known neurobiological processes, not only fails to capture the relationships between the problems, but it fails to give one an idea how to intervene with the individual patient.

Perhaps the major drawback in the emphasis of formulation over diagnosis is the sacrifice of consistency. On the other hand, there is also a potential to invigorate the field by reawakening an interest in the unique features of patients, over the reduction of their problems to a five-line diagnosis. It would be unthinkable to ditch the DSM at this point, and probably unwise if it even could be done. Instead, the radical proposal here is for interested clinicians to create their own alternative nosologies. Use the DSM for bean-counting, but when making clinical judgments or teaching, apply some creative effort to the development of a scheme that makes the most sense for a clinician's own practice. Table 8 portrays one such scheme, oriented around the nature of a patient's presenting problem.

In Table 8, individuals who have a mental illness primarily of one type (for example, psychotic, affective, neurotic, etc.) will have problems more in common with each other, regardless of their diagnosis, than with individuals who have the same diagnosis but different problems. Also note that patients classed into each problem type may have a variety of distinct diagnostic entities. A psychotic patient who has bipolar disorder likely has more in common with a patient who has schizophrenia, in terms of clinical acuity and the nature of active problems, than with a patient who has the same diagnosis of bipolar disorder, whose problem is primarily maladjustment.

With intervention in mind, the next and final section is a general discussion of treatment modalities, as they apply to the varieties of psychiatric problem.

## 5.2. Mending Mentation

Now that the reader has a better understanding about what kinds of problems psychiatrists treat, what are the tools the psychiatrist can use to help patients who have these problems? This section provides a general overview of the treatment modalities available to help psychiatric patients. This section focuses on how the treatments work, rather than on the specific names of drugs, psychotherapeutic modalities, and so on. The reader may consult one of the general textbooks of clinical psychiatry listed under Additional Readings for specific treatment information.

Successful treatment begins with a thorough understanding of the patient's problem. This requires more than a diagnosis. Two patients who have the same

*Table 8.* Common Mental Illness Presentations,
with Associated Signs, Symptoms, and Deficits

| Mental Illness | Signs/Symptoms/Deficits | Mental Function Affected |
|---|---|---|
| Psychosis (severe incapacity to interpret, process, and use information in adaptive social behavior) | Agitation | Arousal |
| | Hallucinations | Perception |
| | Disorganization | Cognition |
| | Extravolition | Action |
| | Avulsion/intrusion | Attention |
| | Disinhibition, demoralization | Value |
| | Paranoia | Alarm |
| | Ambivalence | Bias |
| | Delusions | Belief |
| | Asociality | Cooperation |
| | Derailment, telemission | Communication |
| | Eccentricity | Affiliation |
| Affective illness (impaired capacity to rouse and modulate internally driven behavior) | Anergia, agitation | Arousal |
| | Sleep, feeding, sexual, visceral dysfunction | Appetite |
| | Suicidality, demoralization | Value |
| | Apathy, anhedonia | Motive |
| | Dejection, excitement, irascibility | Desire |
| | Dread, paroxysms, guilt | Alarm |
| | Impulsiveness, inertia | Bias |
| | Labile personality | Personality |
| | Dysfluency/hyperfluency | Communication |
| Neurosis (persistent maladaptive and self-defeating behavior) | Pseudosensory symptoms, pseudohallucinations | Perception |
| | Pseudomotor symptoms | Motion |
| | Pseudomemory/pseudoamnesia | Memory |
| | Self-injurious behavior | Habit |
| | Demoralization | Motive |
| | Avoidance, impulsiveness | Bias |
| | Overvalued ideas | Belief |
| | Anankastic, histrionic | Personality |
| | Projection, dissolution | Identity |
| | Sociopathy | Cooperation |
| | Misrepresentation | Communication |
| | Overdependency | Affiliation |
| | Psychosomatic complaints, parasuicide | Help-seeking |
| Anguish (angst, acute suffering) | Agitation | Arousal |
| | Obsessions/compulsions | Action |
| | Irascibility | Desire |
| | Dread, paroxysms | Alarm |

*continued*

*Table 8.    Continued*

| Mental Illness | Signs/Symptoms/Deficits | Mental Function Affected |
|---|---|---|
| Maladjustment (mental problems as a reaction or relative deficit in adaptive capacities) | Low intelligence | Cognition |
| | Distraction | Attention |
| | Flashbacks | Memory |
| | Sexual deviance | Habit |
| | Demoralization | Value |
| | Apathy | Motive |
| | Guilt | Alarm |
| | Ambivalence, avoidance, impulsiveness, inertia | Bias |
| | Doubt | Belief |
| | Gender disorientation | Identity |
| | Shame | Cooperation |
| | Grief, overdependency, egotism, eccentricity | Affiliation |
| | Denial | Help-seeking |
| Organic illness (facultative disruption due to physiologic or anatomic pathology) | Delirium | Arousal |
| | Sleep, feeding, sexual, visceral dysfunction | Appetite |
| | Illusions | Perception |
| | Agnosia | Cognition |
| | Dyskinesias | Motion |
| | Apraxia | Action |
| | Distraction | Attention |
| | Amnesia | Memory |
| | Disinhibition | Value |
| Self-destruction (volitional ruination) | Addiction, Restricting/bingeing/purging, self-injurious behavior | Habit |
| | Suicidality, demoralization | Value |
| | Territoriality | Motive |
| | Labile personality | Personality |
| | Parasuicide | Help-seeking |

diagnosis—say, major depressive disorder—might require different approaches to treatment because one is elderly and frail and has become malnourished and confused; the other is college-aged, restless, and fighting suicidal urges. Diagnostic categories do not discriminate between these two, but a smart approach to treatment obviously will, because their problems are so different. Evidence from clinical trials might recommend the same medication for both patients, but if medication is the only intervention, in the time it takes the medications to work, they might each be dead: one from dehydration and the other by his own hand.

Although inadequate as a description of a patient's problem, diagnostic categories are useful to guide treatment, because therapeutic trials rely on them. If one is to apply treatments backed by evidence, one looks for the treatment that resolves the symptoms of people who have a given, orthodox diagnosis. Real-world patients often have just one major diagnosis but rarely have only one problem. Multiple problems require multiple modes of treatment. An uncomplicated case of panic disorder, for example, might demand acute symptomatic treatment to suppress attacks while the definitive preventative treatment takes time to work. The patient may additionally benefit from counseling at least once to assuage feelings of embarrassment about having a mental illness, and behavioral therapy to overcome conditioned fears that have arisen, reinforced by the experience of panic.

## Disease Remedies

Pathological symptoms in psychiatry arise from abnormalities in the physiology of the brain. The pathology may be innate or acquired, and it may arise from brain activity or be imposed on it, as in a structural, toxic, metabolic, or endocrinologic insult. Pathological mental states that arise from an identifiable cause, like alcohol withdrawal, delirium, or excessive thyroid hormone, are remedied when the normal physiologic state is restored. For most pathological mental conditions we have no access to the root cause and may in fact not know how to identify the cause.

Some pathological *symptoms* respond to direct treatment. Acute dread or agitation or catatonia may respond readily to a sedative-hypnotic medication, though the symptom returns as soon as the medication wears off. Other treatments may be addressed to the cluster of symptoms that define a disease *syndrome*, like mania, depression, obsessive-compulsive disorder, schizophrenia, or panic disorder. These treatments are not expected to control the symptoms quickly, but when taken over time are expected to control clusters of symptoms and prevent their recurrence. For some syndromes, such as Alzheimer disease, we have no effective way to remove the deficits or prevent their recurrence, but we can at least mitigate the dysfunction and slow the course of the disease.

This section reviews, briefly, the remedies presently available for the phenomena identified as pathological states, starting with drugs that affect monoaminergic neurotransmission and moving on from there. Table 9 lays

Table 9.  Psychopharmacologic Agents

| Drug Type | Pharmacologic Effect | Clinical Uses | Examples |
|---|---|---|---|
| *Monoaminergic Agents* | | | |
| Catecholamine enhancer | Increases dopamine and norepinephrine availability | Symptoms of diminished alertness, anergia, inattentiveness | Amphetamine, methylphenidate |
| Dopamine antagonist | Blocks dopamine access to receptors | Hallucinations, delusions, symptoms of agitation | Thorazine, fluphenazine, haloperidol, risperidone, clozapine, ziprasidone |
| Norepinephrine antagonist | Blocks noradrenergic neurotransmission, mainly in the periphery | Hypertension, tremor, performance anxiety | Propranolol, pindolol  clonidine (indirect—pre-synaptic inhibition) |
| Norepinephrine/serotonin reuptake inhibitor | Blocks removal of norepinephrine and/or serotonin from synaptic cleft | Major depression, panic disorder, neuropathic pain (norepinephrine), obsessive-compulsive disorder (serotonin) | Norepinephrine: Amitriptyline, nortriptyline, desipramine, doxepine, duloxetine  Serotonin: Fluoxetine, sertraline, citalopram  Both: Venlafaxine, mirtazepine |
| Monoamine-oxidase inhibitor | Prevents elimination of monoaminergic neurotransmitters; prolongs their presence in synaptic cleft | Major depression, some anxiety syndromes | Phenelzine, tranylcipramine, iproniazid, selegiline |

*Other Pharmacologic Mechanisms*

| | | |
|---|---|---|
| Neuromodulator | Interrupts hyperactive neuronal processes | Lithium, valproic acid, lamotrigine, carbamazepine |
| GABA agonist | Stimulates GABA receptors, hence inhibits network activity | Lorazepam, diazepam, clonazepam |
| Anticholinergic | Blocks acetylcholine access to receptor; alleviates motor side effects of dopamine blockade | Benztropine |
| Cholinesterase inhibitor | Inhibits acetylcholine elimination, hence promotes tonic arousal | Galantamine, donepezil |
| Glutamate inhibitor | Blocks glutamate binding; slows excitatory neurotoxicity | Memantine |
| Mixed opioid | Prevents opiate withdrawal while blocking opiate reward, thus inhibiting illicit use | Buprenorphine, naloxone |

| | | |
|---|---|---|
| | Bipolar disorder, epilepsy, neuropathic pain | |
| | Anxiety symptoms, seizure | |
| | Parkinsonian symptoms (muscle rigidity, tremor, etc.) | |
| | Alzheimer disease | |
| | Alzheimer disease | |
| | Opiate dependence, other addictive behaviors | |

out the major psychopharmacological classes, their effects, their indications, and examples.

*Dopamine antagonists (blockers)* (also known as *neuroleptics* or *antipsychotics*) are generally effective in the rapid symptomatic relief of agitation and irritability. Taken over a period of weeks, they begin to resolve most of the pathological manifestations of psychosis: hallucinations, disorganization, catatonia, passivity experiences, thought withdrawal and insertion, paranoia, delusions, thought disorder, and thought broadcasting. Newer-generation dopamine blockers, which have greater specificity of pharmacologic effect, tend to address psychotic syndromes about as well as the older drugs, with fewer neurological side effects but more metabolic side effects (Gardner et al. 2005). The newer drugs also have been used to positive effect in controlling anxiety and syndromes of mania and depression (McElroy and Keck 2000; Gao et al. 2006; Thase 2002).

*Serotonin selective reuptake inhibitor* (SSRI) agents, *norepinephrine reuptake inhibitor* (SNRI agents and *tricyclic antidepressants*), *monoamine oxidase inhibitors* (MAOIs), and other agents that increase serotonin and norepinephrine levels in the synapse have no known utility alleviating symptoms. Thus the popular media image of these *antidepressant* drugs (for example Prozac) as "happy pills" is false and a bit pernicious. Taken over a period of weeks to months, they resolve the pathological symptoms associated with the major depressive syndrome, including dysregulation of sleep, appetite, libido, anhedonia, apathy, and dejected mood (Arroll et al. 2009). At high-end doses, the serotonin-selective drugs remedy the pathological syndrome of obsessive-compulsive disorder (Soomro et al. 2008). Over time, the persistent enhancement of synaptic levels of serotonin and/or norepinephrine produces systemic changes that restore cognitive and emotional functioning impaired in these syndromes.

*Lithium salts* and *neuromodulators* (in other words, *anticonvulsants*) also have limited symptomatic effect, but effectively control and prevent the pathological symptoms associated with the manic syndrome (agitation, dysregulation of sleep and libido, excitement, irascibility, hyperfluency, derailment) (Friedrich 1999). They have a weaker effect, if any, against the major depressive syndrome but can prevent its recurrence in some cases. Pharmacologic effects vary, but the therapeutic effect may come from their protective effect against neuronal cell death and facilitation of neuronal growth in subcortical structures (Bauer et al. 2003). Thus, one might conjecture that they stabilize a cycling mood by providing the brain with more cellular substrate with which to learn to adaptively meld appetite, arousal, and actions.

*GABA-enhancing drugs (sedative-hypnotics)* have potent symptomatic effects on pathological symptoms, but minimal utility to alleviate pathological syndromes. Pharmacologically they enhance inhibitory neurons throughout the brain, thus putting a brake on arousal, and to some extent, cognition. They can bring rapid but transient relief from panic and catatonia (Rosebush and Mazurek 2010). They are also in wide use to ease alcohol-dependent patients through the physiological and mental agony of alcohol withdrawal, which can produce a severe state of delirium, including agitation, hallucinations, and delusions, if undertreated (Ntais et al. 2005).

*Acetylcholine blockers (anticholinergics)* are widely employed against the symptoms of abnormal movements that commonly emerge with the use of dopamine-blocking drugs, especially the older-generation drugs. Overuse of these drugs, or of other medications that mimic their effects, commonly triggers delirium (Campbell et al. 2009).

*Acetylcholine-enhancing (for example, cholinesterase inhibitor)* drugs have been of some use in slowing down the advance of Alzheimer disease, a dementia syndrome of progressive amnesia and cognitive impairment (Shanks et al. 2009). The additional cholinergic activity enhances tonic arousal to subcortical structures central to cognitive function.

Elevated or insufficient quantities of some hormones, in particular, thyroid and glucocorticoid hormones (for example, cortisol), whether a result of disease or induced by medical treatment (for example, prednisone treatment for autoimmune disease, thyroid ablation for Graves disease), may produce anergia, agitation, irascibility, excitement, dejection, and other assorted symptoms, depending on the hormone and whether its level is high or low (Geffken et al. 1998). Definitive treatment begins with restoration of normal physiologic levels of the hormone.

*Electroconvulsive therapy* (ECT) and a variety of new electrophysiologic treatments presently under investigation (transcranial magnetic stimulation [TMS], vagal nerve stimulation [VNS], and deep brain stimulation [DBS]) all address the major depressive syndrome. ECT is particularly effective with psychotic depression and catatonia (Pagnin et al. 2004). Though it can be challenging to talk a manic patient into the ECT suite, ECT may also help alleviate mania. ECT, like neuromodulating drugs, may enhance neuronal growth subcortically as a means to heal a brittle or failed linkage of appetite, arousal, and action.

This was not meant to be an exhaustive or detailed list, but should offer an idea of the varieties of biologically active treatment in use for the control, relief, and prevention of pathological symptoms and syndromes. The astute reader may have noticed that several of the pathological expressions of psychiatric disease show up under none of these treatment modalities: for example, disinhibition and asociality. Although the behavioral effects of these pathological symptoms can be managed, there are no remedies at present that reliably remedy the syndromes.

## Mitigation of Vulnerability

In the treatment of a patient who has excessive trait vulnerabilities, the first task is to manage any symptoms, self-destructive behaviors, or adverse circumstances that prompted the pursuit of treatment. When the crisis has settled, there may be opportunities to strengthen the patient's defenses against future crises, and thus prevent or mitigate future harm.

The treatment of hypertension by general physicians has a similar therapeutic aim. In many cases hypertension results not from pathology in the maintenance of blood pressure, but from a patient's allotment of a trait with a more or less normal distribution across the population. At the low end of the distribution, individuals are at higher risk for syncope, that is, they may be more likely to faint from a lack of blood flow to the brain. At the high end, individuals are at increased risk for heart and kidney disease and for strokes. Prescription of an antihypertensive medication for someone at the high end of the distribution mitigates the patient's vulnerability toward other dire medical problems.

Traits are, by definition, permanent attributes, but as the hypertension example illustrates, their potential for harm can be diminished through biological treatment.

*Catecholamine-like agents (stimulants)* that increase the synaptic availability of dopamine and norepinephrine, when given to school-aged children who have significant inattentiveness and impulsivity (that is, who have the diagnostic syndrome of attention-deficit/hyperactivity disorder), improve school performance (Faraone et al. 2006). Actually, they improve the performance of most children, with or without inattentiveness. If one sees the deficit in attentiveness in some children as a *delay* in cortical maturation rather than a permanent deficit (that is, a vulnerability rather than a disease), then the drug effectively speeds cognitive processing, thus preventing the loss of the opportunity for effective education, and reducing the potential harm from the relative deficit in cognitive ability.

Stimulants have also been used therapeutically in adults to counteract fatigue, for example, in air force pilots, and to suppress appetite as a means of weight loss. They are in widespread use even in civilians who find they obtain a useful boost in cognition. However, there is also great potential for abuse in this class of drugs, and the potential to induce psychotic symptoms when taken in high doses.

Medications used for depressive and manic syndromes have been employed by some to address temperamental vulnerabilities, with mixed success. Peter D. Kramer argued, in his popular book *Listening to Prozac* (Kramer 1993), that SSRI medication soothes temperamental vulnerabilities related to excessive anxiety, above and beyond its benefit against the depressive syndrome. Neuromodulating drugs also have been used to smooth out the temperamental instability that afflicts some individuals who have labile personalities (or, borderline personality disorder, in the diagnostic manual), whose stormy demeanors are suggestive of a "bipolar spectrum" of emotional disorders (Abraham and Calabrese 2008).

Education can mitigate vulnerability by enhancing the patient's insight. An insightful patient makes better choices because she or he places accurate value on their consequences. *Cognitive and skills testing*, including vocational and intelligence tests administered by psychologists, may be of benefit to identify a cause for distress in a patient poorly qualified or overqualified for the job in which he finds himself. *Personality testing* may similarly help a patient in need of greater insight about his or her own emotional blind spots. Patients may feel demeaned by having their limitations pointed out to them, so the optimal therapeutic benefit occurs when there is ample opportunity to work with them to understand and apply the results.

Education may also occur through the course of longer-term psychotherapy. Regular interaction in a healing setting provides the opportunity to learn to perceive one's character as it is reflected in the therapeutic encounter.

## Behavior Management

In the simplest terms, behavior problems are those that would go away if the person would just stop doing something he or she shouldn't, or start doing something he or she should. Easier said than done, of course. Powerful forces drive maladaptive behavior in the face of adverse and often counterproductive consequences. There are three phases to the management of behavior problems: intervention, recovery, and maintenance.

When a behavior has become entrenched, the only means to prevent it long enough to begin to resolve the powerful urges behind it may be to physically *intervene* between the patient and the behavior. A three-day detox program, for example, removes the patient from access to alcohol or drugs and safely nurses (and perhaps medicates) him or her through the withdrawal, but is highly unlikely on its own to help the patient refrain from drinking or drugs in the future. Patients who have active suicidal and self-injurious behavior may require the intervention of round-the-clock supervision to ensure they stay safe, until the impetus begins to wane. Intervention in the case of a patient in the grip of phobic avoidance may take the form of exposure to a feared object or situation, where the therapeutic setting prevents the typical withdrawal behavior.

Abnormal illness behaviors involving psychosomatic and pseudoneurologic complaints may be intervened by first altering the clinician's behavior. To change the patient's behavior, the physician takes a different approach to the complaints. The intervention does not deny the patient access to the clinician, but to the misdirected efforts of the clinician to treat a false or exaggerated symptom.

Intervention also takes the form of medical treatment. A patient who has severe anorexia nervosa may need tube-feeding or intravenous nutritional support at first, to ensure survival. For a patient who has overeaten to the point of obesity, in contrast, the intervention may take the form of gastric bypass surgery or the prescription of an appetite suppressant (such as a stimulant). Again, in each case mere nutritional support or appetite suppression is only effective in the short term; to succeed the focus must turn to recovery.

*Recovery* from addiction refers to a three-part process: identify the motivations for the addictive behavior, diminish them if possible, and teach the patient to respond in different ways when the urge hits again. When the addiction has become highly entrenched, as for most drugs and many eating disorders, the recovery process may also require ongoing intervention between the patient and the opportunity to engage in the behavior.

A clinician may need to treat a disease state or symptom or soothe the pain of an adverse experience in order to weaken the motivation for an addiction. Recognizing the true costs of the addiction may further undermine its motivation. These costs may have been hidden to the patient before intervention, while the patient was drinking to forget the problems caused by drinking. Twelve-step programs such as Alcoholics Anonymous place a particular emphasis on taking responsibility for consequences (Moos 2008). In addition, group treatments introduce the inhibitory influence of peers; if a person relapses, she or he will have to explain it to a group of people who know all the excuses. Recovery has begun to take hold when the patient has experienced an urge and has carried on without relapse into the behavior.

For some addictions, the transition from recovery to maintenance is so perilous—the pull of the addiction is so powerful—that intervention continues indefinitely. Opiate drugs that block the euphoria-inducing effects of heroin are widely used for this purpose, and to ensure continued intervention, patients typically must present frequently, even daily, to obtain the drug. Nicotine patches serve a similar function as substitute drugs in treating an addiction to tobacco. Disulfiram (Antabuse), a drug given to some recovering alcoholics, offers a self-imposed form of intervention, in which the presence of the drug in the body causes acute discomfort if the patient drinks. As long as the recovering alcoholic has the motivation once in the day to sustain recovery, and takes the disulfiram, he or she has intervened against any urge that would lead to relapse.

Aims in the *maintenance* phase of treatment otherwise vary widely according to the patient and the nature of the behavior. Relapse prevention may mean the continuation under less closely supervised conditions of the methods employed in the recovery phase, such as a 12-step program. Or, it may require ongoing treatment of a disease syndrome that provoked the behavior, or of counseling to gain greater insight into the life circumstances that triggered and sustained it. For example, delayed functional recovery after a severe or chronic mental illness may signify the acquisition during the state of illness of negative or self-defeating attitudes—habits of thought-toward the resumption of life roles. To address it, the cognitive-behavioral therapist elicits from the patient the specific, reflexive, habitual thoughts as they occur, such as the pernicious, recurrent, passing thought, "There's no point in trying, and I'll only fail." Once identified, the salience of such thoughts weakens when they are exposed as distortions of reality.

## Reinterpretation of Adversity

A clinician typically addresses the consequences of adversity by removing the source of the adversity, whenever possible. Treatment of a disease state, mitigation of a vulnerability, and management of a maladaptive behavior all accomplish this task. Sometimes this is all it takes to restore a patient's confidence. But often the adversity persists, and often it turns out that the patient's experience of living in pain under adverse conditions reflects a problem in the way the patient looks at life, as much as or more than it reflects the bad things that have happened to the patient.

In the movies, it often appears that the most effective way to address a patient's feeling of demoralization, or victimization, or hopelessness, or grief, or anxiety, is to shake the patient by the lapels, administer a few sharp slaps to the cheeks, and order him or her to snap out of it. Alternatively, the therapist may spell out for the patient how some dimly remembered event from the past has continued to plague the patient, and this revelation alone restores the patient's positive attitude toward life. Or, worst of all, the patient finds healing only in the loving arms of the sexy clinician. In real life, these methods are not only ineffective, but they are likely to alienate the patient and perhaps lead to professional sanctions over the serious ethical lapse in patient care.

Jerome Frank, a pioneer in the empirical study of *psychotherapy*, theorized that there are three essential elements in effective psychotherapy (Frank and Frank 1991). First, a patient and therapist must engage in a procedure in which the expectations are understood and shared by both. Second, the procedure must induce emotional arousal in the patient—without this element there is insufficient motivation to change the patient's attitudes. Third, the procedure must take place in a healing setting—some place removed from the distractions of everyday life. It is not so important what is the theoretical basis of the treatment, as long as the healer and patient agree that it should work.

This last point is significant, because it suggests that psychotherapy predates Sigmund Freud by many thousands of years. These essential elements are seen also in the rituals of shamanistic healing known from archaeological evidence of ancient cultures, and observed by anthropologists in isolated, indigenous cultures up to modern times. A designated shaman, or healer, performs in a medicine hut a ritual emotionally exhausting both to sufferer and healer, and thus the evil spirits are released. Similarly, in an evangelical tent, a faith healer among an excited crowd lays hands on a person wheelchair bound by pain (this doesn't work if the patient is truly paralyzed by spinal cord injury), drives out the devil, and the patient walks.

The emotional charge in medical psychotherapy, in general, derives from the patient's projection onto the therapist of power, moral judgment, parental affection, or some other quality of authority (and views these qualities with fear and rage, at times, mixed with the awe). In some therapeutic modes, the authority may be used to motivate a patient directly to change behavior. In other, insight-oriented modes, the aim may be to help the patient see how these feelings for the therapist resemble the patterns of a patient's feelings toward real-world parents, spouse, and other significant people. Part of the process of healing is to help the patient see how, in the Petri dish of the therapist's office, these forces of projection operate, and to provide the patient an opportunity to apply more mature judgments, not immature projections, to the therapist as to significant others in life. So it is by working through the drama of the patient's projected feelings about the therapist—the *transference*, as it is called—that the emotional charge is engaged.

Whatever the method, psychotherapy helps the patient reimagine his or her life story. The patient changes from the hapless, helpless, hopeless victim of adverse circumstances, subject to the whims of authority figures like the psychotherapist, to become an active protagonist in life, capable of choosing among goals, and of anticipating accurately how the consequences of decisions are likely to play out based on knowledge rather than wishes and fears.

## 5.3. Summary: Psychiatric Mind

Our trip from brain cells to bouncing balls, to belief and beyond explodes the conventional psychiatric diagnoses. This text has rearranged each fragment of psychopathology to understand it as a disruption of a specific function of the mind. In place of artificial diagnostic categories, an array of symptoms, propensities, experiences, and behaviors comprises the simplest forms of mental illness. How can one reconstruct these pieces into something useful and enlightening?

To begin, a person in need of psychiatric help has one or a combination of four types of problem. The brain may malfunction due to a disease state. Trait vulnerability may hamper a person's adaptability. The person may behave maladaptively. Or, adversity may induce feelings of despair and defeat. The type of problem points to the method best suited to identifying the specific nature of the problem, and to the treatment most likely to help.

Many of the symptoms and deficits described throughout this book can best be understood as consequences of abnormal or pathological brain activity. When one or a combination of them occurs in a person, one can generally identify them as a *disease* syndrome. To sort out which disease syndrome a patient has, one can employ a roughly hierarchical approach. Disruptions of tonic arousal, for example, may perturb mental activity at all levels. Agnosia, apraxia, loss of memory perturb not only cognitive powers, but also emotional stability, as fear and frustration foster bursts of phasic arousal. Primary disturbances of phasic arousal in the context of normal tonic arousal and memory undermine motivational balance and may interfere with integrative mental activity, hence induce psychotic symptoms such as hallucinations and delusions. Primary psychosis may render one constitutionally asocial. Any of the above may contribute to disabling fear. Pathological anxiety also occurs, often, in the absence of any higher disturbance.

Clinicians remedy disease states via biological interventions that relieve symptoms directly, or that resolve a syndrome at its pathological source. Medications that increase the amount of serotonin and norepinephrine in the synaptic cleft prove useful in alleviating syndromes of emotional dysregulation. Agents that block dopamine transmission tend to alleviate psychosis and agitation. Lithium and other neuromodulators have a greater influence on the stability of arousal than on the prevailing intensity of arousal. GABA-enhancing drugs relieve arousal acutely. Drugs that block acetylcholine neurotransmission alleviate the neurological side effects of dopamine blockade; drugs that enhance acetylcholine slow the cognitive deterioration of progressive dementia. A variety of hormonal replacements or enhancements can correct pathological mental states produced by endocrine failure. Repeated electrical stimulation, as in electroconvulsive therapy, powerfully resolves syndromes of depression.

Trait *vulnerabilities* in mental life reflect an individual's relative efficiency of cognitive integration, as well as the sensitivity of a person to experience fluctuations of motivation and emotion. With respect to cognition, a slowly developing capacity for cognitive integration limits academic progress. Low intelligence limits the range of life challenges that can be mastered with ease. With respect to emotion, hypersensitive or insensitive responses, over time, can lead a person to develop rigid, erratic, or otherwise maladaptive, learned patterns of reactivity. These range from inflexible attitudes of ambivalence and impulsivity, to pervasively troublesome patterns of interpersonal relationships that characterize histrionic, anankastic, labile, and sociopathic personalities, and egocentric, eccentric, or overdependent styles of attachment. In the clinic, one may parse traits through formal testing, but mostly one comes to know them by perceiving patterns in the person's response to stress.

One may mitigate the effect of vulnerabilities by treatment, but can rarely change them outright. Education prepares a vulnerable person to anticipate and manage difficult situations, and appreciate the freedom to act on reason rather than emotion. Pharmacology also may help diminish the degree of vulnerability. The use of a medication like a catecholamine enhancer, or stimulant, may enhance cognitive performance. The use of an antidepressant or antianxiety drug may alter the capacity to engage emotional resources at a level appropriate to a given situation.

Psychiatric problems related to *behavior* all follow from voluntary action on the part of the person with the problem, though the motives may emerge from disease, trait, or adversity. This text describes a variety of maladaptive behaviors that come to psychiatric attention. Many behavioral problems involve the excessive, impulsive, or idiosyncratic choice of means to fulfill one's natural drives. In others, like addictions, the destructive consequences of fulfilling a conditioned or artificial drive constitute the clinical problem. Destructive and self-destructive behaviors may arise from misdirected defensive impulses. Individuals who exhibit abnormal help-seeking behaviors exaggerate or mimic symptoms in pursuit of non-therapeutic ends. There is one common denominator in most maladaptive, habitual behavior: the consequences of the behavior tend to exacerbate the symptoms, stress, and life circumstances that provide its motivation.

The therapeutic management of behavior occurs in stages. First, intervention removes access to the behavior and breaks the cycle of habit that has perpetuated it. Next, recovery aims to weaken the influence of stimuli that once triggered the desire for the behavior. Finally, maintenance sustains recovery, as the suicidal or addictive or somatizing or otherwise behaviorally troubled person develops better strategies to prevent the recurrence of the conditions that fostered the behavioral problem.

Virtually anyone can experience psychiatric problems under *adversity*. This text describes several common painful or maladaptive patterns in the response to adversity: for example, demoralization, dissolution, and denial. Some adversity victimizes a person, some adversity reflects a painful but natural loss, some adversity seems like bad karma. Painful responses to adversity tend to share the common element that they leave the person feeling overwhelmed and hopeless; not incapable of pleasure but unable to find the opportunity for it. They change the narrative of an individual's life story into an incoherent, meaningless, or tragic tale.

One may be able to help a person suffering from adversity if one can remove obstacles, restore losses, or otherwise directly alleviate a source of agony. However, where circumstances are unalterable, therapeutic intervention aims to rewrite the person's incoherent, meaningless, or tragic life story narrative. This is the aim of psychotherapy. Successful psychotherapy, whatever the method used, leads or guides the patient toward a new understanding of the adverse life circumstances, in which the outcome is not so inexorably painful or hopeless.

This text has disassembled and reconstructed psychiatry in order to provide the reader with better cognitive tools to discern the major problem afflicting a patient. The reader may see a psychiatric problem as a certain kind of disruption (disease, trait, behavior, adversity) of a specific aspect of mental life (arousal, appetite, perception, cognition, motion, action, attention, memory, habit, execution, motivation, desire, alarm, bias, personality, belief, identity, cooperation, communication, affiliation, or help-seeking). At our current, limited, state of knowledge of the ultimate causes of mental illness, it may be useful to think beyond diagnostic categories, toward a more practical view of the common problems that afflict psychiatric patients: psychotic thinking, affective disturbance, neurotic reactions, anguished feelings, maladjusted responses, organic failure, or self-destructive acts. The needs of patients who have different diagnoses but share the same mental problem are generally more alike than are the needs of patients who have the same diagnosis but different problems.

So, fundamentally, psychiatry begins when a person comes to a psychiatrist with problems. The psychiatrist ascertains the symptoms, propensities, choices, and experiences that constitute these problems. Applying the orthodox diagnostic system, the psychiatrist then reduces the problems to a multiaxial diagnosis that, in turn, points to empirically validated therapies. If this evidence-based therapy fails, the psychiatrist may apply an algorithm, or a hunch, to plot a new course. But within the bounds of diagnostic orthodoxy, there is little a psychiatrist can do to apply reason to the patient's problem, in order to identify and remove a therapeutic obstacle. If the psychiatrist instead employs a psychological perspective such as the one described in this text, the aim is not to render a conclusive diagnostic reduction, but to relate the patient's problems to specific failures of specific mental functions. Having iden-tified a problem in a mental function or set of functions, the psychological psychiatrist can usefully trace the connections between the components of the patient's problem. For example, it may in some cases prove less important to resolve the symptoms that constitute a diagnosis than to induce a change in habits or outlook. The thoughtful selection of a specific pharmacologic agent helps, but the patient's welfare may depend on the psychiatrist's ability to untangle complex problems the orthodox texts fail to mention.

To borrow, once again, from Paul McHugh: "Psychiatry is medicine with-out a Harvey." William Harvey changed the way doctors think about the body as a system when he explained the circulation of the blood—and he did so without having the whole picture, as no one in that era prior to the invention of the magnifying lens had ever seen microscopic capillaries; the essential conduit between arterial and venous systems. Psychiatry has tried to study and treat mental illness without the benefit of a similar organic understand-ing of the nature of mental functioning. The fact that there are gaps in our data, as there were for Harvey, should not deter the effort to try to develop such understanding. I am no Harvey, and perhaps no one can be in an age when all the money is on molecules, not theories. But I hope I have suggested what Harvey might come up with were he to embrace the work of a multitude of modern psychologists and neurobiologists to make sense of mental ill-nesses as the products of failure somewhere in the information-processing functions of the brain.

# Appendix A

If the standard approach to psychiatry provides a map of the human-made boundaries that define diagnostic entities, this book has offered the corresponding topographical map. A topographical map portrays mountain ridges, rivers, valleys, plains, and other aspects of nature. Some of these features comprise the borders between states and countries, sometimes they are contained within the borders, and sometimes they cut across the artificial borders.

In the topographical map of the mind portrayed in this book, some phenomena are contained within a single human-made diagnostic construct, some define a diagnostic construct, and some cut across diagnoses. If one is to make use of the topographical map in real applications, one needs to be familiar with the human-made boundaries, whether or not they reflect nature. When a highway builder aims to build a highway across several states, in addition to the features of the terrain that concern the road engineer, the builder must be aware of state and local laws in order to obtain the proper permits. For the same reason, in order to treat patients it is essential to know something of the official diagnoses, whether or not they represent valid constructs. Figure A.1 suggests how part of a topological map of mental illness might look.

Thus, this appendix provides a brief guide to the human-made boundaries of mental illness now in use, to link the topographical map of mental function, as laid out in the main text, to the practicalities of research and clinical work. It focuses on the facts and factors that help to define these diagnostic entities. Note that in this appendix diagnoses are given unequal attention. The amount of space given to the diagnoses selected for description in this appendix is a function of the public health significance of the diagnosis, its complexity, and its associated controversies.

## A.1. What Is a DSM Diagnosis?

Psychiatric diagnosis is based on collective opinions about patterns in the clinical presentations, course of illness, and treatment responses of patients. Because psychiatry uses a common reference for diagnosis—the *Diagnostic and Statistical Manual of Mental Disorders* (DSM)—patients who have similar patterns of signs and symptoms are reliably given the same diagnosis by clinicians anywhere and in any setting. However, in the absence of definitive tests of the biological basis of disorders, there is no way to validate a diagnosis in a given patient, nor is there a way to prove the integrity of the diagnostic definitions that lump and split clinical problems into a set of conventional clinical diagnoses.

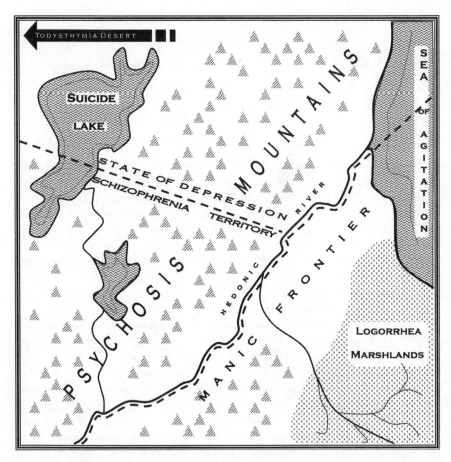

*Figure A.1.* Topographical maps, like psychiatric diagnoses, reflect both manufactured and natural boundaries.

A diagnosis can be thought of as a shorthand label for a pattern of signs and symptoms associated with a patient's clinical problems. Clinical and epidemiological investigations based on these pattern definitions have yielded valuable information to inform predictions about a patient's likely prognosis and treatment response. So, while the most important considerations in the assessment of a patient are the patient's signs, symptoms, and problems, it is useful to be able to assign a name to the patterns observed and to identify treatments that are likely (compared to placebo) to be helpful. There are hundreds of diagnoses in the current version of the DSM, and thousands of variations. In this appendix the focus will be on the diagnoses that one is most likely to encounter in general medical or psychiatric practice.

As of this writing, the fourth edition of the DSM (DSM-IV), established and published originally in 1994 by the American Psychiatric Association, is still in use. The fifth edition is in preparation, and not expected to employ neurobiological concepts to alter the diagnostic criteria or their application (Hyman 2007). It is likely that the DSM-V will serve a purpose similar to the DSM-IV by providing a common reference point to make reliable diagnoses, for the purposes of research and the need to apply a code in order to be reimbursed by insurance companies and governmental agencies.

The DSM-IV system uses five axes, all denoting a different aspect of diagnosis.

Axis I is the diagnosis that explains the patient encounter. It can be a major mental illness, like schizophrenia or bipolar disorder; behaviors like alcohol dependence or pathological gambling; or a reactive state, like adjustment disorder. If a patient is assessed not to have a mental illness, a V-code can be assigned, that is, one of a set of codes that begin with the letter V that describe common life problems that might bring someone in for treatment, such as relationship conflicts. V-code diagnoses are rarely the focus of research and are unlikely to meet criteria for insurance coverage, so are rarely used. We will bypass them here.

Axis II is an optional diagnosis applied to enduring patient traits that modify the presentation and treatment of the Axis I diagnosis. The two kinds of diagnosis that fit here are diagnoses related to intellectual disability (mental retardation) and personality disorder.

Axis III is a list of somatic medical disorders that may affect the presentation and treatment of the Axis I diagnosis.

Axis IV is a description of acute and ongoing life events that may affect the presentation and treatment; these may include acute problems like divorce, bankruptcy, medical illness, or death of a loved one, and ongoing problems like social isolation, poor coping skills, and substance misuse.

Axis V is a numerical estimation of the severity of the patient's acute problem, as well as of the patient's best level of functioning over the preceding year. To offer a rough idea, a score between 91 and 100 is ideal: "superior functioning in a wide range of activities, life's problems never seem to get out of hand, is sought out by others because of his or her many positive qualities. No symptoms." In contrast, 71–80 describes someone who has minor and transient problems and symptoms, 51–60 is a person who has moderate symptoms and difficulty in functioning, 31–40 is major impairment in communication and incapacitation from life functioning. A person who scores in the range of 11–20 has demonstrated some risk of harm to self or others, or incoherence in communication, or failure to maintain even minimal personal hygiene.

## A.2. Childhood Disorders
### Intellectual Disability (Mental Retardation)

Intellectual disability (formerly known as mental retardation) is an Axis II diagnosis defined by an IQ more than 2 standard deviations below the mean (< 70, where the mean is 100). The Axis II designation implies that low IQ is an enduring trait that predisposes a person to clinical problems (diagnosed in Axis I). Thus, intellectual disability is not a primary reason for psychiatric consultation; early in life, it tends more to concern teachers, later in life social workers. The Axis I, or primary problems that affect people with intellectual disability tend to arise out of a high vulnerability to stress from life challenges most would not find overwhelming, combined with a limited repertoire of effective ways to cope. At very low end of the IQ scale, psychiatric intervention may be needed to quell agitation behaviorally or pharmacologically because the patient's limited cognitive skills do not respond to reason. One additional concern for any clinician: the same treatment plan that may work for most adult patients may not work for those who have intellectual disability unless special care is taken to ensure that the plan will not require the patient to calculate dosages or monitor treatment effects.

*See* Cognition: low intelligence

### Autism and Pervasive Developmental Disorders

Autism is part of a group of pervasive developmental disorders that includes also Rett syndrome, childhood disintegrative disorder, and Asperger syndrome. These disorders profoundly affect interpersonal and social functioning from childhood onward. They severely impinge on the behavioral elements of social interaction, including gaze modulation, facial expressiveness, and nonverbal gestures. Consequently, individuals with these disorders fail to develop appropriate peer relationships. Their interactions with others lack social or emotional reciprocity, and they seldom if ever engage in spontaneous conversation about shared interests and events. Often such individuals have difficulty recognizing faces, expressing emotions, and integrating affect with appropriate gaze and communication. There is a fundamental impairment in "theory of mind," meaning difficulty understanding the intents, beliefs, tastes, preferences, experiences, background, and emotional responses of other people. Often there is a profound delay in the development of spoken language, behavioral stereotypy such as hand flapping, an inability to sustain give-and-take conversation, and a lack of spontaneous and varied play with peers. There may be a marked tendency to have intense preoccupations with arcane knowledge, inflexible adherence to specific routines or rituals, stereotyped and repetitive motor mannerisms, and persistent preoccupation with parts of objects.

Known causes include congenital rubella, tuberous sclerosis, neurofibromatosis, specific chromosomal abnormalities such as fragile X syndrome, and abnormal neurochemistry. The common pathophysiologic thread appears to be an early peak in gray matter development, between the second and fourth years, whereas normally this occurs between the sixth and eighth years. During this time normal learning and experience influence the shape of neural architecture and connectivity, but children with pervasive developmental disorders appear to lack sufficient reserves of plasticity-capable neurons to be able to integrate experience into a workable cortical map of the social world (O'Hearn et al. 2008).

*See* Cooperation: asociality

### Attention-Deficit Disorders

Attention-deficit/hyperactivity disorder (ADHD) causes behavioral as well as cognitive problems in about one in 20 school-age children; the condition is present in about half of children in outpatient psychiatric treatment. Although inattentiveness is the essential component, and many children also manifest hyperactivity or impulsivity, the core functional deficit is arguably distractibility. Children with ADHD make frequent mistakes out of carelessness, daydream, fidget, lose focus, are disorganized, and show poor follow-through and forgetfulness. Hyperactivity/impulsivity is apparent via fidgetiness, restlessness, talking, inability to sit still, noisiness, interruptiveness, and impatience taking turns. Many children manifest one or more of these traits at one time or another, but when many of them occur persistently in the same child, with sufficient severity to impede academic progress, then the diagnosis applies. Besides academic difficulties, children who have this disorder may have social and emotional problems as well.

ADHD can be confused with rambunctious behavior on one hand, or inattentiveness as a result of distraction by mood or anxiety problems on the other. Yet, there is no evidence of systematic over- or underdiagnosis (Sciutto and Eisenberg 2007). The diagnosis tends to be controversial first, because it leads to the prescription of controlled substances—amphetamines—to children. Second, it has become commonplace to diagnose it in adults, whether or not the symptoms were present in childhood. In some cases the symptoms in adults may have been overlooked in childhood (Faraone et al. 2000), but in other cases where no school problems existed, the diagnosis may reflect confusion between the symptom of inattentiveness, which can occur for many reasons, and the diagnosis of ADHD. The misdiagnosis thus becomes a license to take stimulants as performance-enhancing drugs rather than to address a true functional deficit.

ADHD is associated with diminished cerebral and cerebellar volumes and with abnormal frontal lobe morphology, suggestive of a deficit in frontal-striatal circuitry (Valera et al. 2007). There appears to be a delay in the maturation (myelination) of the relevant circuits, hence children who have ADHD may manifest age-inappropriate behaviors and capacities because their brains effectively function at a level beneath their years (Willcutt et al. 2005).

*See* Attention: distraction

### Disruptive Behavior Disorders

Two diagnostic varieties of disruptive behavior disorder are recognized.

Oppositional-defiant disorder characterizes a pervasive pattern of disruptive behavior toward parents, teachers, and other authorities. It tends to arise under conditions when parenting either is ineffectual or is competent but not up to the challenges of a temperamentally difficult child in a difficult situation. Power struggles flare up frequently. To view the problem empathically: stress can make anyone feel uncooperative. Children suffer more from this because they have little power over the inescapable demands of authority hence conflict often seems inevitable (Mones 1998). An adult often can just call in sick, no questions asked; a child who might prefer to take a "mental health day" has to deal with a parent who is dead set against it.

Conduct disorder characterizes a pattern of destructive, larcenous, violent, and exploitative or predatory behavior that begins early in life. It can be a precursor to sociopathy (DSM diagnosis: antisocial personality disorder). Conduct disorder tends to have one of two outcomes. In some individuals, the criminally disruptive behavior in childhood is an early sign of the absence of moral sensibility that will form the basis of sociopathy. Others "grow out of it" when they reach maturity and leave behind the harsh environment in which criminal behavior was adaptive (Raine 2002).

*See* Cooperation: sociopathy

## A.3. Cognitive Disorders

### Delirium

The term *delirium* means, literally from the Latin, "off the path." A person with delirium is grossly disoriented not just to time and place, but to situation. Other medical disciplines employ different terms that essentially describe delirium, such as *encephalopathy* and *delta MS* (change in mental status). Delirium is always suspected when there is an obvious change in the level of consciousness—alternately somnolent and agitated at odd times of day. In a hospitalized patient, especially a frail, sickly, or elderly patient, or one who has just undergone surgery, a new onset of agitation, hallucinations, delusions, and the like should be considered delirium until proven otherwise.

Delirium is the most common preventable complication in hospitalized elderly patients, yet is often overlooked or misdiagnosed. Delirium increases the intensity of nursing care and number of inpatient hospital days. While not itself life threatening, it is a sign of systemic illness that itself may produce death, and is as potent an indicator of mortality as other hospital complications such as myocardial infarction and sepsis.

Risk factors include having a complicated medical condition or set of medical conditions, taking many prescription medications, being older, and suffering higher levels of physical debilitation. Among iatrogenic causes, anticholinergic side effects of medications play a major role (Rovner et al. 1988).

Diagnosis of delirium is clinical, based on observation. The diagnosis can be verified by EEG, which will detect generalized slowing of background activity in some cases (Romano and Engel 1944). However, a normal EEG does not rule out clinically evident delirium. It is worth noting that symptoms of delirium may linger after a contributing medical cause has waned.

*See* Arousal: delirium, agitation; Perception: illusions

### Dementia

Dementia is a common, acquired, global decline in cognitive functioning that can affect memory, orientation, attention, speech, praxis, and executive functioning. Minor decline in cognitive function is typical in an aging brain; however, impairment to the point of gross disorientation or loss of capacity for competent self-care is not a normal part of aging. Most dementias are incurable at this time, but their ravages can be mitigated through proper intervention. The few known reversible causes of dementia include depression, certain metabolic disorders, normal pressure hydrocephalus, vitamin B12 deficiency, hypothyroidism, and neurosyphilis (rarely).

Because dementia often has an insidious onset, it is not uncommon for it to become clinically apparent only in the context of a major life change, such as a hospitalization or the death of a spouse who previously had filled in the gaps in the patient's function. A person developing dementia may suspect the diagnosis, but family members most often initiate the assessment. Two features define dementia apart from other conditions affecting cognition: first, there is no altered level of consciousness, as in delirium (Rabins and Folstein 1982); second, there is a significant decline in cognitive capacity to the point of an impact on self-care. It may be tricky to differentiate dementia from depression in elderly people, in whom severe depression can present with profound cognitive impairment (Wells 1979). This has sometimes been called "pseudodementia," but there is nothing "pseudo" about the loss of cognitive function, even if it is a consequence of a treatable mood disorder.

Clinical assessment to establish a dementia diagnosis is essentially a careful evaluation of cognitive functioning. As a screening tool, the mini-mental status examination described in Appendix B is a good place to start (Folstein et al. 1975). A positive screen or clinical suspicion can be followed up with comprehensive neuropsychiatric testing to establish the diagnosis.

The best-known form of dementia is Alzheimer disease, named after the German psychiatrist who first reported a case (Boller et al. 2007). A clinical diagnosis can be made with 90 percent accuracy while the patient is alive; confirmation requires autopsy, which reveals neurofibrillary plaques and tangles. Several genetic tests are available; however, they reveal only the presence of a risk allele, not diagnostic confirmation, and moreover the known genetic risk alleles are found in only a small minority of cases.

In contrast, vascular dementia caused by a series of "mini-strokes" (infarcts from blockage of small blood vessels) throughout the brain may have a similar presentation cross-sectionally, but over time the decline will be seen to be more step-wise than gradual, as in Alzheimer disease. There are likely to be more pronounced focal deficits, and neuroimaging is likely to reveal the presence of lesions suggestive of cerebrovascular disease.

Although the loss of cognitive function is the hallmark of dementia, the most pressing problems at any given time may be emotional and behavioral. Many people with dementia develop a clinically diagnosable, treatable depressive syndrome. Hallucinations and delusions are not uncommon, though at times they may reflect confusion rather than true psychosis. People who have severe dementia may become aggressive and agitated, disinhibited (wandering, grabbing, calling out), or apathetic (more common in advanced cases and certain "subcortical" dementias that primarily affect deep brain structures). Sleep disturbance is particularly hard on caregivers, who lose sleep themselves trying to keep their loved one from wandering away from home or leaving the stove on—hence the title of a popular book for families of people who have dementia, *The 36-Hour Day* (Mace and Rabins 2001).

*See* Perception: agnosia; Action: apraxia; Memory: amnesia

## A.4. Substance-Related Disorders
### Intoxication and Withdrawal

Acute intoxication is a special form of delirium. Like delirium, it can manifest as agitation and anergia, though emotional lability is more common than psychosis or confusion, and the state generally resolves over a matter of hours (sometimes many hours).

Withdrawal from "depressants" like alcohol, benzodiazepines, and barbiturates is potentially dangerous, as the absence of pharmacologic inhibition leaves the brain hyperaroused and vulnerable to seizures, and the body prone to dramatic fluctuations in autonomic tone. Withdrawal from opioids produces a state opposite of the pharmacologically calming intoxicating effect they have; it is a state of acute distress and discomfort, as well as alterations in autonomic functions, but it is not dangerous to life. Withdrawal from cocaine and amphetamines tends to produce anergia and a depressive picture.

A drug's potential to produce intoxication and addiction is a function primarily of the neurotransmitter system it affects, but also of its pharmacokinetics. That is, a drug's rapidity of access to the brain and the rapidity of clearance have significant effects on a drug's abuse potential. The more rapid rise and fall of pharmacologic impact, the more potent the psychological effects and the likelihood of addiction tend to be (Farre and Cami 1991). For example, cigarette smokers are more likely than cigar smokers to develop a dependence on nicotine to the point that abstinence produces withdrawal symptoms. Cigarette smokers introduce nicotine to the brain by direct entry from lungs to arterial blood; with cigars, the nicotine is absorbed through the tissue in the mouth, thus enters the venous system and gets to the brain more slowly. As refined forms of drugs have been developed, including distilled versus fermented alcohol, morphine from the poppy, cocaine from the coca plant, hashish from hemp, and so on, the intensity of the psychological effect is increased, and further potentiated by the more rapid onset kinetics of inhalation or injection versus oral ingestion.

The diagnosis of intoxication is made when recent ingestion of an intoxicating substance produces mental symptoms and maladaptive behavior, accompanied by specific signs for each class of substances. Diagnosis of withdrawal also has components common to all substances, related to the cessation of heavy substance use and the clinical significance of the syndrome, as well as specific signs and symptoms for each substance.

*See* Arousal: delirium; Habit: addiction

### Alcohol

Alcohol has complex effects on behavior. At low levels of intoxication, alcohol is a "social lubricant." It diminishes vigilance about the potentially risky aspects of social embarrassment. At the same time, alcohol, like other drugs of abuse, feels pleasurable, and can enhance other pleasures.

Alcohol intoxication is characterized by slurred speech, unstable gait and coordination, cognitive impairment, and at the extreme, loss of consciousness. As a general rule, consumption of more than a drink per hour is likely to produce clinical intoxication. Some individuals seem to have a diminished sensitivity to the subjective effects of alcohol intoxication, though equal impairment in objective measures of cognition and response time, at a given concentration of blood alcohol. The "official" alcohol content of blood to be declared intoxicated (for example, if pulled over by police while driving erratically) in most of the United States is 0.08 percent. Alcohol is metabolized in the liver and removed from the bloodstream at a steady pace of approximately 0.01 percent per hour down to the normal level of 0. Hence, busy emergency departments on a Friday night often have a few gurneys occupied by drunken people "sleeping it off" and leaving sober, if worse for wear, the next morning.

Alcohol withdrawal is common and potentially dangerous. For someone who has a physical dependence on alcohol, abrupt cessation from drinking, as often happens during a medical hospitalization or incarceration and less often by the patient's own decision, can escalate over several days to a state of frank delirium, complete with confusion, altered consciousness, and hallucinations, and accompanied by autonomic instability (elevated pulse and blood pressure), seizures, and potentially death. Withdrawal can be averted if consumption is tapered gradually, or benzodiazepines or barbiturates are substituted for alcohol.

### AMPHETAMINES

Drugs in the class of amphetamines raise dopamine and norepinephrine levels in synapses and thus stimulate arousal. They are often used therapeutically to enhance alertness, attention, and performance, and have also been used to promote weight loss. Prescription stimulants can and are abused; hence their use is controlled. The most dangerous form of amphetamine prevalent today is methamphetamine. This is a chemical that can be mixed in a home laboratory, using readily available materials (though controls have been placed on the over-the-counter availability of the decongestant pseudoephedrine, to block its use in creating methamphetamine).

Amphetamine stimulants produce a heightened arousal of both reward- and fear-based motivational and emotional states. Depending on which kind of motivational state predominates at a given time, the effect may be euphoria or irritability, expansive sociability or paranoid withdrawal. Significant stimulant intoxication tends to have physiologic effects that mimic sympathetic arousal: increased heart rate, dilated pupils, psychomotor agitation, and other signs of autonomic instability. Stimulant withdrawal is an unpleasant but not dangerous condition marked by fatigue, lethargy, and low mood.

### CANNABIS

*Cannabis sativa*, the hemp plant, produces the psychoactive chemical tetrahydrocannabinol (THC), which is used principally for its euphoric effects. Like most drugs, THC activates a subset of endogenous receptors. Endocannabinoid receptors are

found in neuronal pathways that detect and respond to stimuli that produce the pleasure response, and thus reinforce reward-motivated behavior, possibly by facilitating
plasticity and learning in reward pathways (Chevaleyre et al. 2006). Cannabis use is
allowed in some cultures and under some circumstances, but is rarely permitted in
the United States, and then only for physician-indicated therapeutic purposes (such
as appetite stimulation, nausea suppression, and pain management). In some cultures it has assumed ritual importance in religious observance, whereas in Western
cultures it tends to be used purely for its pleasure-inducing properties.

Clinical intoxication with cannabis is characterized by affective and cognitive
changes, diminished behavioral inhibition, but also heightened arousal of fear ("paranoia") and physiologically by dry mouth, reddened eyes, and increased appetite. A
cannabis withdrawal syndrome is not recognized as a diagnosis.

### COCAINE

Cocaine is derived from the leaves of the coca plant, which grows primarily in
South America. It was used traditionally by natives of the Andes, who would chew the
leaves to combat fatigue. It is still used clinically as a topical anesthetic, in limited
applications. Methods to extract the psychoactive ingredients of the coca plant have
produced inhalable cocaine powder and smokeable crack cocaine. Less common
forms of cocaine abuse include injection and freebasing (in which the cocaine is
vaporized before inhalation). Both of the latter methods are extremely dangerous,
the former because cocaine induces vasoconstriction, thus putting tissue at risk for
necrosis and the development of ulcers and abscesses, the latter because of the flam-
mable nature of the vaporized cocaine preparation—it was through the latter method
that the famous comedian Richard Pryor suffered severe burns. The use of refined
forms of cocaine produces rapid-onset euphoria.

Cocaine is a dopamine reuptake inhibitor, so it effectively increases synaptic levels of dopamine. Cocaine intoxication and withdrawal syndromes are similar to the
syndromes observed with amphetamine stimulants. Intoxication generally arouses
sympathetic nervous system-like activation of cognitive, emotional, and physiologic
volatility; withdrawal tends to produce the opposite: lethargy and depression.

### OPIOIDS

Drugs derived from the poppy plant include morphine and a host of natural derivatives; the class of opioids includes also synthetic imitators of morphine. Derivatives of the poppy were known from ancient times to induce euphoric and worry-free
states. Medicinal uses to relieve suffering and recreational use via opium smoking were
known worldwide by the dawn of the modern era. An ingestible extract of opium,
laudanum, was widely used beginning in the sixteenth century. Morphine was first
isolated as the psychoactive component of the poppy in the nineteenth century and
introduced into battlefield medicine in the wars of that era. Morphine is in general
poorly tolerated in the digestive system, and its psychoactive effects are potentiated

by parenteral administration, so its use for its euphorigenic properties has mainly been by way of inhalation (snorting or smoking) and direct injection intravenously. Modern derivatives of morphine include heroin, a slightly altered morphine molecule that is readily packaged and self-administered, and synthetic opioids like codeine and oxycodone, which are more readily tolerated in the digestive tract, hence are commonly used therapeutically in pain management.

Opioid intoxication is characterized by a euphoric feeling that gives way to apathy and inertia, along with typical physiologic effects such as pupillary constriction and diminished alertness, attention, and motivation. Opioid overdose can result in death by respiratory drive inhibition. Opioid withdrawal is among the most notoriously unpleasant experiences known to humankind, and is characterized by severe dysphoria (low, irritable, or anxious mood), gastrointestinal disturbances (nausea, diarrhea), runny nose and watery eyes, pain, and restlessness.

### SEDATIVES/HYPNOTICS/ANXIOLYTICS

Like amphetamines, sedative/hypnotic/anxiolytics are drugs developed by the pharmaceutical industry and have medicinal purposes. They do not tend to produce euphoria directly, but they can produce a highly reinforcing experience of relief from dysphoric and anxious arousal. They are similar to alcohol in many ways, including their effects to depress brain arousal, but also in the patterns of intoxication and withdrawal. Older sedatives, in the barbiturate class, had the unfortunate and often deadly effect of inhibiting respiratory drive, along with arousal; newer-generation drugs in the benzodiazepine class are more selective in their effects. Most problems with drugs in this class at the present time stem from the misuse of prescription benzodiazepines.

### OTHER DRUGS

Diagnoses of caffeine intoxication and withdrawal and nicotine withdrawal can be but are rarely made in psychiatry, as they are rarely a cause for seeking treatment. Hallucinogens, inhalants, and phencyclidine produce severe states of intoxication, albeit are used to this extent far less frequently than other drugs.

### Abuse versus Dependence

Chemical addiction is the problematic use of intoxicating substances, but "addiction" is not a DSM diagnosis. Psychiatry recognizes two major classes of addiction diagnosis: abuse and dependence. The criteria for making a diagnosis of abuse versus dependence are the same regardless of the substance. Substance abuse is a pattern of problematic drug or alcohol use despite adverse consequences. Problems that typify substance abuse include driving while intoxicated, and allowing substance use to interfere with work and relationships. Substance dependence is a pattern of *persistent* use despite adverse consequences; additionally, a substance dependence diagnosis implies that the person has tried and failed to stem the addiction and has developed signs of tolerance and withdrawal—a state in which habitual and escalating use is needed to avoid lapsing into physiologic symptoms of withdrawal and psychological symptoms of craving. The line between the two diagnoses is sometimes indistinct.

*See* Habit: addiction

## A.5. Psychotic Disorders

### Schizophrenia

Schizophrenia is a chronic mental illness in which patients are plagued by psychotic symptoms (hallucinations, delusions, thought disorders, disorganized speech and behavior) and by a progressive failure to function in occupational and relational roles. The diagnostic term encompasses patients who have a variety of chronic symptom sets, so may be an umbrella diagnosis for several distinct pathologies of mental function.

Patients who have schizophrenia seek treatment for any of a number of problems, ranging from suicidal and explosive behaviors to social withdrawal and erratic behavior, to distress from tormenting ideas and intrusive thoughts. Schizophrenia is characterized by persistent abnormal mental experiences (psychoses), by loss of mental energy and efficiency, and by subtle but disabling cognitive impairment (not gross dementia). The abnormal mental experiences such as hallucinations and delusions are considered "positive symptoms" and the behavioral disorganization, apathy, and impaired social function are considered "negative symptoms." The chronic impairment in the cognitive aspects of the functions of perception, thought, belief, cooperation, and communication support the idea, originally encapsulated by German psychiatrist Emil Kraepelin, who termed the disorder *dementia praecox*.

Although the existence of a syndrome of chronic psychotic symptoms is unquestionable to anyone who has observed it, it has proven difficult to identify aspects of the syndrome that are universal to all who have the diagnosis, or unique to those who have the diagnosis. Eugen Bleuler attempted to whittle the essential features of schizophrenia down to four: ambivalence, asociality, emotional blunting, and derailment. However, these criteria proved so broad that they often were applied to people who were only slightly idiosyncratic in their presentation. Much later, Kurt Schneider tried to identify symptoms that would clearly differentiate schizophrenia from other disorders. Not everyone who has Schneider's "first-rank symptoms" would be diagnosed with schizophrenia by every diagnostician, but the presence of several of these symptoms makes it more likely (Mellor 1970). These symptoms include, essentially, a variety of specific kinds of hallucinations and delusions that tend not to be seen in mood disorders, delirium, or states of intoxication, such as hearing voices commenting aloud on one's actions or arguing with one another; thought withdrawal (avulsion) and insertion (intrusion) and broadcasting (telemission); and delusions of passivity (extravolition; the experience of literally feeling one's actions under control by an outside force).

Schizophrenia occurs in between 0.5 and one percent of the population worldwide. A variety of subtypes of schizophrenia are recognized, some characterized more by the positive symptoms such as hallucinations and delusions, some by negative symptoms such as passivity experiences and disorganized behavior. The typical onset occurs in the late teens or early twenties, somewhat earlier in males than females. A second peak of incidence occurs in midlife, primarily in women. These later-onset cases are sometimes classified as "paraphrenia" and often express primarily positive symptoms, with social and interpersonal function remaining relatively intact. About half of patients diagnosed with schizophrenia may have a mild course, or may recover, while the other half tends to have persistent and severe problems. One caveat when interpreting outcome studies is that, with older data, there is the possibility that the index diagnosis was based on an archaic concept of schizophrenia before the development and consistent use of diagnostic criteria in the 1970s (Cooper et al. 1988).

Schizophrenia produces distress, dysfunction, and dangerousness. Hallucinations are often relentless, painful in content, and distracting; patients seek relief from them. Patients experience destructive urges such as a drive to use illicit drugs, or inflict self-injury. The state of fear and alienation related to many delusional beliefs is a source of desperation and misery. Social dysfunction is profound—poverty, homelessness, social isolation, criminal victimization are common; mortality rates are high and life expectancy is short. The risk of suicide is high—purportedly 10 percent. Although most patients never become violent, violence is far more common among patients who have schizophrenia than in the population at large.

Schizophrenia is a complex phenotype. No single, simple cause accounts for it (Lewis and Lieberman 2000). It is widely accepted that the ultimate cause is pathology in brain function, possibly neurodevelopmental in origin, albeit the specific source of the dysfunction remains unknown. There is strong evidence of familiality and several suspected risk alleles. Studies of monozygous twins discordant for schizophrenia demonstrate greater brain atrophy (larger ventricles) in the schizophrenic twin, and pathological studies find thinner cortex, fewer and smaller dendritic spines are associated. Factors that may adversely affect the prenatal environment, including season of birth, birth complications, and maternal malnutrition, raise the risk. Most investigators believe in a "multiple hit" model in which biological predisposition and environmental insult combine to produce the development of the syndrome.

*See* Perceptions: hallucinations; Cognition: disorganization; Motion: catatonia; Action: extravolition; Attention: avulsion/intrusion; Belief: delusions; Communication: derailment, telemission; Cooperation: asociality; Affiliation: eccentricity

### Other Psychotic Disorders

Many patients have some symptoms of schizophrenia, but do not fit the full syndrome. When the symptoms of schizophrenia are present, but have persisted less than the arbitrary six-month cutoff required for a diagnosis of schizophrenia, then the patient is said to have schizophreniform disorder. When patients have the full syndrome of schizophrenia and, at times, the full syndrome of mania and/or major depression, then the diagnosis is assessed as schizoaffective disorder. The presence of delusions without the full schizophrenia syndrome may be diagnosed as delusional disorder if they are persistent; as brief psychotic disorder if they are of recent onset; and as shared psychotic disorder if they appear to reflect the delusional ideas of someone else on whom the patient is emotionally dependent.

## A.6. Mood Disorders

The diagnostic category of mood disorders includes depression and mania, and variants of these two syndromes of persistent and pervasive changes in mood. The diagnoses included under the umbrella of "mood disorders" were formerly called "affective disorders." Psychiatrists worldwide officially stopped using the term *affective disorders* in the 1980s, and substituted the term *mood disorders*. However, the term *mood* still obscures the essential feature of these disorders, which is not the mood. Many people who have depression do not feel "depressed," and for people who have mania, the problem is not an enviably high mood, but the heedless behavior that follows. To classify a disorder by a symptom is at any rate uninformative, as it would be to diagnose angina as a "chest pain disorder." The one functional deficit most specific to and ubiquitous among people who have a mood disorder diagnosis is a deficit in hedonic function, that is, a deficient or excessive capacity to be motivated by the anticipation of satisfaction.

Disorders in this category are characterized by significant disturbances in mood, self-worth, and feelings and functions of physical well-being that can lead to occupational and interpersonal impairment, even incapacitation. Suicide is an all-too-common outcome of a severe mood disorder. According to the United Nations World Health Organization, the major mood disorders are among the leading causes worldwide of lost time from work and lost health (Ustun et al. 2004). Mood disorders routinely wreck families and careers, and trigger and sustain substance abuse.

### Major Depression

The term *major depressive episode* describes a persistently low, sad, anxious, irritable, or flattened mood that lasts at least several weeks, associated with anhedonia and altered patterns of sleep, appetite, energy, concentration, and self-attitude, often leading to suicidal thoughts and actions. The term *depression*, though entrenched in the vernacular, is an imprecise and often misunderstood term for what is in reality a severe mental illness. The older term *melancholia* was perhaps better at suggesting the alien and alienating experience that is the major depressive syndrome. *Depression* trivializes the problem because everyone has some idea what it is to *feel* depressed, for a few hours or days.

Moreover, *depression* does not describe the prevailing mood in a great many cases of "major depression." Feelings of pervasive sadness are common, but so are feelings of anxiety, irritability, or even the sense of having *no* emotions. The symptoms that typically accompany depression largely revolve around the inability to become moved by the prospect of reward. Thus, the patient may sense a drive to eat but have no interest in food, may feel tired but be unable to embrace sleep, may avoid stimulating activities; may lose the anticipation of pleasure altogether and become hopeless. Attention wanders, as nothing engages it. The person with depression can muster no enthusiasm even for self-reflection, as the salience of past experiences and future plans has been lost. Tragically, suicide may begin to appear to be a legitimate response to the misery; nothing of value holds the person to life and life has become unremittingly painful.

Depression is a common and vivid enough experience that writers have represented it well, in literature ranging from Anna Karenina to Harry Potter, who entered into a depressive state after his encounter with the "dementors" who suck all good experiences from life. Lifetime prevalence estimates for major depression range widely, to as much as 20 percent in some countries. Surveys also find women to consistently be more likely to have depression than men. Age of onset tends to peak in the twenties to thirties and again in old age (Weissman et al. 1996). There is a high risk of recurrence. Of people who have recovered from a significant depressive episode, about half will relapse within five years. If depression is accompanied by delusions, they tend to be consistent with depressive themes, such as a belief that one is dying of cancer, or has committed a horrible crime, or smells bad. Nihilistic delusions (for example, that the world is coming to an end) are also congruent with the depressive mood. Evidence from genetics, functional neuroimaging, and bioassays supports the existence of biological determinants of major depression including disruptions in monoamine and hormone activity in the brain, but the details of the process remain to be discovered (Nestler et al. 2002).

*See* Arousal: anergia; Appetite: sleep, feeding, sex; Attention: distraction; Value: suicidality; Motive: anhedonia; Desire: dejection

### Mania and Bipolar Disorder

Mania defines the diagnosis of bipolar disorder. Manic episodes are periods of a week or more of markedly altered mood—elated, irritable, or some combination—accompanied by elevated drive, speech, distractibility, restlessness, and self-confidence, as well as a diminished drive for sleep. Manias tend to occur episodically, often alternating with episodes of major depression.

Bipolar disorder (traditionally called manic-depressive illness) afflicts approximately one to 2 percent of the population in its most severe form and an additional 3 to 4 percent if one includes variants in the bipolar spectrum (Akiskal and Pinto 2000). It generally begins earlier than major depression, with first signs in the teens and twenties, but also involves a longer lag time to treatment (Lish et al. 1994). Males and females are equally likely to have bipolar disorder. It may appear primarily as major depression at first; the manic element can emerge either through careful history-taking or by accident, when antidepressant treatment unleashes a manic response.

Problems from mania typically include explosiveness and erratic behavior. Patients in the midst of a manic episode, if they perceive a change in their functioning at all, tend to see it as a change for the better, and fail to perceive the increases in risk to themselves and harm to others that occur as collateral damage. While a few experienced patients may come for help at the earliest sign of illness, which is often a lack of drive to sleep, it is more common for the alarm to be sounded by family and friends who see the patient wasting resources, taking risks, and alienating others by poor social judgment. If delusions are present, they tend to be grandiose in theme, consistent with manic overconfidence. Patients who have mania and delusions may come to believe that they have special knowledge or abilities superior to those of most mortals; if paranoid, they believe that the motives driving their persecutors stem either from jealousy or from fear of the manic patient's self-perceived power.

The exact pathophysiology of mania is unknown, but genetic (Farmer et al. 2007) and functional neuroimaging (Strakowski et al. 2005) point to a biological basis. Individual variation in the capacity for recovery argues against a pathophysiology based on a degenerative process, but the fact of residual impairment suggests long-term dysfunction can be a consequence or correlate of the illness. Cognitive symptoms are common in active states of mania and depression, and in bipolar disorder specific cognitive deficits have been documented in patients after symptoms have resolved, most consistently in executive functioning and verbal learning, but also in tests of attention (Schretlen et al. 2007). Although there is some evidence that greater illness severity correlates with greater cognitive dysfunction, causal connections are not established.

*Bipolar* is a poor term for the mental illness surrounding the manic syndrome. It reflects the fact that most patients who have episodes of mania also have episodes of depression—hence, at each polar end of the world of moods—but many patients also experience mixed or anxious mood states that can be classified as neither manic nor depressed.

*See* Arousal: agitation; Attention: distraction; Desire: excitement, irascibility; Bias: impulsiveness; Personality: labile personality; Communication: hyperfluency; Affiliation: egotism

### Mood Disorder Diagnosis

A hierarchical approach is used to diagnose a mood disorder. With one exception, if a full manic episode is or ever has been present, the diagnosis is bipolar disorder, whether or not the patient has ever had major depression. The only exception is when the manic or major depressive episode is superimposed on the full syndrome of schizophrenia. In that case the diagnosis of schizoaffective disorder applies.

When the full manic syndrome is present, the diagnosis is bipolar disorder type I. If the impairment from the manic syndrome is only mild at worst, if there is no psychosis, nor troublesome behavior or inability to follow through successfully with educational, occupational, and interpersonal affairs, then the episode is considered a hypomania (below mania), and the patient is diagnosed with bipolar disorder, type II. Although some investigators have suggested a more expansive "bipolar spectrum" of disorders, including bipolars III and IV, officially the subtypes stop at bipolar II (Akiskal et al. 1999). Nevertheless, the bipolar spectrum idea suggests, with good reason, that there is a relationship between full bipolar and major depressive syndromes and other milder forms of mood variability. These include dysthymia, which is defined as a chronic mild depressive syndrome in which the mood is low most of the time and a few symptoms of major depression are present; and cyclothymia, defined as a persistent state of "moodiness" in which there are frequent swings from mildly elevated to mildly depressed moods, most of the time.

## A.7. Anxiety Disorders
### Panic Disorder
Panic disorder, historically known as neurocirculatory asthenia, anxiety neurosis, and a dozen other names, afflicts the one to 2 percent of the population that has recurrent, severe, debilitating panic attacks.

A panic attack (or paroxysm, in this book) is a sudden, self-limited, and generally unprovoked sense of fear accompanied by a variety of visceral symptoms, including palpitations, dyspnea, nausea, or parasthesia. Panic attacks can be severe enough to bring patients to the emergency room, convinced they are about to die. Particularly severe or frequent attacks can contribute to a patient's avoidance of any public outing (agoraphobia). Panic attacks are frequently found among individuals who have major depression and bipolar disorder (Kaufman and Charney 2000). The high rate of comorbidity of panic with mania and depression is not well understood, but may point to a common pathophysiologic cause in the common mechanisms of emotional regulation (MacKinnon and Zamoiski 2006).

*See* Appetite: visceral functions; Alarm: paroxysms

### Phobias
Phobic disorders are among the most common diagnosable mental disorders in community settings. They are characterized by intense feelings of fear in the presence, or at the prospect of being in the presence of, a specific situation or object. In addition to the fearful state that is experienced transiently, there is avoidance of the situation or object, and that avoidance leads to impairment in some sphere of life. The symptoms are similar across the different phobia types—a sense of alarm, catastrophic thoughts, sympathetic activation—but the different types differ somewhat in their objects, subjective experiences, and functional effects.

There are three main types: agoraphobia, social phobia, and specific phobias. The specific phobias concern objects—dogs or knives, for example—or environments such as tight spaces, heights, or bridges. In some cases, the phobia involves an object or location that is easily avoided, such as snakes or roller coasters, and so the degree of impairment is marginal, but when the object is something commonplace, then the avoidance of that object/environment can be relatively disabling. In social phobia there may be a variety of settings or activities that trigger the feeling of fear, but the common element is that the person is afraid of being scrutinized and embarrassed. The intense self-consciousness produces awkwardness when the person is among people, hence the fear becomes self-reinforcing, as the awkward behavioral response is more likely to place the person under embarrassing social scrutiny. Agoraphobia, literally the fear of the marketplace, may resemble social phobia in its effects; the agoraphobic person also fears and avoids public settings and groups of people. The difference is that the agoraphobic person fears not so much embarrassment, as a sense of being trapped in a crowd, away from safety. This is of course an irrational and empty fear, but it is worth keeping in mind that agoraphobia tends to go with panic disorder, and often is a residual aversive effect of having suffered panic attacks in public places.

*See* Alarm: dread; Bias: avoidance

### Acute and Post-Traumatic Stress Disorders

In the event of a traumatic experience—something threatening to life, limb, or property-there can be such a strong feeling of fear that, for a time afterward, it is normal to "flash back" to recall the intense emotional reactions to the incident whenever the person is reminded of it. The emotional intensity of these episodes of recall tends to fade over time. However, some people experience a failure to extinguish the conditioned fear response. This, essentially, is what occurs with traumatic stress disorders.

Robust evidence exists for a biological basis of this problem (Heim and Nemeroff 2009). Normally, cortisol secretion—the stress response—terminates the acute, norepinephrine-mediated fear response. Elevated brain cortisol levels have been associated with diminished hippocampal size. Diminished hippocampal size implies a lack of substrate for new learning. In the absence of such learning there is impaired capacity to experience the memories of a traumatic experience as anything other than horrific, and the terror upon being reminded of them merely reinforces the conditioned response to those reminders.

The observation that some aspect of fear conditioning and the psychological correlates of stress have normal, adaptive functions argues that the experience of a traumatic event alone does not sufficiently account for the risk to develop a traumatic stress disorder. Frequently, mood, anxiety, personality, and substance abuse disorders preceded the traumatic event. Moreover, when there are incentives against confronting and overcoming the conditioned fear response, such as a disability claim or lawsuit, the normal work of healing from a traumatic experience may be hindered (McHugh and Treisman 2007).

*See* Memory: flashbacks; Alarm: dread; Bias: avoidance

### Obsessive-Compulsive Disorder

Obsessive and compulsive symptoms are fairly common but significant impairment from them less so. Between one and 3 percent of individuals have persistent problems with obsessions and compulsions to the degree that they are highly distressed, or even suffer dysfunction as a result. Distress may come directly, as a result of disturbing intrusive images or impulses, or of dry, cracked skin as a result of excessive hand washing, or indirectly, as a cost of being late for or missing out on social engagements or work because of the need to spend excessive amounts of time conducting compulsive rituals. This also is the source of much of the impairment from obsessive-compulsive disorder. If someone must spend hours a day washing, counting, checking, and so on, it is hard to conduct a full and satisfying life.

There are varieties of presentation of obsessive-compulsive disorder (Mataix-Cols et al. 2005). Among the more prominent subtypes are obsessive fears of contamination and uncleanliness and by the time-consuming process of repeatedly and ritualistically cleaning whenever the feeling of contamination hits. Another subgroup (with a poorer prognosis than others) is characterized by disturbing intrusive thoughts and images of aggressive, sexual, and religious significance. A third subgroup includes people preoccupied with counting, ordering, symmetry, and repeating; perfectionism run wild. If a person in this group makes a small mistake, he or she may feel the need to undo the problem by repeating the entire process—a highly effort-intensive and time-wasting approach. Many individuals with obsessive-compulsive disorder suffer from inescapable urges to check and recheck things that might conceivably cause danger if left undone. For example, a person who has this affliction might check the lock on the front door or the burner on the stove, but having checked and found no danger, the experience of uncertainty that the task was accomplished fuels the urge to return to recheck, ad infinitum. Finally, some people engage in hoarding, feeling compelled to save almost any item that comes into the house, despite the accumulation of worthless items that impedes the functional (and at times safe) use of the household.

Obsessive-compulsive disorder tends to begin in childhood. Some cases have known biological causes, for example, traumatic brain injury and a poststreptococcal infection autoimmune response. The basal ganglia appear to be involved, consistent with the idea that the basal ganglia structures are involved in the regulation of simple motor programs.

*See* Action: obsessions/compulsions

### Generalized Anxiety Disorder

The diagnosis of generalized anxiety disorder describes individuals who are, as the name suggests, generally anxious. They tend to have chronic worry and chronic symptoms of high autonomic arousal: muscle tension, restlessness, distractibility, irritability, easy fatigability, and sleep disturbance. This tends to be a persistent, but not incapacitating disorder that causes sufficient distress to induce a person to seek treatment.

The diagnostic rules for generalized anxiety disorder establish it as a diagnosis of exclusion. If the symptoms occur in the context of a mood disorder, or active substance use disorder, or schizophrenia, or a developmental disorder, the diagnosis does not apply. If another psychiatric disorder is present and the content of the person's worries can be explained by that disorder, for example, worry about public events in a person who has social phobia, or worry about food in a person who has an eating disorder, then the diagnosis is not applied.

*See* Appetite: visceral functions; Alarm: dread

## A.8. Somatoform, Factitious, and Dissociative Disorders

Somatoform and factitious disorders are forms of maladaptive help-seeking behavior in which patients seek medical attention for complaints, diagnoses, or pathological signs that have no basis in physical disease.

### Somatization Disorder

The diagnosis of somatization disorder is made when a (usually depressed or anxious) patient complains of many physiologically unfounded or unexplained symptoms, over a period of years (Lipowski 1988). Patients who have this disorder tend also to have excessive medical treatment that results in high costs and greater risk of injury because of unnecessary surgical procedures and side effects and dependence on medications that do not treat pathological causes. They also tend to become disabled occupationally and socially by self-identification as a person afflicted with sickness, someone overdependent on help from others. Persistent somatization is a behavioral disorder in which the person seeks a reward from the emotional gratification of a medical visit. The behavior of presenting to physicians with physical complaints is established and sustained to the extent that the dependency on the attention of physicians becomes a form of maladaptive attachment (Stuart and Noyes 1999).

People who have somatization disorder can be hard to spot, as their symptoms, taken one at a time, are usually the symptoms of actual diseases, and the people seem distressed by them. Further complicating matters, medicine legitimizes a number of diagnoses for syndromes that often have no known pathological basis and that can therefore apply a diagnostic label to at least some of the symptoms that beset patients who have somatizing behavior, for example, chronic fatigue syndrome, fibromyalgia, systemic candidiasis, or environmental hypersensitivity.

Patients who have somatization disorder may be differentiated from patients who have legitimate, complex physical diseases by the improbably widespread nature of symptoms, across many bodily systems. The diagnosis is more likely the more systems are affected and the wider the variety of symptoms, including pain, gastrointestinal problems, sexual problems, and pseudoneurological symptoms, that is, symptoms suggestive of a neurological deficit, but without a known neurological basis. Conversion, or pseudoneurological, symptoms are among the defining expressions of somatization disorder.

*See* Appetite: visceral functions; Perception: pseudosensory symptoms, pseudohallucinations; Motion: pseudomotor symptoms; Help-seeking: psychosomatic complaints

### Other Psychosomatic Diagnoses

In general, patients who have somatization disorder are unaware of or have limited insight into the lack of physiologic validity to their symptoms. Their behavior differs from that of patients who fabricate signs and symptoms in order to gain some advantage from treatment, such as a prescription for opiates to fulfill a specific craving for narcotic intoxication. The distinction may seem subtle at times, as the patient who has somatization disorder may also seek opiates, but the motive is not a craving to be intoxicated; it is a craving to alleviate anxiety about a symptom.

To knowingly fabricate signs and symptoms in order to gain some material benefit is malingering. A small subgroup of psychosomatic patients feigns signs and symptoms of illness not for material gain, but in a conscious effort to be treated as patients. They seem to be motivated by an attraction to some aspect of the experience of being confined to bed, subjected to tests, tended to by nurses, and so on. These patients are said to have factitious disorder, popularly known as Munchausen syndrome, after the famous eighteenth-century adventurer and fabulist.

Hypochondriasis specifically applies to patients possessed of a strongly overvalued idea of having a serious disease, or many serious diseases. In contrast to somatization disorder, in which the focus is on symptoms and their relief, the hypochondriacal patient is preoccupied with the diagnosis itself. Hypochondriacal behavior is organized not so much around a specific reward for being ill, but around the overvalued idea that the cause of all kinds of stress and physical suffering can be attributed to a disease.

*See* Belief: overvalued ideas (hypochondriasis); Communication: misrepresentation (malingering and factitious disorder); Help-seeking: psychosomatic complaints

### Dissociative Disorders

A patient who has a dissociative fugue, amnesia, or identity disorder presents with a profound disturbance in the cognitive apprehension of reality. The patient may be unable to provide information about her or his identity or personal history, or she or he may appear at times to switch to an alternative identity, sometimes without insight about the multiplicity of identities. A hallmark of these symptoms is that they do not adhere to any established patterns of memory or cognitive processing. Like patients who have pseudoneurological symptoms, patients who have dissociative syndromes lack insight about the psychological factors that may have caused them intense distress. They are focused on the presenting symptoms.

The symptoms of dissociative disorders are cognitive in nature, but unrelated to cerebral pathology or to known functions of the brain (Jureidini 2004). Like pseudoneurological, or conversion, symptoms in somatization disorder, they may best be understood as a severe form of abnormal help-seeking behavior (Fahy 1988). Models of dissociative behavior are prevalent in popular culture, where a character who has "multiple personalities" presents a psychologically fascinating narrative device. A distressed person, convinced that such a thing not only is possible, but also explains a state of distress or conflict, may spontaneously present with these symptoms. However, when the symptoms are treated gently, as the behavioral expression of distress in a vulnerable and suggestible individual, the cognitive complaint is likely to resolve more quickly than if it becomes a focus of intense therapeutic fascination.

*See* Memory: pseudomemory/pseudoamnesia; Identity: dissolution

## A.9. Eating, Sexual, and Sleep Disorders
### Anorexia Nervosa

The diagnosis of anorexia nervosa is made on the basis of persistent behavior aimed at reducing the caloric intake below physiologic needs, and of the physical consequences of that behavior in terms of weight loss and altered physiology. Specifically, a patient who has a diagnosis of anorexia nervosa will practice self-starvation to the point of a reduction of body weight below 85 percent of the ideal. The prevalence is between one and 10 per 1000 girls and women (much rarer in boys and men). Patients who have anorexia nervosa tend to have a distorted sense of their body size and an overvalued idea of the importance of being thin. Anorexia nervosa is strongly associated with mood, anxiety, and personality disorders. These disorders all confer the vulnerability to the kind of behavior that places health at risk in pursuit of an ever-receding ideal of thinness. Psychological intervention is rarely helpful until the malnutrition can be resolved, and can be challenging even at that point.

*See* Habit: restricting/bingeing/purging; Belief: overvalued ideas

### Bulimia Nervosa

Bulimia nervosa is diagnosed when a patient habitually binges on food and compensates for the dreaded weight gain that might result by inducing vomiting or otherwise attempting to sweat, starve, or void the weight away. Bingeing and purging episodes tend to be driven by stress, often related to a mood or anxiety disorder. Frequent cycles of binge eating and purging are physiologically damaging, in that they cause fluctuations in blood chemistry and expose one to the risk of aspiration pneumonia. Moreover they are psychologically maladaptive as they take the form of an addictive behavior that is practiced to the exclusion of problem-solving behaviors that might alleviate a source of stress. Bulimia is also predominantly a disorder of women and at least two to three times more common than anorexia nervosa. Bulimic activities are often observed in patients who have anorexia nervosa. Bulimia tends to be a more stable and sustainable condition than anorexia. Non-anorexic bulimic patients tend to be older, to have a lower death rate, and to have a lower preoccupation with body image; however, they also tend to be more impulsive and so prone to other self-destructive behaviors.

*See* Habit: addiction, restricting/bingeing/purging

### Sexual Disorders

Diagnoses of disorders in sexual activity come in three varieties: dysfunctions, paraphilias, and gender identity disorders. Diagnoses are straightforward and descriptive, with the general criteria to be a specific disturbance of performance or desire, of significant severity that it is clinically problematic. Sexual dysfunctions include problems with low arousal or desire, inadequate orgasmic response, pain, and impairment in sexual function related to other medical conditions. Paraphilias are literally, para-(beside) plus philia (love), alternative forms of erotic expression and are not necessarily problematic. Paraphilic disorders, on the other hand, are diagnosed when the sexual behavior is either exploitative of people who are unable or unwilling to consent, as with *exhibitionism* (display to others), *frotteurism* (sexual pleasure by furtive erotic contact with unwitting strangers), *pedophilia* (sexual attraction and activity with children), and *voyeurism* (secretly observing others having sex), or when the paraphilic interest supplants other cooperative and mutually satisfying activity, hence interferes with relationships. This category includes *sadism* (desire to inflict pain or humiliation), *masochism* (desire to receive pain or humiliation), *transvestic fetishism* (cross-dressing for sexual pleasure), and *fetishism* in general (sexual fixation on an inanimate object like an undergarment, or on a specific body part, like feet). *Gender identity disorders* are diagnosed when a person persistently feels disturbed by the overwhelming feeling that her or his anatomic gender does not match her or his psychological gender—that is, a girl who identifies much more strongly with boys than with female peers, or a "man, trapped in a woman's body."

*See* Appetite: sex; Habit: sexual deviance; Identity: gender disorientation

### Sleep Disorders

The two major classes of sleep disorder in psychiatry are dyssomnias and parasomnias; neurologists also treat a variety of sleep disorders. Dyssomnias encompass the various inadequacies of sleep and of sleep regulation. *Insomnia* and its opposite, *hypersomnia*, are diagnosed as primarily sleep disorders if they occur outside the context of another disorder associated with sleep changes, such as a mood or anxiety disorder, or substance intoxication or withdrawal, or normal hormonally driven perturbations in sleep that accompany development, such as adolescent early morning hypersomnolence. *Narcolepsy* is a disorder characterized by frequent, sudden attacks of sleepiness throughout the course of waking hours; it turns out to probably be related to a genetically linked disruption in the hormonal control of arousal. *Breathing-related sleep disorder* would be diagnosed in someone who has sleep apnea syndrome, a common disorder in which the muscle relaxation that occurs in deepest sleep allows airways to close. The loss of air flow allows carbon dioxide to build and oxygen to fall, which alarms the nervous system sufficiently to override sleep in order to ventilate, hence the patient never truly falls into a deep, satisfying sleep. Such patients are often identified by their loud snoring, and by persistent daytime sleepiness. The parasomnias include problems with dreams (*nightmare disorder*), fear (*sleep terror disorder*), and behavior performed during sleep (*sleepwalking disorder*).

*See* Appetite: sleep

### A.10. Impulse-Control, Adjustment, and Personality Disorders

### Impulse-Control Disorders

This group of diagnoses is a grab-bag of behavioral disorders, all motivated by separate impulses. In practice, these troublesome behaviors occur most often in the context of other mental disorders, and are not assigned a primary diagnosis. *Intermittent explosive disorder* is a diagnosis applied to people who express violent or destructive behavior out of proportion to circumstances. *Kleptomania* is applied to individuals who steal, repeatedly, primarily for the stimulation of the experience rather than material gain. *Pyromania* is similarly driven by the anticipated pleasure of watching something burn. *Pathological gambling* is an addiction to gambling, characterized by patterns of craving, difficulty stopping, and escalation of behavior similar to those observed in substance dependence. *Trichotillomania*—habitual hair-pulling—stands apart from these other diagnoses in that the behavior is not driven by strong emotion, as intermittent explosive disorder, or by pleasure-seeking, as with kleptomania, pyromania, and pathological gambling; rather it more strongly resembles obsessive-compulsive disorder phenomenologically, epidemiologically and genetically, as well as Tourette syndrome (a disorder of repeated motor and vocal tics).

See Habit: addiction (pyromania, pathological gambling); Action: obsessions/compulsions (trichotillomania); Bias: impulsiveness (intermittent explosive disorder); Personality: labile personality (intermittent explosive disorder)

### Adjustment Disorders

A variety of *adjustment disorders* can be diagnosed, differentiated only by the form of expression: depressed, anxious, or mixed emotions, or disturbed conduct. These diagnoses may be applied when a person experiences significant and maladaptive distress or dysfunction in the aftermath of some stressful life event. They are not diagnosed when another major mental illness is present. This is conceptually a problem for the class of adjustment disorders, as having an episode of mental illness is itself an enormously stressful event, and people clearly struggle to adjust to the loss of psychological functioning. Adjustment disorders can best be understood as forms of demoralization or experiential difficulty.

See Motivation: demoralization; Alarm: guilt; Bias: inertia; Belief: doubt; Cooperation: shame; Affiliation: grief; Help-seeking: parasuicide

### Personality Disorders

These diagnoses, in general, are meant to describe enduring patterns of inappropriate emotional responsiveness and maladaptive behavior that contribute to the vulnerability to mental disorder, but are not acutely the focus of treatment. There are significant areas of overlap between personality disorders, and strong relationships between some personality disorder diagnoses and major mental illnesses, such as between schizotypal personality and schizophrenia (Battaglia and Togersen 1996), avoidant personality disorder and social phobia (Brandes and Bienvenu 2006), or borderline personality and bipolar disorder (MacKinnon and Pies 2006). Epidemiologic and genetic data support causal connections between some personality disorders and major mental illnesses. A personality disorder diagnosis is not, by definition, a reason to seek treatment—it is a way to characterize the individual traits and behavioral propensities that complicate the course of illness and response to treatment.

The personality disorders for which diagnostic criteria have been established fall into three clusters:

*Cluster A:* "Odd and eccentric." This cluster includes diagnoses that apply to individuals within the broad spectrum of schizophrenia. Individuals diagnosed with *paranoid* personality disorder are suspicious and grudge-bearing sorts of people, but their suspiciousness does not cross the line to the outright certainty that characterizes true delusions. *Schizoid* personality disorder applies to people who seem not to need people; rather they adhere to solitary activities, avoid intimacy and emotional expression, and show little interest in social pleasure or sexual relationships. *Schizotypal* personality disorder applies to people who tend to be cognitively disorganized and to exhibit social dysfunction as a result of highly idiosyncratic ideas, habits, and relationships, but who are not formally psychotic.

*See* Cooperation: asociality; Affiliation: eccentricity

*Cluster B:* "Erratic and dramatic." This cluster includes *antisocial* personality disorder: individuals who manifest persistent sociopathic traits from childhood into adulthood, including failure to maintain adult responsibilities, criminal activity, and a lack of conscientiousness or empathy about the consequences of their behavior for other people. *Borderline* personality disorder is a diagnosis applied to people who manifest persistent emotional and behavioral instability. These individuals tend to veer from crisis to crisis, from relationship to relationship, often acting recklessly and even self-destructively when driven by the perceived relationships with other people. In practice, this diagnosis tends to be used less precisely to denote that a patient is extremely difficult to manage. *Histrionic* personality disorder also is applied to people who have excessive emotionality, though in contrast to borderline personality, the behavior tends to be not so much self-destructive as aimed to draw attention from others. *Narcissistic* personality disorder applies to individuals who demonstrate a pervasive pattern of self-importance, or self-centeredness, along with a fragility of self-attitude such that a perceived criticism or rejection meets not with a constructive effort to improve, but with rage and despair.

*See* Habit: self-injurious behavior; Personality: histrionic, labile; Cooperation: sociopathy; Affiliation: egotism; Help-seeking: parasuicide

*Cluster C:* "Anxious and fearful." The diagnoses in this cluster all apply to individuals who tend to bias behavior toward fear-driven responses. *Dependent* personality disorder applies to people who manifest clinging, needy, and submissive behavior; the behavior is driven by an intense fear of losing the rewards of a relationship. *Avoidant* personality disorder describes people who tend to flee even minor social risks, hence develop a highly circumscribed life—the final product of an avoidant personality is often agoraphobia, seclusion to the home. *Obsessive-compulsive personality* disorder mainly applies to people whose bias toward rigidity and orderliness impedes their capacity to make decisions and partake of healthy relationships. Obsessive-compulsive traits, on the other hand, induce the sorts of detail-oriented, highly conscientious behavior found among many professionals.

*See* Bias: ambivalence, avoidance; Personality: anankastic; Affiliation: overdependency

# Appendix B

Demonstration complements description in any teaching endeavor, and more so in psychiatry, where the phenomena of interest cannot readily be photographed, diagrammed, or dissected. One has to encounter mental illness in actual patients if one is to flesh out the concepts conveyed in books and lectures. To truly know a thing, one must work with it to see how it performs; to truly know a person, it is best to engage the person in an active, goal-directed discussion or activity. You have, I hope, found the portrait of mental life and illness described in this book an enlightening way to think about these most human of biological functions and dysfunctions. I hope also that you will have ample opportunity to test this way of thinking with actual patients.

To derive something meaningful from interaction with patients, it is useful to approach the interaction with a method in hand. This provides a framework for guiding the conversation to productive areas, sorting out the many and various facts that emerge, and understanding their significance. Of equal importance, a method is needed to put a patient at ease so the patient will trust the interviewer with sensitive, intimate, often shameful and painful information.

This appendix is intended as a guide for the student in his or her first encounters with psychiatric patients and as a supplement to the book's discussion of mental life and psychopathology.

The overall question to be answered in the psychiatric assessment is: Why is the patient there? What is the patient's problem? The first clue may come from the circumstances of the encounter. Where, how, and with whom the patient shows up for treatment says much about the acuity and nature of the problem. From here, the aim of the interview is to help the patient tell the story. Some patients need little help with this, but often it will be necessary to encourage a timid patient to elaborate or an overly loquacious patient to rein it in. It will also likely be necessary at some point to steer the interview in the direction of a question-and-answer discussion to test hypotheses about the nature of the patient's problem. All the while, try to attend not just to the content of patient's words but to how they are delivered, along with the patient's appearance and actions in the interview, simultaneously.

The goal is to develop a diagnostic formulation for the patient. This is not the same as a formal DSM diagnosis; quite the contrary. One may or may not derive adequate information from a single interview to be able to assign a meaningful formal diagnosis.

But even with sketchy information one can provide a summary description of the patient's problem and dissect its components. Specifically, the formulation lays out what parts of the patient's problem arise from a disruption of normal cerebral processes, what parts are the direct result of the patient's behavior, what parts suggest enduring traits that cause trouble for the patient, and what the problem means for the patient (alternatively, how other meaningful events in the patient's life contribute to the problem). Table B.1 summarizes the stages of a psychiatric assessment.

## B.1. Psychiatric Problems

Patients see psychiatrists for one or a combination of three kinds of problem: dangerousness, dysfunction, and distress. Dangerousness encompasses suicide and nonlethal acts of self-destruction as well as violence and threatened harm against other people. Dysfunction refers to problems of performance, including cognitive impairment or confusion, erratic or unpredictable behavior, and failure to engage successfully in life roles. Distress comes in the form of pure suffering and also of chaotic emotional states that almost inevitably accompany chaotic lives. Assessment of the salience of each kind of problem for an individual patient, and of the specific nature of the problem, guides the rest of the interview.

For each variety of presenting problem, a brief description is provided and some illustrative scenarios. Suggestions about the interviewer's approach for each sort of problem are given later, under the heading "The Patient's Problem."

### Dangerousness

Danger is both extremely significant and overrated in its importance in the psychiatric setting. On the one hand, the risk posed by a truly dangerous patient trumps all other concerns, including the patient's autonomy; all states provide for the involuntary hospitalization of patients who present an unmanageable threat to public or personal safety (Large et al. 2008). On the other hand, dangerousness has become de facto a more important consideration than severity of illness in determining the intensity of treatment that will be offered to a patient (and paid for by insurers) (Simon 2006). This is not only a poor way to assess the need for treatment; it unjustly skews treatment resources toward patients who have poor impulse control and deprives care to patients who have equally or more severe symptoms but excellent impulse control.

Four common scenarios in which patients present a threat or risk of harm to self or others are suicidality, self-destructive acts, menacing behavior toward others, and uncontrollable violent urges.

#### THREAT OF SUICIDE

Suicidal patients have either survived a recent attempt—in which case they remain at risk until proven otherwise—or have expressed an intention to kill themselves or a strong desire for death in the abstract (Pompili et al. 2009). Some common scenarios follow.

- Police bring a homeless man to the emergency room after they find him darting in and out of traffic.
- A woman threatens to kill herself if her social worker does not get her admitted to a detox center.
- After a stroke, an elderly man awakens from stupor and says, "I might as well die."
- During an office visit, the wife of a patient pulls the doctor aside to whisper that she is terrified because her husband is depressed and has just bought a gun.
- The middle school nurse calls parents to inform them that their daughter has confessed to taking a handful of aspirin.
- In the intensive care unit, a man awakens after being resuscitated from a hanging attempt but insists it was an accident and demands to be allowed to go home.

## RISK OF VIOLENCE

Patients may pose a risk of physical injury to other people through intention or recklessness. Emergency department staff must frequently assess the risk of violent escalation in an agitated patient (Beck et al. 1991). When violence, especially of the latter kind, is an active threat, the interviewer is encouraged to take precautions for his or her own safety and the safety of others, as safety is a more urgent concern than gathering information.

- An intoxicated patient kicks and bites emergency transport personnel as they attempt to place the patient on a stretcher.
- A patient awakens after surgery, yanks out intravenous lines, and attempts to force his way past nurses to leave the ward.
- A patient in the waiting room has just punched a hole in the wall.
- A married patient asks for help with "anger management" to stop abusing his spouse.
- A patient admits to fantasies of killing co-workers and sending packages of poisonous material to strangers.
- Police bring in a homeless man after he abruptly stabs a total stranger in the leg on a bus.

## SELF-DESTRUCTIVE BEHAVIOR

Ruinous or self-destructive behavior is often brought to clinical attention by people other than the patient. There is an addictive quality to these behaviors; the immediate reward for the patient has come to outweigh the costs and risks. Patients who practice them may wish not to have to give them up. Thus, they may be of lesser concern to the patient than to the patient's family and so the patient's visit might be the result of a planned intervention (Copello et al. 2006).

*Table B.1.*  Stages of a Psychiatric Assessment

| Stage | Method | Goal |
|---|---|---|
| Pre-interview | ✔ Observe patient behavior<br>✔ Examine available clinical record<br>✔ Interview interested other parties | ✔ Assess the acuity/dangerousness of the situation<br>✔ Assess the possible ulterior motives of the patient<br>✔ Begin to think about the available options for intervention |
| Introductions | ✔ Establish a safe and quiet space for an interview<br>✔ Identify yourself and state your intentions<br>✔ Gather or confirm essential vital statistics (age, marital status, occupation, etc.) | ✔ Set a context for the interview for both patient and interviewer<br>✔ Put the patient at ease about the professional nature of the interview |
| Mental state (performed simultaneously with interview) | ✔ While speaking with the patient, be aware of specifics of:<br>○ patient's level of consciousness<br>○ appearance<br>○ behavior<br>○ form and content of speech<br>○ stated and apparent mood / emotional state<br>○ cognitive capacity<br>○ specific signs of disorder (e.g., tics, tremors, rituals, distractedness, restlessness) | ✔ Provide additional dimensions to the patient's story<br>✔ Gather clues to nature and acuity of the patient's problem |

| Stage | | |
|---|---|---|
| Initial assessment | ✓ Ask open-ended questions<br>✓ Ask vague patients for more detail and overly specific patients for more explanation<br>✓ Aim to know enough to say why the patient is present now and what the patient expects to happen | ✓ Assess the acuity/dangerousness of the patient<br>✓ Form hypotheses about the nature of the patient's problem: danger, distress, and/or dysfunction |
| Biographical background | ✓ Explicitly state that you intend to come back to the patient's problem after you have gathered some background information that will help you understand it<br>✓ Work methodically through a structured life story to cover high points of early life, education, occupation, relationships, social status, habits, and health | ✓ Communicates to the patient interest in the patient's entire life<br>✓ Provides essential information about the impact of the psychiatric problem on the patient's life<br>✓ May provide clues about the source or nature of the problem |
| Hypothesis testing | ✓ Ask focused questions to determine the type and probable cause of the problem<br>✓ Draw linkages between symptoms, deficits, or actions and adverse changes in life function<br>✓ Establish through queries that the problem is not due to another common cause | ✓ Gather sufficient information to be able to construct a case formulation<br>✓ Gain insight into the kind of treatment needed and the patient's likely acceptance of treatment |

- A young woman is brought to a clinic by family members who are concerned about the patient's wasted physique and refusal to eat.
- A patient who has frequent mood swings has been cutting her arms and legs at an escalating pace.
- A middle aged man, miraculously alive after another auto accident, refuses alcoholism counseling and demands discharge against medical advice.
- A married, upper-middle-class mother of three is arrested for shoplifting and confesses to her husband that she has been doing it off and on for years.
- A homosexual male continues to have unprotected sex, despite recently enduring an HIV scare when a former partner turned up positive.
- An intravenous drug addict, hospitalized for a blood-borne infection, goes missing for several hours and turns up later intoxicated and with a fever.

## Menacing Behavior

Menacing patients see clinicians because they have threatened or frightened other people. They tend to be either "mad" or "bad" (Kamphuis and Emmelkamp et al. 2000). The "mad" patients are delusional or cognitively impaired or gripped by abnormally intense drives; the "bad" patients, in contrast, are primarily uninhibited by ethical concerns for the suffering their actions bring to others. Either way, such patients are likely to arrive at treatment by force or under threat of punishment.

- A middle-aged man is court-ordered to undergo psychiatric assessment after he violates a restraining order to prevent him from stalking a local newscaster.
- An aging business executive is fearful of punishment after nearly being discovered sending anonymous emails to corporate superiors to try to sabotage a colleague.
- A female middle school teacher seeks help after she is fired from a job over accusations of flirtatious behavior with a male seventh grader.
- A reclusive, unemployed pharmacist admits to a plan to plant poison-tainted bottles of cold medicine in stores across the country as a way to alert the public to the danger of the hospital/insurance/pharmaceutical industry conspiracy.
- A worried mother brings in her mentally retarded adult son after he is arrested for exposing his genitals to schoolchildren.

## Dysfunction

Problems of dysfunction encompass a spectrum that ranges from involuntary impairment of mental faculties to willing avoidance of activities that produce distress. Normal functioning may be either impossible or merely difficult. A patient who has dementia, delirium, intoxication, brain injury, or psychosis clearly cannot practice sound judgment and operate normally. Such patients' deficits occur at the foundations of mental life: arousal, perception, cognition, memory, and executive planning. If the source of a functional problem occurs at a higher level, as a deficit in motivation, emotion, bias, belief, or social cooperation, the foundations remain intact but are not implemented adaptively. For these patients, it is difficult—perhaps unimaginably difficult—but not impossible to function.

## IMPAIRED PERFORMANCE

The functional problems of a patient who is impaired may hinder success or portend outright failure, but stop short of causing acute danger. They vary along a spectrum between inability and disability; the degree of functional loss is only partly correlated with the severity of the psychiatric disorder (Sanderson and Andrews 2002).

- After the death of his spouse, a widower is no longer seen at church and is later found home alone, half-starved and living in squalor.
- A 35-year-old lawyer seeks help to overcome shyness that has held her back from promotion in her firm.
- The aging parents of a 40-year-old woman who has never lived independently worry that she has progressed from merely having a prickly demeanor and odd behavior to being mute and withdrawn, occasionally adopting odd postures.
- A postoperative surgical patient is alert but refuses to converse with the treatment team on morning rounds.
- A middle-aged former high school principal who has chronic lower back pain seeks a prescription for narcotic analgesics and also wants a disability form filled out.
- A couple presents for marital counseling over conflict related to the wife's seeming inability to throw out useless objects; the husband complains he has to navigate a labyrinth of stacks of old newspapers to get from one room to another.
- A 22-year-old college dropout, unemployed and living in his parents' basement, is brought in by his parents, concerned that his "depression" has not been adequately treated; however he spends most evenings out with friends (smoking pot), is surly with his parents and sleeps all day at home.
- An adult patient diagnosed with autism and intellectual disability is admitted from his group home, as he has begun to argue with staff and to refuse to perform household chores.
- The parents of a second grader worry that their son has fallen into academic and conduct problems at school and wonder if he may have a learning disorder.

## ERRATIC ACTIONS

Erratic patients may be driven by forces similar to those of violent or self-destructive patients, but at a diminished level of intensity, so there is less risk the patient will commit violence. Delusional patients often act on their false beliefs, hence may act on motives unfathomable to others around them and thus will appear unpredictable, though their motives are fixed (Wessely et al. 1993). Although erratic patients often are at risk of being harmed, the risk is indirect, a result of placing themselves in harm's way rather than being the cause of harm.

- A 50-year-old grandmother is brought to the emergency department after reportedly wandering through her inner-city neighborhood, naked.
- A 75-year-old man who lives in a nursing home has barricaded himself in his room and can be heard shouting about a "communist invasion."
- A middle-aged woman politely asks for a referral to a surgeon to remove the transmitter implanted in her left ear.
- A young man is referred by his family doctor after asking for the name of a surgeon who would be willing to remove his perfectly functioning right leg.
- A formerly stable business entrepreneur and father of six has over the past year plunged his family into debt through bad investments, been indicted for check fraud, and moved in with a stripper.
- An oddly dressed man forces his way to the podium at a city council meeting and denounces the mayor as the murderer of Michael Jackson.

Confusion

Confusion is not intrinsically dangerous, but can be a signal of imminent danger. A confused patient is impaired by a lack of accurate information to guide adaptive behavior. Outwardly the confused patient, whatever the cause, seems lost. In some cases this occurs due to gross cognitive dysfunction, and in others the confusion is more a matter of the patient's delusional misinterpretation of information, than a global error in processing. Clinicians may separate the delirious from the delusional by clinical judgment or assessment tools (Wei et al. 2008).

- A hospitalized patient is unable to say why he is in the hospital, or what hospital he is in, or perhaps even that he is in a hospital.
- A worried husband reports that his wife has become lost while driving several times in the past month.
- A patient who has chronic mental illness tends to stare into space for hours on end and seems befuddled by normal activities or human interaction.
- A downcast-appearing woman mutters that she is ready for the medical staff to put her to death for her sins.
- A middle-aged man expresses concern that his aging father has twice been found in the middle of the night, wandering many blocks from home, and wonders if he needs to be admitted to a nursing home.
- A patient walks into an emergency room with the chief complaint, "I have lost my memory. I don't know who I am or where I live."

**Distress**

Distress compels an individual patient to call for help. A patient who presents in mental distress resembles the patient who seeks help for almost any other painful or worrisome medical symptom. As a rule, any patient who seeks help independently, whether in the emergency room, in consultation, or in ongoing psychotherapy, is motivated by a desire to relieve or avoid some form of distress, if only by reaching the comfort of a safe therapeutic island in a sea of troubles. However, distress can be an elusive target. In many cases it seems attached to some life circumstance or event, and in others it seems to float free. The circumstances associated with distress may change from visit to visit. For example, a recovering alcoholic patient may be distressed about the pervasive anxiety that arose soon after quitting alcohol. A few months later, this may give way to feelings of lonely despondency in the absence of old drinking buddies.

### SUFFERING

Adverse experiences of many kinds cause pain to most people, but not always suffering. On top of pain, suffering adds anguish, an active state of anxious arousal that tends to make the problem seem far more urgent. Emotional distress drives treatment seeking in both medical and psychiatric settings (Follette and Cummings 1967). Patients transform feelings of anguish into problematic behaviors of all kinds and may fall into danger or dysfunction; those who manage to steer clear of such behaviors may nevertheless seek help for their suffering.

- A patient has just come into the emergency department for the third time in a month with abrupt onset of pounding heart, shortness of breath, lightheadedness, chest tightness, dizziness, and an intense fear of dying. All laboratory studies are normal.
- A fellow physician confesses that, despite the fact that he shows up at work and maintains a marriage, he sobs uncontrollably after his wife has gone to sleep and prays that he might die in his sleep.
- A patient who has previously been treated for aching joints, irritable bowel, and headaches now presents with lower back pain.
- An unemployed 30-year-old woman admits that she constantly hears voices that demean her appearance, intelligence, personality, and hygiene.
- A young, married accountant complains that he has not had a good night's sleep or felt content since he got drunk with friends and went to a strip club during a business trip six months ago.
- A visibly distraught, middle-aged woman in the emergency department asks the nurse for a tranquilizer after being informed that her son has just died of his gunshot wounds.
- A patient describes with horror the things she has done to obtain money for crack cocaine and pleads for help to find drug addiction treatment.

### CHAOTIC FEELINGS

Some people suffer helplessly in silence, others wax and wane chaotically and behave in maladaptive ways when there is a shift for the worse. Their intense emotional reactions tend to destabilize their relationships and alienate people who might otherwise be supportive. Thus, emotional distress induces provocative behavior, which causes interpersonal conflict. Conflict, in turn, yields more distress, and so a self-perpetuating cycle of chaos ensues. The difference between a patient who has chaotic feelings and one who behaves erratically or self-destructively is largely a matter of degree and sometimes a matter of time.

- A 30-year-old graduate student goes from catastrophe to catastrophe on almost a weekly basis; a month ago she fought with her mentor, two weeks ago she crashed her car, last week she argued with her sister, this week she learned her boyfriend is sleeping around.
- A middle-aged homeless man is brought into the emergency department on a snowy night, intoxicated and screaming threats, but is calm and eager to depart the next morning.
- A young woman who has sickle-cell anemia and a disrupted home life has presented to the emergency department at least twice a week for months, in a sickle-cell "crisis," requesting narcotics.
- A new patient complains of anxiety and stress on the job and goes on to describe a 20-year history of bad marriages and short-term employment. In all cases, the spouse or the co-workers were blamed as the source of the problem.

Now that the reader has some idea what to look for, it is time to discuss how to gather the information to decide which problem the patient has, what caused it, how serious is it, how has it affected the patient, and what can be done about it.

## B.2. Clinical Context
### Setting

The irony of a psychiatric encounter is that the person in the best position to describe the problem—the patient—is sometimes impaired in the very faculties needed to recall, identify, describe, and make sense of the problem. Therefore, it is particularly important to know something about the patient before the encounter. Before a word is said, the interviewer always knows one essential thing about a patient: the setting of the encounter. Patients arrive at different settings for different reasons. The most common clinical settings for a psychiatric encounter are the emergency department, the psychiatric unit, an office, or an institution like a general hospital, nursing home, or prison.

- Emergency department: Patients almost always arrive at the emergency department in crisis. Often the patient is brought to the emergency department by other parties concerned for the patient's safety and well-being, or that of others. The emphasis in an emergency assessment is disposition: is the patient to go home, stay in the hospital, or be placed in another appropriate setting? Assessment of behavior and immediate context, of mental status, and prediction of risk are more important than diagnosis in this setting.

- Psychiatry unit: Patients are admitted to psychiatric units, in general, because of a crisis that is not easily resolved or problems that cannot effectively be managed in an outpatient setting. At the time of admission, the principal aim of assessment is to establish a treatment plan, based on the salient factors that prompted the admission. On subsequent inpatient days, the aim is to assess the progress of treatment and readiness for discharge to home or to a subacute (supervised, but not secured) facility.
- Outpatient office: During an initial office visit, the aim is to gather information and to formulate at least a preliminary idea about the nature of the patient's problem so that a plan of treatment can be discussed and initiated. It is important to use the initial visit to provide the patient with an overall blueprint for treatment, including the justification, if it is necessary, for the patient to return for a follow-up visit. In subsequent visits the aim is not only to clarify the problem in depth, but also to assess treatment progress in terms both of symptom resolution and enhanced functioning.
- Institution: Psychiatrists are frequently consulted in institutional settings, such as medical units, prisons, and nursing homes, to evaluate the causes and management of psychiatric symptoms in patients sequestered for reasons of medical care or safekeeping. These consultations are rarely initiated by the patient, so the aim is generally to provide an expert opinion on the nature and causes of a patient's psychiatric problems and to recommend a course of action.

Of course, in any setting another aim may be to intervene to modify the situation, and treatment may include medication, education, advice, behavioral measures, or psychotherapy.

### Outside Information

It is usually a good idea to read any documents that may have accompanied the patient to the treatment setting, such as a legal order to compel assessment or an emergency department note, as well as past records when available. You should also speak with any parties who have accompanied the patient, upon first meeting the patient or even before that. Information from third parties may suggest the proper approach to the patient, and practically, if you don't catch them before they go home, you might miss your chance.

Before you start a face-to-face assessment, you should take a quick glance at the patient's appearance, demeanor, and behavior. A disheveled, agitated patient who shouts threats and bangs on walls is probably not going to tolerate a prolonged cross-examination over facts of the history. Conversely, a sobbing, morose patient may require gentle, persistent probing to bring out the story. The incongruity of a calm patient, well-groomed and overdressed for the setting, or a patient who smilingly reports intense pain or suicidal urges, or a provocatively dressed, flirtatious patient should warn you to be cautious about the facts of the story, as the patient may have a hidden aim to disarm your best judgment. An obviously intoxicated patient needs more time to sober up; forgo the full assessment until the drugs or alcohol wear off.

With this preliminary information, you may already have some idea about the severity and nature of the problem and about what approach to take in the assessment. Now the task becomes to gather information to see if your initial impression of the problem is accurate and complete and to learn what is needed to initiate treatment. In general, an assessment has three phases. Note that these are not necessarily done in this sequence and that no method works for every patient in every setting, but it may be helpful to have a structure to organize the assessment.

### General Approach to the Patient

Keeping the setting in mind, the next most significant bit of information may or may not come directly from the patient: the reason for the encounter. This can be broken down into two parts. First is the question of agency: who wants the patient to see a psychiatrist? Patients may walk in, be forced in by police, or be led in by relatives or friends. Second, what kind of problem does the patient have? There are three principal problems, as discussed in the previous section: dangerousness, distress, and dysfunction.

The linkage between agency and the presenting problem can be straightforward. Logically, a patient forced to treatment is dangerous until proven otherwise; someone must have believed the patient to be dangerous in order to legally compel or be motivated to coerce the patient in for an assessment. A successful encounter will contain or negate the danger. A patient who walks into treatment is probably motivated by distress; whatever the problem turns out to be, a successful encounter will leave the patient less distressed. A patient led to treatment by others is likely to have some form of disordered function, by process of elimination—if the patient were dangerous, he or she would probably not have been easily led, and if the patient were in great distress, he or she would have needed little prompting to seek help. A successful encounter will set up a viable plan of action.

If your job is to assess the patient, the general procedure is as follows:

1. Encourage the patient to narrate, in the patient's own words and with emphasis on the facts the patient finds most relevant, the story of how the patient came to psychiatric attention. Why did the patient come in today, and not yesterday or last month; or why not wait longer to seek help? What was it about the problem or the context of the problem that made it necessary to be seen today? If the visit was planned in advance, what motivated the appointment? If someone else initiated the visit, why does the patient think the psychiatrist has been called? In the latter case, the instigator of the visit must be queried as well.

2. Gather context about the patient's background, educational, occupational, and relationship history and functioning, and health. Also ask about other factors that might complicate the illness or its treatment, such as addictive

behaviors, signs of temperamental vulnerability, and other symptoms of mental illness not already discussed.

3. Probe the patient to test the hypothesis that the initial impression of the problem is accurate and, if not, whether another problem is more salient. Thus, if a patient complains of anxiety (distress) and it turns out the patient has been too frightened of leaving home to be able to work (dysfunction), then the latter may be the most important problem to resolve. If you then discover that the patient has been harboring suicidal thoughts, the focus may shift again to dangerousness as the major problem.

All the while as you gather information you perform another, parallel assessment of the patient's mental state as you observe the patient's appearance, attitude, behavior, speech patterns, emotional responsiveness, knowledge, and cognitive performance. These are the raw materials of the mental status exam, which validates the historical information, much as a medical history and physical examination record complementary information in the assessment of general medical problems.

### B.3. The Patient's Story

Every patient has a story but many cannot or will not tell it without some help. Beyond whatever distress-related angst or raw agitation is attached to the psychiatric encounter, patients often are in a highly self-conscious state when confronted with the symbolic authority of a clinician, even a trainee. The first task is to convey to the patient that his or her story is of professional interest and that any sensitive information revealed will be heard without moral prejudice and will be kept private. You may state this explicitly and may demonstrate it by seeing the patient privately, behind closed doors, maintaining a sober demeanor and minimizing outside interruptions, and practicing active listening. In active listening, the examiner frequently repeats back to the patient elements of the patient's story. This can alleviate the patient's worry that you have failed to understand the patient's perspective or, worse, have secretly formed a harsh judgment about the patient.

A few patients will provide an articulate and focused narrative account of their problems, but most of the time your job is to keep the patient talking and at the same time ensure the narrative does not veer off into unproductive areas. An inexperienced trainee may fail to realize when an interview either has failed to produce a coherent narrative or has begun to go astray. To be confident that you have adequately addressed the patient's primary problem, you can stop and think whether the story the patient has told satisfies the five W's of journalism.

- Who is the person seeking help—the patient or someone else?
- What is the complaint? Also, what is the problem, if the two are not identical.
- Where (or, more generally, in what setting) does the problem occur?
- When did the problem begin, when did the patient decide to seek help, and what motivated help-seeking?

- Why does the patient (or other interested party) believe the problem has occurred?

If these questions have not been adequately addressed, then you may need to return to them, prompting or interrupting the patient's narrative (politely, of course) if necessary. The issue to keep in mind throughout this phase of the assessment is the timing. What made the patient come in today, not yesterday, not next week, not last year? When you have a sound and plausible answer to that question, you have achieved at least the minimum amount of narrative necessary to make an informed hypothesis as to the nature of the patient's problem.

When histories go off track, they tend to deviate either toward the "what/where" aspects of the situation, with a focus on play-by-play chronology unenlightened by other context, or toward the "why" aspect, which attempts to explain (or explain away) rather than describe the problem. A patient who veers toward a "what/where" kind of story may need to be prompted to explain *why* events seem to the patient to have occurred, as the patient's own perspective is likely to bring out clinically relevant details that a simple fact-based chronology would overlook. Why, for example, did the patient cut herself, why did this other patient give away his money? Conversely, patients who focus on explanation ("why" questions) may need to be probed frequently to tell *what* happened ("What were the events that led up to the fight?" "Before you tell me more about why you went back to using cocaine, I wonder if you could tell me more about what you were doing that day before you had your relapse?"). Patients tend to accept these forms of redirection to help them to tell their stories. Clients and users, who have agendas beyond help-seeking, are more likely than patients to become irritated when the examiner redirects the conversation.

Other forms of active listening that encourage patients to provide a richly layered and detailed account of their problems should also be employed liberally. As a rule, whenever a patient says something that stands out as disturbing, provocative, evocative, revealing, or simply surprising, it is a good idea to ask the patient to say more about it. This can be done through a direct, general request, such as "Tell me more about that," or can be encouraged by repeating back to the patient the statement in need of elaboration, such as "So, a moment ago you were saying you carved your boyfriend's initials in your thigh . . ." It is encouraging to the patient when a follow-up question is preceded by a restatement of something said earlier: "You mentioned that you were hearing voices yesterday. Can you tell me more about that?" When the interviewer is unsure whether to move on or to wait for the patient to provide more information on a topic, there is nothing wrong with waiting in silence, expectantly, to see what the patient may think to add without prompting. Thirty seconds of silence feels like a long time—long enough to recall many overlooked thoughts; try it sometime. Sometimes this yields highly useful information that would never have emerged in the give-and-take of a fully structured interview.

As the problem takes shape, it is time to move from a general, journalistic interview about the patient's path to the assessment, to questions tailored to elicit essential details about that kind of problem. Lists of these are provided with the descriptions of each of the nine major kinds of problem described in a previous section.

## B.4. The Patient's Problem

So far in the assessment you have taken note of the treatment setting, the manner of the patient's arrival, documentation and other informants, if available, and the patient's demeanor. You got the basic story from someone, if not the patient directly—the essential who, what, when, where, and why that explain the patient's presence today, and not some other past or future time. From these sources, you should have a basic idea whether the patient is dangerous, distressed, or dysfunctional.

### Risk Assessment

The more careful and conscientious among the readers may find that it never feels comfortable to declare that a patient is not at risk for danger, because, after all, people can be surprising. On the other hand, it is neither practical nor legal to keep patients under protective custody without cause.

Rather than attempt the hopeless task of proving a negative assessment of danger, you can make a positive assessment by examining the patient for the common varieties of dangerousness: threat of suicide or violence, self-destructive acts, and social menace. But first, one caveat about dangerousness in general. It is particularly important to keep the question of agency at the forefront when dangerous patients are brought in, rather than arrive on their own. The patient brought by others out of concern for danger is apt to deny or minimize the risk of dangerous behavior, to claim it was a misunderstanding, that he is the victim of lying and persecution, or that she did not mean what she said or no longer has an intent to do harm. Keeping in mind that the patient was not the one who sought help, and in fact may be motivated to conceal harmful intentions in order to be released to carry it out, you should always weigh carefully the observations and concerns of the other interested parties.

Another caveat: many patients who have attempted or threaten suicide or violence are intoxicated at the time. Although the impetus to dangerous acts may fade when the patient sobers up, the risk of a dangerous act in the future hinges somewhat on the generally high likelihood that the patient will once again become intoxicated.

#### THREAT OF SUICIDE

To assess the threat of suicide when a patient has not taken action, you must aim to establish the seriousness of intent. Does the patient think of actively taking his or her life, or rather does the patient have an indifferent feeling about living (a passive death wish)? How persistent are the suicidal thoughts? Do they take the form of specific ideas about methods? Are those methods available to the patient? Has the patient taken steps to make them available (such as buying a gun or stockpiling old medications)? What is the patient's attitude about the thoughts—are they resisted and regarded as horrifying and alien, or are they embraced as a solution to an emotional problem or even romanticized? Is the threat of suicide linked to thoughts of vengeance against others? What has kept the patient from acting on suicidal impulses so far?

After a failed attempt, the threat is assessed partially in retrospect, on the principle that a line crossed once is likely to be crossed again. To assess the seriousness of the intention to die in the failed attempt, have the patient narrate the act, from its planning to the arrival at the psychiatric encounter. Had the patient researched the method (for example, to learn what would be a lethal dose of a particular drug)? What kept the patient from acting on it sooner, and what made it an opportune time to act when the patient did? Were any precautions taken to prevent or delay discovery? How exactly was the patient discovered and brought for assessment? Finally, to assess the likelihood of a recurrence, you will want to know about the intensity and quality of suicidal thinking now, as described in the previous paragraph.

### Risk of Violent Behavior

Containment of violent agitation is an advanced clinical skill; the trainee is cautioned to await the patient's sedation and seclusion before attempting a close interview. When the patient has calmed, it may be possible to probe a little into the patient's mental state and propensity for violent action. Are there any specific violent intentions? Does the patient acknowledge a need for help? Is there a past history of violence? Can the patient recognize a trigger for violence and negate or avoid it? Is there anyone in the patient's life with reason to fear the patient who, legally, may need to be notified under the Tarasoff rule? That is, based on the legal finding in the case of *Tarasoff v. the California Board of Regents* in 1976, a clinician has a duty to warn the police and/or the identified victim of violence threatened by a patient, or else confine the patient; safety overrides confidentiality in these circumstances. If the patient is to be released, does the patient have access to a weapon at home? If the patient was intoxicated, what are the prospects for intervention to prevent a recurrence?

In a calmer patient who has made violent threats, the aim is to learn whether the patient wants to harm someone or wants help to resist the impulse. It may also help to know whether the patient has taken any steps, such as obtaining a weapon, and it is particularly important to know whether there is anyone in the patient's life who can vouch for the patient when the patient changes his or her story and denies intending to harm anyone. Just knowing that the patient has others willing to support the patient is a fair indicator that the patient has at least enough self-restraint to be able to sustain close relationships.

### Ruinous (Self-Destructive or Addictive) Behavior

The assessment is focused on learning as much as possible about the behavior: what is it, how does the patient perform it, what triggers it, how does the patient feel before, during, and after, and what consequences has the patient experienced as a result? When did the patient begin to do it, and how often is the patient doing it now? Has the patient tried to stop; what was the patient's experience during that time? Was there craving? What events preceded the relapse? If the patient has come in for another problem or is brought in by family, the hidden agenda of the assessment is to discover and nurture whatever motivation the patient might have to stop.

As you gather information about the behavior, you can also examine the patient for signs of specific mental dysfunctions that produce the pain or fear the behavior is aimed to alleviate. Dejection, irascibility, dread, shame, relationship, personality, or temperamental problems that produce frequent interpersonal conflicts, and demoralization are common motivations. The anhedonic inability to experience pleasure by normal means can motivate the patient to take extraordinary and destructive means to feel relief. It helps engage the patient more effectively in the therapeutic endeavor if the patient can expect relief to come from another source, in return for the surrender of the addiction.

## SOCIAL MENACE

Whether a menacing patient is "mad" or "bad"—impaired cognitively, motivationally, or ethically—one primary aim of the assessment is to determine what leverage there may be to help manage the threat. The degree of potential dangerousness may be assessed via interview. Does the patient comprehend the threat he or she poses to others? Has the patient tried to resist; does the patient even wish to resist? How does the patient feel when prevented from acting on these drives? Are there situations or experiences that ignite the drive or that can deter it? What has provoked or compelled the assessment? What could happen if the behavior is not stopped?

If the patient is not driven by delusions and is not obviously asocial or clinically eccentric or intellectually limited, then some gentle probing into the details of the patient's appetites is warranted (it may be warranted for other patients too, just harder to get). For a sexually menacing patient, this means learning what you can about the patient's patterns of sexual activity, including frequency of orgasm, pornographic interests, and history of prior sexual abuse, consensual activity, and inappropriate activity.

### Degrees of Decline

To comprehend the nature and severity of functional impairment, you need to know mainly what the patient could do before the onset of the problem, what the patient is capable of doing now, and the milestones along the path from baseline to the present, including the pace of decline, the steady or jerky course of decline, new symptoms, and new life circumstances.

## IMPAIRED PERFORMANCE

In addition to the standard questions for any dysfunctional patient about the nature and course of the functional decline, it is particularly important with the underperforming, undermotivated patient to obtain a detailed account of the facts of daily living. From the time the patient wakes up in the morning—or afternoon—what is the structure of the patient's day? When, if ever, does the patient dress and bathe? What is a typical breakfast, and what does the patient do next? These questions should cover a typical day up to when and how the patient typically sleeps.

In addition, the basic material facts of life should be probed. Who buys groceries, cooks, and cleans? Is the patient expected to pay rent or do chores? Does the patient have access to a car or Internet or cell phone, and who pays for that? When and why does the patient get out? The aims of this detailed line of questioning are twofold. First, it provides a rich source of data to establish the nature and severity of the patient's impairment. Second, it may reveal therapeutic opportunities to motivate a higher level of functioning. For example, parents of an underachieving college dropout might take the position that if the child is too "depressed" to contribute to the household work and welfare, then the child is too depressed to drive the family car to meet friends at a bar.

### Erratic Actions

The major question to be addressed in the assessment is how aggressively to intercede to keep the patient out of harm's way, while attacking the source of the problem. Motivation, and what arouses it, is the key question. Is the motivation diffuse and unfocused and aroused by intoxication or delirium? Or is it pleasure- and excitement-directed, uninhibited by normal constraints by mania? Or is the erratic behavior fixed and focused on a paranoid theme, aroused by the fear of (nonexistent) threats? In the latter case, the tasks of assessment are to gauge the power of the idea that drives the patient, to determine if it is delusional beyond reason or remains open for debate, and, perhaps most important, whether other people in the person's life are aware of and disturbed enough by the person's idea to help to reinforce the need for treatment.

### Confusion

The key question is what capacities are disrupted, and how badly they are disrupted? From there, you can work out the cause of the disruption and predict what problems are likely to occur for this patient in the near future. An organized approach to the assessment begins with the hypothesis that the patient may primarily be confused by delirium. If the patient is agitated or sleepy, or unexpectedly becomes agitated or sleepy, delirium is the most important cause of confusion to address. If consciousness is clear, then performance on a variety of cognitive measures can suggest whether dementia is a likely cause. A quick screening evaluation of cognitive performance can be done in the office (see the later description of the Mini-Mental State Examination). A low score suggests dementia as the cause of confusion. Inattentive confusion can also occur with severe states of malaise and excitement, and bewildered confusion is often observed in frankly psychotic patients who have an idiosyncratic view of things.

### Acuity of Pain

It is not difficult to see that a patient is distressed; the challenge is to find out if the patient is also either dangerous or dysfunctional. If the patient is also dangerous, then safety must come first. If the patient has a significant dysfunction, then it may be necessary to focus on the source of dysfunction in order to relieve the distress.

When the focus is primarily on distress, the task of the assessment is to understand what it feels like to have that patient's experience of distress. The distress can be approached from two different directions. The direct approach is systematic. Every distressing symptom can be described from a finite set of qualities. It may help to have a mnemonic device in mind: an easily memorized word or phrase that cues recall of a list of items. For the delineation of a symptom, "OLD CARTS" is a useful mnemonic anywhere in medicine.

ONSET: When and how did the symptom or distress start?

LOCATION: Where does it hurt? More specific to psychiatry, what mental faculty is affected—emotion, cognition, or behavior?

DURATION: How persistent is the symptom or distress?

CHARACTER: What kind of pain or distress is it? In psychiatry, is the distress angst, or sadness, or rage, or something else?

AGGRAVATING FACTORS: What makes the symptom or distress worse?

RELIEVING FACTORS: What makes it better?

TREATMENT: What has been tried so far? What were the effects?

SEVERITY: How bad is it? How does it compare now to when it was at its worst?

From this short list, you often will learn enough about the distress to be able to identify its nature.

The other approach is empathic. A patient in distress may find it more amenable to describe its quality in poetic images. "My depression is like a black cloud" or "I feel like I could explode!" or "It's as if I was encased in a thick plastic bubble." This is the case not only in psychiatry but in all of medicine—any time a patient talks of shortness of breath "like an elephant sitting on my chest" or stabbing pain "like someone jabbed a knitting needle in my forehead" it is the same phenomenon. Unless you have literally been caught in a black cloud, a plastic bubble, or an explosion (or been sat on by an elephant or impaled by a knitting needle), there is no rational way to know what these expressions mean. But, of course, most of us know exactly what these expressions mean. They add color to the description of symptoms and distress that may be lacking from the systematic approach.

The systematic and empathic approaches are complementary. Their effective use together will allow the examiner to have a comprehensive and nuanced understanding of the patient's experience. The systematic approach is initiated by the clinician. The empathic approach emerges spontaneously and can be encouraged as appropriate when you ask the patient to elaborate on the image and also when the image is paraphrased and repeated back to the patient to ensure that the message has been grasped accurately. One may ask: "So do you mean you feel a black cloud hovers over you and blocks out the sun, or do you mean you feel you are immersed in a thick, lightless fog?" or "Is the fuse already lit, or are you afraid one more jolt will trigger the explosion?" or "If you feel yourself in a bubble, then it must seem the world is far away from you, not real."

One occasional pitfall in the assessment of distress is when the patient uses the specialized jargon of psychiatry to describe symptoms. Many of these terms are in common usage and mean something quite different from one person to another. A "depressed" person may be merely sad or stuck in hopeless misery; a person "obsessed" could be addicted, preoccupied, or truly experiencing the symptom of intrusive thoughts. The use of these terms is a red flag to stop and say to the patient, "People may mean different things when they use that word. What does it mean to you?"

The end result of these queries and efforts at clarification is a rich picture of what the patient is going through. This becomes a source of data when you begin to reason through the possible sources of and solutions to the patient's problems. Thus, the patient may not have said outright, "I have a low self-attitude," but you learned about it when the patient said, "My family would be better off if I was no longer a burden to them." Only someone who has a low self-attitude could say such a thing.

### Suffering
Having elicited the patient's account of the quality and supposed reasons for the suffering, the aim of the assessment of a patient whose problem primarily is that he or she is in emotional torment is to identify what the patient dreads losing.

### Chaotic Feelings
As with the assessment of suffering, in the course of a one-time assessment of a patient who has problems related to a chaotic life it can be futile to try to find a definitive cause of the problem, though the patient may wish to focus on little else. Often the emotional cores of chaos and suffering are the same: pain of loss or threatened loss, and fear of more pain and loss. The critical difference between suffering and chaos is that intense, painful, chaotic emotions will evaporate in a few hours.

## B.5. The Patient's Biography
Ideally, the patient has been able to provide a full and rich story that explains exactly what problem motivated the psychiatric assessment, and the sequence of events that led to it. But there is still at best insufficient information to come up with a meaningful formulation of the salient factors that caused and sustain the problem, or complicate it, and thus a limited potential to select and evaluate good treatment. Or if the patient's best effort to lay out the problem and the story leave fundamental questions unanswered, then the clinician must take an organized approach to fill in the gaps. Information about the patient's background, hypothesis-testing cross-examination to probe elements of the story and background, and an examination of the patient's mental status are all essential.

With increasing clinical experience, you may come to realize that the sharpest tools are in your head. These tools are the sets of questions to ask patients. You should develop queries that are efficient, sound natural, and effectively start an informative conversation about a topic. In time and with much practice, it will become natural to phrase questions suited to a specific context, to aim for precisely the information needed to fully answer a question, and to have reasonable expectations about what kind of answer the patient will give.

It may be useful to have a list of all the qualities of life experience one might need to know; for example, "What age did you start school? What age did you graduate? Did you skip any grades? Were you held back? What school did you go to? What kinds of grades did you get in school?" and so on. But once you have a general idea which qualities are salient, it is time to toss out the fill-in-the-blank approach and instead to open with a general question "How was school for you?" from which you may then move to the relevant particulars. But first, in training, it may be helpful to run through the list in order to know what kinds of things might be important to ask about school, or in a review of systems, or about other components of a history. The development of a comprehensive checklist of questions is an important exercise that can be left to clinical skills instructors. Here is a moderately advanced approach.

### Background

To gather context, conduct a tour through the major facets of life: origins, roles, habits, and clinical history.

- *Origin* topics include family history, the circumstances and environment in childhood, education, and any childhood problems experienced by the individual (social, medical, behavioral, or developmental).
- *Role* topics include primarily occupational and marital history.
- Questions about *habits* gather primarily information about the use of alcohol and drugs.
- *Clinical background* includes medical and past psychiatric history (origin of symptoms, prior treatments, and when the patient last felt well). If possible, include in the psychiatric history a description of the patient's temperament, attitudes, and typical behaviors when the patient has been free of illness, that is, "premorbid personality."

It is best to gear questions of background to the individual patient. A college-age patient may have little important information to offer about occupations ("Oh, I worked part-time at the college library last summer") or marriage, but much of clinical importance to say about educational aspirations and limitations and about sexual explorations with individual boyfriends and girlfriends. For a middle-aged, disabled, separated person who has chronic mental illness, details about college major and early dating will be of far less importance than information about employment history, the onset and nature of disability, and the quality of and problems in the marital relationship.

Some skill with memory is helpful as well. When it comes time to run through the questions about context, it is good to remember the incidental facts the patient introduced while spinning the clinical narrative. Thus, if the patient has already mentioned conflicts with her children, you don't want to ask her, "Do you have any children?" Instead, ask "Can you tell me more about your children?"

The major areas to explore for historical context, and some key introductory questions to explore, are as follows.

## Origins

The goal in queries about family and childhood history is primarily to discover genetic or developmental factors that explain a patient's risk for mental illness, illustrate its impact during formative years, and document the state of function, if possible, before the onset of the problem at hand.

### Family History

- Are your parents living? If not, when did they pass away and how? If so, where do they live? What is their health status?
- Tell me about your mother/father. What kind of person is/was she/he?
- Do parents depend on you for care or provide support and care to you?
- Are they together? If not, when and why did they separate?
- What did/does your father/mother do for a living?
- Do you have brothers or sisters? Where are they in life?
- Is there any sign of mental illness in family members? Suicide? Are any diagnoses known? Can you describe their symptoms or problems?

### Childhood

- Were there any problems with your birth (pregnancy complications, prematurity), childhood health (hospital stays, long or frequent school absences), or development (did you walk and talk on time)?
- What was it like for you growing up? Was the household peaceful or chaotic? Bitter or warm?
- Where were you born and raised?
- Did your parents both raise you? If not, who did, and why?
- Did your family move? Why? How did you adjust?
- How was school for you?
- What sort of grades did you make? Did you have to study?
- What did you do in school besides study?
- (If college-educated) Where did you go to college, and why did you choose that school?

## Roles

The roles a patient has performed in jobs and relationships is a document either of the patient's prior capabilities, or of longstanding problems that disrupt the fulfillment of roles, or of the progress or loss of function that has occurred. Secondarily, knowledge of the patient's present roles provides a template for recovery, that is, specific functional issues to be addressed in treatment.

*Occupation*

- What do you do for a living?
- What other kinds of jobs have you had?
- What responsibilities do you have?
- Have you had good performance reviews / advanced over time?
- (If disabled or unemployed) When did you last work? How are you supporting yourself?
- (If disabled, unemployed, or retired) How are you spending your time?
- (If many jobs were held) What was the job you did the longest? Why did you change jobs (fired, quit, moved, became ill)? What was the best job?
- Have you been in the military? What assignments did you have? Did you see combat? What was your highest rank? Circumstances of discharge?
- Have you been in prison? How long? How many times? What were you convicted of? What are the circumstances around your release? Any pending legal issues or court dates?

*Relationships*

- Have you ever been married? How long? More than once? If so, how many and what happened with prior marriages?
- How did you meet your spouse?
- How do you get along? Any separations or counseling?
- How has your illness affected your relationship?
- Do you have children? How are they doing? Where are they now?
- (If unmarried) Any serious relationships? What was the longest?
- Have you been sexually active? When did you start?
- Are you exclusively interested sexually in men/women?
- Do you have any sexual problems?
- Do you live alone or with other people? Describe your home.
- Are you religiously inclined?

## HABITS

The goal here is to delineate the contribution of habitual drug or alcohol use, or of other maladaptive habits like gambling and eating disorders, to the patient's past and ongoing problems. If time is limited, an oft-used brief screen for alcoholism may be used, such as the CAGE questions ("Have you often felt you should Cut back on your drinking? "Have people often Annoyed you by criticizing your drinking habits?" "Have you often felt Guilty about your drinking?" "Have you often felt the need for an Eye-opener [a drink first thing in the morning] to steady your nerves or treat a hangover?").

- Do you drink alcohol? Why?
- When did you start? (If drinking stopped or diminished) What made you stop / cut back?

- How much? (If the answer is "socially," ask the patient to define "social")
- Have you had problems with alcohol?
- (If alcohol use seems to be or to have been heavy) Have you had blackouts where you can't recall what you did when drunk? Have you ever had shakes the morning after? Have you had serious withdrawal: DTs (delirium tremens) or seizures?
- Have you ever wished you could stop drinking but been unable to do it?
- How much, if any, do you smoke? For how long?
- Have you used other drugs?
- Have you injected drugs?
- (If any drugs) What did you use? How did you use it (smoked, sniffed, huffed, shot, ate, drank)? Where did you get it? How did you afford it? What problems did it cause with school, work, relationships, health, or the law?
- What effect did the alcohol/drugs have on your mood?
- Have you been in treatment for an alcohol or drug problem? Been in any 12-step programs (like Alcoholics or Narcotics Anonymous)?

## CLINICAL HISTORY

Regarding physical health, it is of particular interest to know whether the patient has health problems that require treatment with drugs that may have psychiatric side effects, like prednisone. It is important to know about health in general; is the patient otherwise hale and hearty, or a sickly person? What are the active issues, active symptoms, and current medications? Regarding psychiatric background, the aim is to trace the trajectory of the patient's present problem, to determine whether the problem is new and stereotypical, or something strange and unexpected. If the former, how was it managed before?

### General Medical Background

- Have you had any health problems? What were they? How serious (in terms of aggressiveness of treatment or impact on life functions)?
- Do you take any medications now?
- Are you having any physical symptoms now?
- When did you last have a check-up?
- Do you have any drug allergies?
- (Women only) When did you reach menarche? Have you been pregnant? How many times? How many live births / miscarriages / therapeutic abortions? Are your periods regular? Do you have mood or other symptoms with your periods? Have you had signs of menopause or reached menopause?

### Psychiatric Background

- When did you first notice problems (like the primary problem)?
- When did you first have psychiatric treatment? What first brought you to treatment?

- (If the diagnosis is known) When did you receive the diagnosis, and why did the doctors think you had that diagnosis?
- How many hospitalizations have you had? What was the longest? Most recent?
- Have you had any suicide attempts in the past? What were the circumstances?
- What other treatments have you had for psychiatric problems in the past?
- Have you had success with past treatments?
- Have any past treatments been intolerable, or made things worse?
- Have there been any psychiatric problems unrelated to the present primary problem?

## B.6. The Patient's State of Mind

The initial mental status examination occurs at the outset of a psychiatric assessment, as a rapid triage of a patient's problem, and the risk of danger at that moment. If a patient appears dangerous, to other staff members if not obviously to the junior clinician, then safety precautions are indicated, such as seeing the patient in an open room or with a colleague and giving the patient ample "space."

Beyond the initial assessment for dangerousness, you will continue to conduct a mental status examination for the duration of the assessment. Beginners would do well to keep the mental status items in mind as part of their hidden agenda in the assessment process, and run through them from time to time as the patient speaks. To do so may require the development of what is probably a new and unnatural skill. The new skill is to attend not only to the content of what a patient is saying but also pay attention to how the patient says it. At first, it may be helpful to "tune out" briefly at times once you have heard the gist of the patient's narrative and take a "mental snapshot" to come back to later when it is time to reconstruct the patient's mental state.

The how of communication, or its form, is often more important than content to identify the nature and severity of a patient's problem. For example, if a person said, "Bad people are planning to attack us! We are all in danger!" assessment of this statement would differ vastly depending on the appearance, behavior, and manner of speaking of the person who said it. These words, grumbled by a grubby person on a street corner, convey different meaning there than if the exact same words were spoken to a roomful of reporters by a well-scrubbed secretary of state.

The aim of the mental status examination is to complement the history. Having gathered the content, look to the objective facts of the patient's presentation to provide the final validation or to shed doubt on the adequacy of the patient's story. In addition, there are certain symptoms, events, experiences, and intentions that are important to touch on if they have not already been a focus of the history. They may be placed under the heading of the mental status examination because they are of such high importance that the narrative and the examination should always be compared.

## The Mental Status Examination

The major items in the mental status examination are, by convention, appearance, behavior, speech, mood and risk assessment, other mental phenomena, and the cognitive exam.

### APPEARANCE/BEHAVIOR/SPEECH

Appearance includes body habitus (youthful or aged, heavyset, thin, mesomorphic, etc.), grooming (neat or unkempt, clean or malodorous), dress (casual, soiled, formal, mismatched, provocative), expressiveness (blunted, constricted, full-range, labile, animated). Avoid the word *normal* here and in other parts of the mental status examination. The idea is to communicate to someone not present in the room at the time of the examination some idea how the patient actually presented; what the patient looked like, how he or she acted and spoke. *Normal* conveys no useful information about that.

Behavior includes attitude (cooperative, guarded, sarcastic, hostile, flirtatious, overly familiar), posture (upright, slouched, standing), movements (fidgety, motionless, pacing, gesticulating), unusual activities (tics, rituals, tremors), eye contact (fixed, avoidant, downcast).

Speech includes rate (slow, rapid, delayed, retarded), tone (sarcastic, hostile, flirtatious, overly familiar, soft, loud, shrill), fluency (mute, monosyllabic, telegraphic), spontaneity (unresponsive versus latent versus responsive versus pressured), logic and associations (verbigeration, word salad, loose associations, flight of ideas, tangentiality, circumstantiality, intact).

Logic and associations in speech can be tricky to detect and describe. By habit, listeners tend automatically to make sense of patterns. To read a verbatim, unedited transcript of actual conversation is to understand that in normal talk we continuously and seamlessly filter out leaps in logic, sentence fragments, nonverbal grunts, repetitions, and so on in order to make sense of it. It takes special attention to ask whether the speech makes formal sense.

A major clue that the patient has a disruption in the form of speech is the experience, while listening attentively, of feeling lost or confused. A feeling of being repeatedly perplexed and wondering "Does this answer my question?" suggests that the problem is not a lapse in attention, but the patient's disordered thinking and speech. When this occurs, pay particular note to the connection between the patient's words and sentences, and be alert for discontinuities.

Speech disturbance can be described along a spectrum. Ranging from closest to farthest from cogent and logical, this includes:

- circumstantiality (aka overinclusiveness), or speech that deviates from the main topic but ultimately returns
- tangentiality, or speech that wanders in a logically traceable way from the main topic to some unrelated topic
- loosening of associations / flight of ideas, in which the connection of one sentence to the next is tenuous at best

- word salad, in which grammatical connections between words is lost
- verbigeration, in which non-words or neologisms are introduced into speech

Any time you assess a patient's speech as thought-disordered in one of these ways, it is highly useful to jot down an exact quotation of a few sentences, to note for the benefit of others the nature and severity of the disordered speech.

### MOOD AND RISK ASSESSMENT

Mood is the next element and consists of an assortment of elements.

- Stated mood is the qualitative self-assessment of a patient's persistent and pervasive emotional state. Happy, upbeat, excited, elated, down, blue, sad, worried, angry, irritable, are moods. "Fine" or "okay" may describe a normal mood, or may be used to deflect the question: probe further.
- Rated mood is a quantitative assessment (often used in hospital settings, and in patient's serial self-ratings) that allows changes in mood to be tracked over time; a useful and simple rating system would be a 1–10 scale, where 1 is deeply morose, 10 is highly elated, and 5 is perfectly okay.
- Apparent mood, also sometimes known as the "affect," is how bright or sad or irritable or nervous the person appears to be, as well as how widely these presentations of emotional state vary across the course of an evaluation (flat or constricted versus labile versus reactive). You should also take note when the apparent mood seems incongruent with the subject matter, for example, if the patient laughs while describing a tragic event.
- Self-attitude is the person's sense of self-value, and particularly important in mood disorders; implicitly notable when patients report feeling "worthless" or like a "burden on my family" or when a manic patient spontaneously reports being the "smartest one in the room." The patient can be asked explicitly as well ("What are your thoughts about your value as a person? How is your confidence?").
- Vital sense is implicit in the patient's statements about the patient's capacity for action; a low vital sense is reflected in statements of hopelessness and resignation; an elevated vital sense describes someone who feels "hyper" and ready for anything. Questions about "energy" also serve as a proxy for vital sense.

Because suicidal behavior is closely linked with depression and low mood, a focused examination of the patient's propensity for suicide is routinely included in the mental status examination. To screen for suicidal thinking can be as simple as asking: "Have things gotten so bad that you've thought you don't want to live?" It is unlikely to the extreme that posing this question to anyone would put the intention in mind if it is not already there, so there is essentially no risk, and the benefit is that you may uncover dangerousness where it was unsuspected. On the other hand, some tact is called for: if you hear a patient's sad story and your next question is: "Have you considered killing yourself?" it might suggest that *you* think the patient *ought* to be thinking about it. A better way to frame it would be to say, "Some people who have had experiences like yours have had thoughts of suicide. Has that been the case for you?"

Suicidality can be classified as active or passive.

- Passive suicidality refers to the thought that life is not worth living, or that the person thinks he or she would be better off dead, and may range from a fleeting, vague feeling of wishing not to have to wake up in the morning, to a tormenting wish to be killed in a violent accident or crime.
- Active suicidality crosses over from merely wishing for death, to the contemplation of action to bring it about. Qualities of active suicidality include intensity, frequency, and vividness.
- Active suicidality occurs over a wide range. Many patients have no real desire to do themselves in, but have fleeting images of suicidal acts, which are resisted. Other patients, who are particularly worrisome, have not only done the research to discover what acts are likely to prove lethal (for example, what drugs are likely to be deadly in overdose, and how much one would need to take), but have also worked out how they would arrange not to be discovered in the act.

It is important to be as specific as possible about the active or passive nature of suicidality, and its frequency, intensity, and vividness, as this information can be critical in the decision to take measures to ensure the patient's safety.

Other Mental Phenomena

The topic heading of "other mental phenomena" includes other symptoms that may or may not have been a part of the history or presenting problem. Because these are clinically significant symptoms if validated, it is noteworthy when they are part of both the history and the mental status examination, so routinely covered in both places.

*Hallucinations:* "Have you had the experience of hearing voices when no one is around? Seeing visions others could not see?" These are unlikely to come up positive unless stated in the history; however, active hallucinations can be validated if the patient appears to be responding to sights, sounds, and other unshared sensations.

*Delusions:* It is a challenge to construct a graceful query about delusions in general, as by definition a delusion occurs without insight; a patient who agrees in full that she or he is delusional probably does not have a true delusion. Delusions are generally detected when the patient's explanations include factors that are unlikely or incredible to the observer, but accepted wholeheartedly by the patient and defended on cross-examination. If delusions are suspected, it is worthwhile to ask about a variety of specific delusions. The following covers many of them.

- "Have you experienced persecution?" or "Have you felt you were the focus of an investigation?" (persecutory, or paranoid)

- "Have you felt that you have caused some great calamity, or that you should be punished for a crime or sin?" (depressive)
- "Have you felt that you had superior talents, plans, ideas, or abilities compared to other people?" (grandiose)
- "Have you ever been convinced that someone you have never met was in love with you?" (erotomanic)
- "Have you been convinced that your body was going through changes that doctors could not detect?" (somatic)
- "Have you been convinced that your spouse or significant other was unfaithful, without evidence to prove it?" (jealousy)
- "Have you had the experience where messages you read or saw on television were meant only for you to see or hear?" (reference)

*Anxiety Symptoms:* Anxiety symptoms are extremely common. Some are indicative of pathology and add immensely to suffering when present, yet may have been over-looked if they were not part of the main presenting complaint. Positive responses to these questions do not establish a firm diagnosis, but are suggestive of one.

- Panic attacks: "Have you had sudden feelings of panic, along with physical symptoms, when there was nothing to fear?"
- Compulsions: "Do you have irresistible, irrational impulses, such as to wash your hands repeatedly, or count things, or check things?"
- Obsessions: "Do you experience intrusive, annoying or disturbing thoughts, worries, or urges that you can't seem to get out of your head?"

*Insight:* Insight is accurate knowledge of one's own mental state, and recognition of its abnormality. In terms of the mental status examination, it can mean several things. In a psychotic patient, insight refers to the patient's capacity to see the hallu-cinations or delusional ideas as false; one might ask a patient whether she or he has considered that the psychotic symptoms might be the result of "your mind playing tricks on you." A patient without insight will deny this vehemently.

In non-psychotic patients, insight principally reflects the level of agreement be-tween the patient and clinician about the nature and severity of the patient's problems. This knowledge may be implicit in the conversation between patient and clinician throughout the evaluation, or it may be gauged explicitly by a direct question such as "What do you think is wrong?" A patient who lacks insight may have no idea, or a fanciful idea, or an argumentative idea about the reason for the encounter. It is useful to record a lack of insight in the mental status examination, as it indicates an obstacle that must be overcome in order to ensure agreement and adherence to treatment.

*Judgment:* Judgment may also be established implicitly, in the clinician's assess-ment of the accuracy of a patient's predictions about the consequences of his or her actions, as revealed in the history. Otherwise, it can be examined formally by asking how the patient would handle a theoretical situation. Standard queries include "what would you do if you were in a crowded theater and saw smoke?" (calmly get up and inform the manager) and "what would you do if you found a stamped, addressed, sealed envelope on the sidewalk?" (pick it up and mail it).

### The Cognitive Exam

The cognitive exam encompasses intellectual capacity and knowledge base as well as a screen for impairment in attention, memory, abstract processing, and language. Intellectual capacity is often estimated based on the sophistication of vocabulary used and comprehended by the patient. If one has to frequently explain terms that a literate layperson should know, you may conjecture that the patient has a limited intellectual capacity, or at least a limited education.

Similarly, intellectual limitation is suggested by a patient's "concrete" understanding of abstract concepts. This can be assessed quickly and formally by asking the patient to interpret proverbs like "people who live in glass houses shouldn't throw stones" and "a stitch in time saves nine" or comparisons like "how are a chair and a table the same?" and "how are a dwarf and a child different?" The concrete answers would be on the order of "because you might break the glass," "because one is less than nine," "they both have legs" (not all chairs or tables have legs), and "they're both small" (missing the valence of the comparison).

The patient's knowledge base can be assessed implicitly based on the degree to which the patient and clinician share common cultural points of reference, if appropriate, and specifically by asking about points of common knowledge, such as "Name the nation's vice president " or "What happened on September 11, 2001?"

Before asking about cognitive capacities, it is helpful to the patient to frame it with a statement like "I'm going to ask you a few more questions to check how your brain is working." The Mini-Mental State Examination (Folstein et al. 1975), a brief and effective screening tool follows.

- Orientation to time: "What is today's date (month, day, year)? day of the week? season?" (5 points)
- Orientation to place: "What is our location: state, city, street, building, floor?" (5 points)
- Registration: "Repeat these three items and try to remember them because I will ask you again later." Name three objects, preferably unrelated to one another, for example, "nickel, pony, cactus." (3 points)
- Calculation: "I want you to count backward from 100 by 7's." If uncertain, suggest "start by taking 7 away from 100, then 7 from that, and so on." If the patient is unable to calculate, ask the patient to spell the word world, and then ask for it to be spelled backward. (5 points)
- Recall: "Can you remember those three items I asked you to remember a minute ago?" (3 points)
- Language output: Hold up a pen and ask, "Can you tell me what this is?" Do the same with a watch. (2 points)
- Language repetition: "Repeat after me: 'No ifs, ands, or buts.'" (1 point)

- Language comprehension: Write the words "Close your eyes" on a piece of paper. Say "I want you to do what this says" and hold up the page. Don't forget to tell the patient to open his or her eyes after. (1 point)
- Spatial comprehension / graphic output: Draw a set of interlocking pentagons on a page. Ask the patient to copy the picture on the page. (1 point)
- Language graphic output: While the patient still has the page, say "write any complete sentence that comes to mind." (1 point)
- Praxis: Ask the patient to perform a three-step command, such as "I want you to take this piece of paper in your right hand, fold it in half (with both hands), and place it on the table with your left hand." (3 points)

The points may total up to 30. A healthy and well-educated adult person middle-aged or younger should have no trouble scoring a near-perfect 29. The average "normal" score declines with advancing age and is lower with lower education. An unimpaired, well-educated 80-year-old might be expected to score a 27; a cognitively intact 80-year-old who has an eighth-grade education, 25 (Crum et al. 1993).

## B.7. Hypothesis Testing

Having established whether the patient is primarily in need of protection from danger, assistance with dysfunction, or relief from distress, the task turns to determining the causes of the danger, dysfunction, and distress. There are two levels to consider: which mental phenomena contribute to the psychiatric problem, and whether these phenomena constitute disease states, trait vulnerabilities, maladaptive behaviors, or adverse experiences.

When the patient has reported phenomena strongly linked to a particular problem the task is to confirm one's impression by asking about other phenomena likely to be associated with it. Then, whether you have formed a strong impression or not, make a systematic run through the common problems of each kind by either reviewing the notes and observations or inquiring of the patient.

After the reviewing these questions, you will be prepared to summarize the case in a diagnostic formulation.

### Disease Syndromes

If the patient has any of the following, then the patient has a diagnosable disease syndrome, rooted in pathological brain functioning.

*Delirium* (including severe intoxication): Does the patient have an altered level of consciousness (is the patient agitated, disoriented, obtunded)? If not, the patient is unlikely to have delirium or to be clinically intoxicated.

*Dementia*: Does the patient have normal cognitive performance, that is, can the patient state where and when the encounter is taking place? Can the patient repeat and recall several items? Can the patient perform mental arithmetic? Can the patient follow commands, name objects, write a sentence, copy a figure? If the patient can do all of these, the patient probably does not have dementia.

*Mild alcohol/drug intoxication/withdrawal*: Has the patient been taking alcohol or drugs on a regular basis, and has the patient recently ceased or cut back on using them? If not, then mild drug intoxication/withdrawal is probably not the explanation for the patient's problem. A patient who is severely intoxicated or in active withdrawal is likely to fit the definition of delirium.

*Depression/mania*: Is the patient's mood in its usual state versus depressed, elevated, or irritable? Is the patient getting the same enjoyment from normal activities as usual? Is there a change in energy, sleep, or appetite? If there is no change in mood, enjoyment, arousal, or appetite, then there probably is not a mood disorder.

*Schizophrenia*: Does the patient have hallucinations or delusions (in the absence of any of the above)? Have they persisted for a long time (at least six months)? Has the patient lost significant capacity for interpersonal, social, educational, or occupational function? If not, then the diagnosis of schizophrenia is doubtful. If the problem is limited to a psychotic symptom (such as a hallucination, delusion, or inexplicable behavior), or has newly emerged, then one would not call it schizophrenia (yet), though it is still most likely a result of a similar pathological problem.

*Autism* (or other pervasive developmental disorder): Does the patient demonstrate a persistent insensitivity to the emotional content of communication? Is there an indifference to or fearful avoidance of physical and interpersonal intimacy with other people? Is this a lifelong problem? If not, then there does not appear to be any sign of autism or autism spectrum disorders.

*Obsessive-compulsive disorder*: Does the patient spend significant amounts of time performing senseless, repeated activity like handwashing, checking doors, counting, or organizing objects; or does the patient complain of disturbing and distracting intrusive thoughts, urges, or worries? If not, the patient probably does not have obsessive-compulsive disorder.

*Panic attacks*: Does the patient experience sudden attacks of intense fear or anxiety accompanied by at least several physical symptoms consistent with sympathetic arousal, like shortness of breath, heart palpitations, shaking, feelings of unreality, feelings of doom, lightheadedness, and so on? Do they ever occur when the patient is not under stress? If the patient never has attacks like this, the patient does not have panic attacks.

Patients often have symptoms from a variety of categories on the list. As a rule, take a hierarchical approach. The disorders near the top take precedence, but any other phenomena suggestive of another syndrome may also be mentioned in the formulation.

### Trait Vulnerabilities

Because these constitute the potential for trouble rather than the trouble itself, the interviewer aims to establish whether the present problem, of whatever sort, is one incident in a larger pattern of problems in the patient's life. A patient who becomes discouraged or takes to drink during major life changes all through life is likely to have problems when she or he moves, divorces, or retires from working. A patient who cuts his or her arm or threatens to kill someone when faced with a romantic breakup is probably more emotionally unstable than the average person. Both the vulnerability and the recent stress or challenge that produced the psychiatric problem should be elicited and confirmed.

One of the clues that a patient who has a psychiatric disease may also have a psychological vulnerability as a contributing factor is that the degree of functional impairment is much greater than the severity of the disease symptoms would indicate. Similarly, if a patient's emotional reaction or behavioral change seems disproportionate to events, it is a clue that the patient is at the extreme end of a distribution for one or more of the temperamental traits.

As it is unlikely you will have access to definitive data on the patient's traits—an IQ test for the trait of intelligence, and a personality inventory for the trait of temperament—trait vulnerability is inferred. There is no substitute for long life experience to conclude with confidence that a person's lifelong problem is, say, inertia versus ambivalence, but a few key questions from the history may offer support for the hypothesis that traits play an important role in the problem.

*Intelligence*: Was the patient placed in special education settings in school? Were grades repeated due to academic underperformance? Has the crisis connected to the problem occurred at a time of increased intellectual demand?

*Temperament*: The best informants about enduring traits of emotional volatility and valence are usually significant others. If no one is available, the patient's self-assessment is at least a start, but will likely need to be confirmed by others. If an informant is available, what to ask? One fairly efficient gauge of temperament involves a series of questions about various characteristics across which people differ. Geared toward the patient's personality before the onset of the acute problem, it provides an overall sense of who the patient is normally. Often, after you have spent time getting to know a patient, you can assess the patient along these axes without running through the list.

A set of trait qualities we teach to trainees at Johns Hopkins follows. You can ask the informant: Do you consider the patient to be more . . .

- optimistic or pessimistic?
- suspicious or trusting?
- even-tempered or moody?
- worrier or carefree?
- controlled or demonstrative?
- dependent or independent?
- cautious or impulsive?
- stingy or generous?
- a leader or a follower?
- solitary or sociable?
- patient or impatient?
- strict or easy-going?
- confident or self-doubting?

- unreliable or reliable?
- easily hurt or thick-skinned?
- neat or messy?
- self-conscious or unconcerned about what others think?

Assessment of trait vulnerability may help explain the reason for the emergence of the patient's problem now, and may help predict the likely response to treatment, whatever the major source of the problem. Another benefit of determining where a patient is in the distribution of intelligence or temperament is to predict likely adherence to treatment and anticipate problems that are likely to emerge.

### Maladaptive Behavior

Start with the assumption that behavior always plays a role in the patient's presentation. If the patient has serious problems of any kind, and is seeking help, then help-seeking is the patient's primary motivated behavior that prompted treatment. You understand the story if you grasp what it took to motivate the patient to come to treatment, and what the patient hopes to gain from it. When the patient has pursued treatment for a legitimate problem (as opposed to a psychosomatic complaint), then treatment-seeking behavior is adaptive.

What of maladaptive behaviors? It would be remarkable for a patient to feel sufficiently motivated for treatment if the patient's disease, trait vulnerability, or adverse experience did not induce some maladaptive behavior. As for patients who are brought to treatment only through the efforts of others, it would be similarly unusual for this to occur unless the patient had behaved in some way that was disturbing or threatening to others. Either way, if the patient can articulate a reason for his or her actions, the interviewer will gain important clues to the other mental disturbances that motivated it.

The common, nonaddictive behaviors that motivate help-seeking include withdrawal from social, occupational, and familial responsibilities; waste of resources and unnecessary risk-taking; disturbing or embarrassing public behavior; manipulative maneuvers in relationships; conflict-seeking behavior; presuicidal behavior; assaultive actions; and many others. In the case formulation, it is important to note these, as they contribute to the assessment of the acuity of the problem.

Maladaptive addictive behaviors often explain directly why the patient is in trouble at this time, or they may be the end result of the trouble. Active addictions, as noted elsewhere in this book, contribute to treatment failure for a number of reasons.

One can gain a clearer sense of whether a maladaptive behavior is reactive, as in an emergent suicidal urge or intermittent drinking binges, or addictive, as in chronic suicidal threats or alcohol dependence, by inquiry about the frequency and circumstances of the behavior, and whether the patient has failed in efforts to stop.

### Adverse Experience

A psychiatric interviewer often cannot help but encounter adverse experience in a patient's problem, as patients tend automatically to see their problems through a lens of personal experience. Indeed, a patient may need to be persuaded that disease, vulnerability, or problematic behavior is the most significant problem, and not life events, as the patient insists. Take as merely a hypothesis the adverse experience the patient may blame for all problems. Loss, conflict, worry, or injury pervade most lives at some point, but do not necessarily explain the immediate problem. On the other hand, a problem of psychiatric disease, trait vulnerability, or maladaptive behavior is likely to adversely affect the patient's view of his or her prospects for happiness in life.

For example, if the patient explains a suicidal threat as the natural outcome of a lover's quarrel, there may be some narrative logic to the explanation, until you realize that this would probably be a rather extreme response for yourself, or almost anyone you know to be a reasonable person. To explain the suicidal threat, you must invoke temperamental vulnerability or a pathological emotional state or a manipulative motivation, to make sense of the patient's motive. As a rule, the more the patient's experience resonates with your own personal experiences, the more likely it is that life, not illness, is the source of the problem—unless, of course, your own life is in disarray or you have been sheltered from experience.

You can approach the issue of adverse experience with a question: how does the patient's personal perspective on the problem contribute to the problem? It is safe to assume the perspective is part of the problem, until proven otherwise. If a patient has never seen a psychiatrist previously, assume the patient is apprehensive and possibly ashamed to be in the role of "mental patient." If a patient has been compelled by family to address erratic behavior, assume the patient is embarrassed, possibly angry, and desperate to minimize the problem in order to protect the one activity that reliably relieves distress. If a patient is overcome with the belief that a squad of killers is intent on assassinating him, assume he is as frightened as anyone would be who believed such a thing for good reason, and keep in mind that the patient may not be so sure of your good intentions.

You may conjecture freely about the patient's personal perspective to help the patient in the short term. For example, you can reassure a patient that it is natural to feel anxious when speaking with a psychiatrist. In all but the most routine visits, the patient's perspective is an essential factor in a successful and helpful encounter.

### B.8. Two Case Scenarios

The following two examples illustrate how the story and the clinically essential information can be gathered in two different scenarios. In the subsequent section, these cases will serve as examples for the development of a clinical formulation (that is, the process of distilling a case into its elements).

#### The Case of Marco M

*The Story*: Marco and Gladys M walk into clinic one morning without an appointment in search of your colleague, Dr. Q, because of an urgent new problem: Marco's bizarre nocturnal behavior. Dr. Q is out of the office today so you agree to see Mr. M. According to the electronic record, Mr. M is a 55-year-old banker who has previously come in for an occasional sinus headache, dyspepsia, and insomnia, nothing serious. Dr. Q has prescribed only a sedative (a benzodiazepine), which Mr. M refills irregularly.

You introduce yourself and ask about the problem. Gladys tells the story while Marco looks on. In the early morning hours last night, Gladys awoke to a crashing noise in another part of the house to find her husband out of bed. She then heard him talking loudly so she called out to him, but he did not answer her. She crept out of the bedroom to find a kitchen drawer and its contents scattered across the floor and the outside door open. By the time she found him, Marco was attempting to crawl under the car, in his pajamas. When she was able to get his attention, he demanded that she help him find his keys. She asked him where he was going, and he said he was late for work and kept palpating the driveway for the keys. Frightened, Gladys coaxed him into the house on the pretense that his keys were somewhere inside.

When Marco saw the mess on the kitchen floor, he forgot about the keys and became alarmed about home intruders. Gladys eventually reassured him and coaxed him to rest on the couch. Marco soon conked out. She shook him, but was unable to revive him to get him back to bed. She spent the rest of the night sitting by him in the living room.

Today Marco recalls none of the events of last night, but he shares his wife's concern about what happened. You notice that she seems haggard, while he is freshly groomed and wearing a suit. He feels fine now and plans to go to work after the clinic visit. She dreads another night like last night. And they both wonder what happened—did he have a seizure? A mini-stroke? Does he need a brain scan?

*The Problem*: Now you have the basic elements of the story: what happened, to whom it happened, when and where it happened, and why the patient came in today. What is the problem? The first concern is danger. Mr. M seems in no danger now, but was he in danger last night or is he likely to be in danger from his problem in the near future?

One negative clue about dangerousness—not definitive, but certainly suggestive—can be derived from the setting of the encounter. You are seeing them in a clinic, not in an emergency department. Had Ms. M been seriously concerned about his (or her) own safety, it is likely she would not have waited; she would have called an ambulance last night. And when Mr. M awoke in good spirits and fully rational in the morning, the level of acute concern further diminished. You might decide that he should have come in emergently, once you get the whole story, but for now any possible danger seems to have passed. Distress is not the major problem for this untroubled patient, so the nature of the problem sits more in the realm of dysfunction.

Mr. M's incongruous behavior last night, and the lack of recollection of it today, points toward cognitive dysfunction, or confusion, as the primary problem. Based on what you have heard, he was grossly disoriented and had fluctuating states of arousal—he was sufficiently agitated to wrest a kitchen drawer off its tracks, and later so somnolent he could not be awakened to shuffle off to bed—which supports the hypothesis that Mr. M had a transient episode of delirium. Now you must try to discover why he was delirious.

*Biographical Background*: Because you know very little about Mr. M, you decide to gather more biographical information. You begin: *I need to know more about you before I can say what needs to be done. Let's start at the beginning. Tell me about your family: your parents, brothers and sisters, and so on.*

Mr. M reports that his parents live independently, but occasionally cause worries. His mother broke her hip last year and his father seems to be losing some memory. He has a sister who's "a little neurotic," is married, and lives in another state. An uncle died young of heart problems and another died in a one-car accident. (He drove into a bridge abutment.) Gladys adds that it might have been suicide, but no one talks about it.

*And where are you from?* He reports that he was born and raised in the Midwest and grew up in various places, as his father relocated a lot for his job as a civil engineer.

*How was school?* He was a fair student but a star football player. He attended a local community college for two years and then transferred to the state university to complete his bachelor's degree.

*And then what?* Mr. M reports with some pride that he is a branch manager for a moderate-sized bank and that he has worked for the bank since he finished college.

*How are things at work?* Mr. M tenses up a bit at this question and murmurs that things are not so good. He was up for promotion to a regional office, but they passed him over for some MBA hotshot he had trained.

*And how about the two of you?* They have a solid marriage. On further probing, they explain that they were both married before and they met because their kids were good friends. You ask about the kids: both have just started college.

Having recently witnessed the high cost of college, you venture to ask if it isn't a burden having to pay for two kids in school. This strikes a nerve. Mr. M blurts out with obvious bitterness that he had been counting on a raise from the promotion to help pay tuition.

You make a mental note that he may have some reason to be under more than the usual amount of stress, and plan to return to the issue later. You ask if he drinks. He says not a lot. You ask what that means. He says about two glasses of wine with dinner; his wife holds up three fingers, out of his line of sight. Taking her cue, you probe more about his alcohol habits. You ask: *Has alcohol ever been a problem for you?* He pauses, glances at his wife, and admits that he and his wife had argued a lot about it earlier in their marriage, and so he had stopped altogether for a few years, but has eased back into a smaller but steady drinking habit that seems to him to be no problem.

Moving on to the medical history, you confirm that he has had no prior problems with his heart, with seizures or other neurological phenomena, or with strokelike symptoms. You then run through a review of systems and find that now he has only a dull headache. What about sleep? He has had some trouble lately, he thinks because of financial worries. The sedatives seem to help a lot. He doesn't know how many he's been using lately, but his wife does—he has gone from an average of less than one a week to at least one pill nightly, and she believes he took at least three last night. Marco explains that he was having a particularly rough time falling asleep, because of his job woes.

Just to be sure, you ask if he has had any prior psychiatric treatment, but he has not. You ask specifically about depression, panic attacks, suicidal thoughts, hallucinations, and paranoia, and he denies all.

*Mental Status:* Having heard the basic story and delved into some background information, you have begun to form some ideas about the cause of the acute episode of confusion last night. He has a new, but transient symptom, in the context of a change in his use of sedatives. As you move your focus toward more specific questions, you take stock of Mr. M. You stop to think specifically about whether his presentation confirms your impression or confounds it, and you run through a mental checklist of other psychiatric indicators that could prove troublesome if they were there and you missed them.

Mr. M, you have observed, is a healthy-appearing man in no acute distress, dressed neatly in business attire. He cooperates fully but at times seems disengaged from the evaluation, deferring to his wife's report, and oddly unconcerned about the implications of his episode of confusion last night. His behavior and demeanor are unchanged when his wife is out of the room, briefly. His speech, when he does speak up, has spontaneity, he is fluent, speaks in a slightly rapid but even pace. Thoughts are generally logical, associations intact, no signs of formal thought disorder. His affect is bright, even jovial, and when you ask, his mood is "great" and he has no signs of any suicidality. He does not appear anxious or, when asked, report any specific anxiety symptoms, such as obsessions, compulsions, or panic attacks. When you ask if he has had unusual sensations (hallucinations) or ideas (delusions), he asks jokingly if you think he's "nuts." He scores 29 out of a possible 30 on a cognitive screening exam, missing 1 point for being off by one day on the date. His inaccurate and incomplete answers to questions about drinking and use of medications suggest his insight is limited.

*Hypothesis Testing:* The biographical context has provided some information that may help to solve the mystery. You have heard about something likely to cause transient confusion in the absence of any other new symptom. Sedatives, especially in the context of moderate, perhaps immoderate, alcohol consumption, can produce transient delirium, or intoxication. And you have heard that he may have been more worried than usual, because of financial concerns, and that he found sedatives useful. You have not confirmed yet that sedative intoxication is the problem, but now you have a hypothesis to test. Also, you have not heard things that would lead you in an alternative direction. No history of seizures, and no cardiac disease that might indicate a risk for stroke. The possible suicide in a family member is significant, but would not explain transient delirium. A remote history of playing football, which might have produced minor head trauma, clearly hasn't affected him much over the past 37 years. He has maintained a relatively stable and successful life—no sign of mood disorder or cognitive decline suggestive of dementia, for example.

To help the patient, and not merely explain his problem, you have to know about the factors that contributed to his apparent intoxication on sedatives. You need to address the circumstances that led to the problem: insomnia, work stress, and over-reliance on sedatives and alcohol for stress management.

It is time now to test your understanding of the story, the problem, and the relevant circumstances by relating back to the patient a summary.

*Let me see if I have the story right, so far. Last night you had an episode of confusion that you don't remember but that alarmed your wife. Now you feel fine. Generally, you're a pretty healthy guy. Occasionally you have had trouble with insomnia. But lately you have been having more trouble. As I glance at the prescription record here, I see that you have been refilling your sedative prescription monthly over the past few months, which suggests you are using it daily. A year ago, a prescription lasted you three to six months.*

Mr. and Ms. M both agree with this summation. As you probe into the question of his insomnia, you note that he has developed some poor sleep hygiene habits—working on his laptop in bed late into the night, then finding he can't settle down to sleep without a sedative. Lately, when he has tried to sleep without a sedative, even on a weekend, he tosses and turns and worries until he gives in and takes a pill. He has begun to dread going to bed. After you take the opportunity to teach him about good sleep habits and some alternatives to using the sedative every night, you ask him more about the stress. *What will you do now about the tuition?* He and his wife agree that in the light of day, tuition still seems a burden, but not one they can't manage, as they had planned all along to manage it, by frugality and strategic borrowing.

At the close of the visit, you explain that you believe the confusion last night was due to intoxication on the sedatives. You add that the alcohol may also have contributed. Mr. M says with some relief that he will certainly never take extra pills again, and his wife adds that she will keep an eye on his drinking. You suggest that if at all possible he should stay away from the sedatives altogether (you don't prohibit them entirely, as he might need to taper from them gradually if he has built up a drug dependence), and that Mr. M make an appointment to see Dr. Q to discuss some alternatives to sedative use, if the simple recommendations for better sleep hygiene do not resolve the insomnia and allow him to cut back on or eliminate the use of sedatives.

How would you compose a brief note to Dr. Q to summarize the acute problem, as well as the other important information you have gathered about Mr. M that might help him in the future?

### The Case of Joan K

*The Story:* On call in the psychiatric emergency department in the wee hours of the morning and just about to lay your head on the pillow for a nap, you are paged by triage. The police have brought in a young woman who crashed her car into an ambulance. Before you can ask why this is a psychiatric problem, the triage nurse adds that she appeared to do this deliberately and that the emergency personnel and police on the scene found her to be agitated and talking nonsensically. You further establish that she is not agitated at the moment, cooperated with blood tests, and provided urine for a toxicology screen, and is calmly awaiting neck films. Suspecting she may simply be drunk and knowing there is little to be learned by assessing an inebriated patient, you ask them to call you back when the labs and X-rays come back, sooner if she becomes agitated. Then you sleep.

Your pager chirps you awake 90 minutes later. The psychiatric nurse in the emergency department has called you to say that the new patient has been cleared of having a neck injury and is in the psychiatry area, but has started to pace and talk to herself. The apparent change in her behavior sounds worrisome. You go immediately to assess the situation. As you observe the patient in the glass-walled waiting area, agitated as the nurse described, you ask the nurse to fill you in.

The patient's name is Joan K. She is 24. No one has been able to get a meaningful history from her. She has an up-to-date student ID from a local university. She has never been a patient in your hospital. Her toxicology screen has come back negative, her vital signs are significant only for a slightly elevated pulse, and all other labs are more or less normal. The nurse was able to find one helpful clue—a prescription for an antipsychotic medication from Dr. Y, a psychiatrist in another state.

The patient stiffens when you enter the waiting room. Who sent you? she asks. You calmly bypass the question, introduce yourself, and tell her that you are here to help. You ask her how she came to the hospital. At first she denies that she needs help and says there was simply a misunderstanding with police. Her gaze darts past you toward the door, repeatedly. You consider asking her why she rammed the ambulance, but experience suggests it would be prudent to quell her agitation before confronting her. Instead, you suggest that she appears anxious and offer her a dose of the same antipsychotic medication on the prescription from Dr. Y. You are relieved when she agrees, readily. You ask if she might be more comfortable in the seclusion room, away from so much light and noise, but she declines and agrees to have a seat. She is not uncontrollably agitated, and no one else is waiting who might stir her up or get into harm's way, so you do not press the point.

As the nurse retrieves the medication, you excuse yourself and withdraw to your desk to look over the scant documentation available (leaving the patient under the supervision of a security officer). The police report provides useful detail. The trouble apparently began when an ambulance came for an elderly neighbor who was having chest pains. As the emergency medical technicians were inside assisting the neighbor, Ms. K bolted from her building, jumped into her car, backed out of a parking space, and then jerked forward, plowing head on into the side of the ambulance, near the rear wheel. When neighbors came out to investigate, she rolled down her window—the door was damaged—and shouted at them not to try to follow her. As someone called 911, she tried to dislodge the front end of her car from the ambulance, and succeeded only in spinning her wheels and hemming herself in between the ambulance and the other cars in the parking lot. Police arrived soon thereafter and were able to help her from the damaged vehicle. She was secured, without violence, in the patrol car. You learn that your first impression, that she might be drunk, was disconfirmed on the scene, as the roadside test revealed zero alcohol in her system.

Nursing notes since her arrival in the emergency department describe her as distracted and jumpy, unwilling to reveal information but generally cooperative when asked to do something. Although you have limited information, you can begin to form an outline of Joan's story: a college student who has a past psychiatric history has behaved bizarrely and dangerously, so has been brought in by police for an emergency assessment.

*The Problem:* The police brought Ms. K to the hospital for her protection and the protection of others because of her dangerous, violent actions. She did not injure anyone, fortunately, and it is not clear that she intended to injure anyone, but because her actions were unpredictable and her motives unfathomable, she remains at risk of inadvertently injuring someone later. There is no question that she must remain under your care, even if she were to demand to leave. Although your major job will be to arrange for her to be admitted to an inpatient unit, you still need to learn what you can about her history and state of mind. The more you can learn about her mental illness now, the more quickly she can be started on the right treatment.

*Biographical Background:* As you peruse the nursing notes, your telephone extension buzzes and the operator announces that a woman has called for you—Ms. K's mother, Marla. You assure Marla that Joan is intact, but that she has not been in a state of mind to talk about what happened. You ask Marla if she knows what has been going on with Joan. Marla can't say much about recent events. Calls from Joan have become stranger and more rare the past few weeks. You confirm with Marla that Joan attends the local university and that she has made slow progress toward a bachelor's degree. Her education has been interrupted by psychiatric hospitalization and inhibited by the fact that, until recently, she has tended to become overwhelmed when she has taken more than one course at a time.

Marla also has valuable information about Joan's biography. First you ask Marla about herself. Marla is a registered nurse and earns a decent living in a hospital—enough to continue to help Joan as she struggles to advance her education. The father disappeared before her birth—he had mental problems of some sort.

You ask whether Joan had any difficulties at birth or in early childhood. In fact, Joan was born a month premature and spent several weeks in the neonatal intensive care unit, but she walked and talked at the appropriate ages. She was always able to maintain decent grades in school. The major area of difficulty was her social life. From her earliest school years, she seemed hypersensitive. Emotional meltdowns became almost a daily occurrence. Marla had taken Joan to see a counselor, and Joan had made gradual progress in managing her emotions. One doctor thought she should take a medication, but Marla had wanted to avoid that. By junior high, Joan had settled a bit. She always had one close best friend and steered clear of activities like band, athletics, and cheerleading, in which there was a large amount of close contact with many other people. By high school she had learned to keep to herself, mostly.

Marla could not recall if Joan had ever dated in high school. Joan has talked of a boyfriend now and then, but Marla has never met one and suspects these have been casual hook-ups or one-night stands, if not simply imaginary. It has been a year or two since Marla has heard of any boyfriends.

Marla didn't believe Joan had ever had problems with alcohol or drugs. Aside from her premature birth and some childhood asthma, Joan has always been fairly healthy, physically.

Marla seems to have only a vague understanding of Joan's psychiatric problems. She thought they must have begun when Joan first went off to university, directly after high school. Joan had seemed excited and eager when Marla had dropped her off to begin freshman year. Joan emailed home daily at first, then began to space out the messages, and by mid-October had stopped replying routinely to Marla's messages. Marla chalked it up to Joan's busy college life. Marla was shocked when Joan showed up at home unexpectedly one day in November to announce that she wouldn't be going back and wouldn't talk about it. All Marla could learn by talking to the student counselor was that Joan had not engaged at all in the typical first-year social functions and that the day she left school she had gotten into a shouting match with one of her professors during a large, introductory lecture.

Living at home, Joan was able to take courses at the local college, and although she had no life beyond school, she made steady academic progress. But then about a year ago Joan had a "nervous breakdown." She had gone missing, and Marla eventually found her hiding in the attic and mute, and so had her hospitalized. They told her it was "psychotic disorder NOS." Joan emerged a week later looking more sedated than well, but gradually seemed to recover, and in a few months looked better than she had looked in years. Last semester, she took a full load of classes at the local college and made good grades. In fact, Joan had seemed so well that Marla readily agreed that she should return to the university to get back on track earning a degree. And when Joan had called soon after starting school to say she no longer needed the medication and felt great, Marla had been persuaded that the nightmare of Joan's mental illness was behind them and had supported Joan's decision.

Before you end the call, you confirm with Marla that Joan had been taking the same drug named on the prescription she had with her. You glance at the unfilled prescription and notice that it was dated three weeks ago—just before Joan must have left home to begin the semester at the university.

Marla promises to make the two-hour drive to the hospital in the morning, once she can arrange coverage for her shifts at the hospital.

*Mental Status:* While you were on the phone, Joan took her medication and grew sleepy, so the nurse let her snooze on a mattress in the seclusion room. By the time you have assembled the story and written it up, the sun has risen, she is awake again and not as restless as she had been last night. You sit down with her in a quiet corner to try to complete your assessment.

Joan appears rumpled, her hair wild from sleep. Her clothes are wrinkled and slightly soiled, and you notice some odd things about them—mismatched socks, misaligned buttons, pockets stuffed with newspaper. She seems to try to avoid eye contact. More than once she pauses before answering a question and cocks her head to one side before responding. She gives no sign of acknowledgment when you make a mildly humorous observation; in fact, she seems tense and guarded throughout the assessment. Her speech is generally spontaneous and fluent. However, many of her answers are distinctly hard to follow. For example, when asked why she did not fill her prescription, she said, after a pause and a somewhat quizzical look in your direction, "You should know. It's all on the website . . . you know, the science-ology page. The guild, of course you're a member of the guild, the guild has plans. You get the insurance and you bury the answers and kill us." Many of her responses are similarly thought-disordered; the statements are illogically connected. She reports her mood as "vindified" but does not elaborate. She denies suicidal or homicidal ideas but adds, as an aside, "That's what I'm supposed to say, right?" She appears floridly delusional, based on her statements, but becomes evasive when you attempt to pin her down to specific forms of delusion. When you ask if she hears voices, she pauses and cocks her head, nods in assent but at the same time says "never." Later, she mentions voices, in passing, without evident awareness of the contradiction. She appears to have poor insight and is uncooperative on a formal cognitive assessment, though she has no trouble describing, in an idiosyncratic way, events of the past few weeks, which suggests her memory is grossly intact.

*Hypothesis Testing:* With gentle probing, you are able to glean the following from her direct answers and from her reactions to various questions about the past days' events:

In all the commotion of starting over at the university, Joan's antipsychotic prescription had run out and she had put off getting it refilled. At first it felt good to break free of the lethargy-inducing effects of the medication. Then it began to dawn on her that there must be a reason she had felt lethargic on the medication. Someone wanted to dull her senses. She did not know who might want to do this. One day, in a political science lecture, the professor spoke about health care legislation and about the pharmaceutical lobby, and the pieces began to fall into place. The professor confirmed this by writing "K Street" on the blackboard—she knew this to be a reference to the Washington, D.C., location of many lobbyist offices, but she also knew that the "K" referred to her, Joan K. She took this as a warning to stay away from the lecture hall and to stay off the medications. She began to think of the medical industry as a guild, out to protect itself by tormenting those who had figured out its secret.

So she was awake at the computer, late at night, investigating the "medical industrial guild," when she saw the ambulance pull up in front of her apartment house. At that moment a voice from somewhere told her to get out, to save herself, and so she fled to her car. She believed the ambulance was there to take her, to drug and kill her. She rammed the ambulance so it could not follow her but the car became stuck. When the police came, she was initially relieved, because they were not part of the guild; then they took her to the hospital. A voice told her to hide her pain, which she took to mean she should remain cooperative and perhaps convince the guild that she was not the person they were looking for, but her resolve had begun to wane by the time you met her. When the nurse arrived with the medication, she took it in the belief that it would provide a quick and painless death rather than the torture she feared. Now she remains convinced she is destined to do battle with the guild, but feels oddly at peace about the prospect, come what may.

This account and her odd presentation convince you that Ms. K was and is indeed, psychotic. She has prominent hallucinations and persecutory delusions. She has long-standing problems of poor social and limited academic functioning. Her appearance reflects behavioral disorganization and her speech demonstrates several kinds of disordered thinking. There is a family history in her father of an unspecified mental illness you suspect must be either severe or chronic or both. These add up to a highly likely diagnosis of schizophrenia. However, the diagnosis alone offers only a broad idea about the best way to help this patient. Knowing the content of her delusions does not give you the power to talk her out of them, but it does raise your awareness of the source of her apprehensiveness toward treatment. This, combined with her mother's ambivalence about medication, portend a struggle at some point in the future when she once again chafes under the burden of medication.

When the time comes to transfer Ms. K to an inpatient bed, she signs in willingly. How will you condense the essential elements of this case into your note so the treatment team upstairs knows how to assess and medicate the symptoms of her schizophrenia, how to anticipate the influence of her specific beliefs on her behavior in the near term, and how to address the factors that have made psychosis re-emerge at this time in order to prevent another recurrence?

### B.9. The Case Formulation

The end result of this process of problem-oriented evaluation is a multilayered case formulation. The formulation restates the critical elements of the case and develops hypotheses or conclusions about the nature of each problem: disease state, trait vulnerability, maladaptive behavior, or adverse experience. The knowledge of the mental functioning of the brain, and of the forms of dysfunction that occur in each component of the mind, informs the assessment of the problem and provides some basis to link the known mechanisms of action of treatment to particular aspects of mental dysfunction.

To build a case formulation, start with the preliminaries: what are the essential demographic factors (age, sex, ethnicity), roles (occupation, marital status), and clinical background (significant known medical or prior psychiatric illness)? Where is the patient being seen, and who brought the patient to psychiatric care? What was the deciding factor that prompted the assessment now? For example, the start of the formulation for Marco M's case, from the previous section, might read *"This is a 55-year-old married banker without prior psychiatric contact, who has requested an assessment because of a disturbing episode of nocturnal confusion.",* Or, for Joan K, *"The patient is a 24-year-old unmarried student brought in by police after she rammed her car into an ambulance."*

Next describe the presenting problem, as a general type (danger, dysfunction, or distress) and as it has emerged in the individual patient (disease state, trait vulnerability, maladaptive behavior, adverse experience). Any given problem may have a number of causes. The formulation then builds a case for or against the likely causes, using evidence from the patient's history, records, other informants, and mental state. This is done methodically, considering whether the patient has a pathological syndrome that explains the problem, or has decompensated due to a psychological vulnerability, or has come to experience the consequences of bad behavior, or, finally, how much the patient's own understanding of events influences the degree of suffering from the patient's point of view.

It sounds complicated, but a thorough formulation in many cases can be constructed using four or five sentences: one to state the presenting facts, and one to lay out the salient features of each problem. For example, for Marco M: *"The confusion appears to be the result of intoxication [disease] that arose in the context of the patient's use of a higher-than-usual dose of a sedative for insomnia. The habitual use of sedatives may pose a problem for the patient, as he has reported he is unable to sleep without them [behavior]. Another factor that has contributed to the insomnia is stress at work related to the promotion of a former protégé to a position as his supervisor [adversity]. The patient's tendency to become rigidly focused on work in times of stress suggests that he may possess a mild anankastic tendency that both motivates him to find pharmacologic ways to control his unmanageable anxiety and at the same time may prove an asset as he conscientiously develops new strategies to cope [vulnerability]."*

And, for Joan K: *"Her erratic, violent action appears to have been driven by auditory hallucinations and florid persecutory delusions; her mood appears stable, so psychotic mania or depression seem unlikely, and there is a family history suggestive of chronic mental illness in the father, all consistent with a provisional diagnosis of schizophrenia [disease]. A major complicating factor for this patient is her failure to adhere to a prescribed regimen of antipsychotic medications, motivated at least in part by the belief that doctors and drug companies are a part of a conspiracy [behavior]. She has no social resources in the city, having just moved here from another state, which suggests a further reason why she may not trust treatment advice from people she only just met [adversity]. Her above-average intelligence may in a way be more of an obstacle than an asset, as it contributes to the sophistication of her delusions and perhaps also provides her with the intellectual confidence to challenge the treatment plan [vulnerability]."*

These rudimentary formulations offer an idea how an organized and organic approach can sort out a patient's problems concisely, prioritize them, and show their interrelationships. Over time, of course, your own formulations will become richer as you gain experience and wisdom. This is one of the beautiful things about psychiatry. The passage of years may make our technical knowledge obsolete, but they enhance wisdom (or so one hopes), so you can get better and better at psychiatry over the course of a career.

# Glossary

*Note:* I have provided these abbreviated definitions in order to give the reader a handy reference to terms I have used in this book and what I mean by them. These definitions should not be taken as complete or necessarily as the most common meanings of these terms.

**Acetylcholine:** a neurotransmitter involved in tonic arousal, autonomic nervous system communication, and activation of muscles at nerve endings

**Action:** purposeful motion

**Action potential:** rapid depolarization of a neuron involving sudden flux of electrical charge

**Action program:** a cortical neural network that encodes a sequence of goal-directed motions

**Adaptive:** facilitating survival

**Addiction:** repetitive consummatory behavior that temporarily subdues emotional distress or satisfies a conditioned craving, but not an actual appetite

**Adversity:** a life challenge that overwhelms adaptive coping

**Affective:** related to the mental functions of emotion and/or motivation

**Affiliation:** the mental function concerned with affective bonding between parent and child, between sexual partners, and between individuals and larger groups to whom they show loyalty and with whom they identify

**Aggression:** hostile motivations; violence or the threat of violence undertaken for defense against a real or imagined threat or for coercive purposes

**Agitation:** severe restlessness; arousal of activity without activation of a specific purpose toward which to direct it

**Agnosia:** the pathological loss of ability to identify things, people, or other objects

**Alarm:** a state of heightened vigilance aroused by surprise or the perception of threat

**Allostatic regulation:** bodily self-adjustment of physiologic state to match changing environmental demands

**Ambivalence:** failure to select a course of action from fear of selecting the less rewarding course

**Amnesia:** loss of memory; retrograde amnesia is loss of past memory, and anterograde amnesia is loss of capacity to remember new things

**Amphetamine:** a variety of stimulant drug that potentiates catecholamine neurotransmission

**Amygdala:** almond-shaped subcortical brain nucleus at the center of networks that transform arousal into adaptive action

**Anankastic:** personality style characterized by rigidity and preoccupation with detail; also known as obsessive-compulsive or anal-retentive personality

**Anergia:** deficiency in the subjective sense of having sufficient arousal to perform necessary actions

**Anguish:** the mental equivalent of pain

**Anhedonia:** lack of ability to experience pleasure

**Anorexia nervosa:** a behavioral syndrome of significant self-starvation in the context of a functioning appetite

**Anticholinergic:** blockade of acetylcholine neurotransmitter receptors; a drug that accomplishes this

**Anticonvulsant:** any drug that stops or prevents seizure; *see also* Neuromodulator

**Antidepressant:** any drug with known efficacy against major depression; includes tricyclics, selective serotonin reuptake inhibitors (SSRIs), and monoamine oxidase inhibitors (MAOIs), among others

**Antipsychotic:** any drug that stops or diminishes psychotic symptoms; generally dopamine-blocking drugs

**Anxiety:** encompasses a diverse class of diagnostic entities, including generalized anxiety disorder, panic disorder, phobic disorders, and post-traumatic stress disorder. Regarding anxiety as a symptom: *see* Dread

**Apathy:** failure to become aroused by the prospect of loss

**Aphasia:** the loss of the ability to construct fluent speech; often considered a special form of apraxia

**Appetite:** desire induced by physiologic signals

**Apraxia:** the pathological loss of the ability to perform practical tasks

**Arousal:** the brain state that differentiates conscious coherence from confusion (tonic); the mechanism by which signals of physiologic need and environmental threat and opportunity mobilize attention and resources for action (phasic)

**Asociality:** deficit in the capacity to navigate cooperative behavior

**Association:** (with respect to neurons) a potentiated connection between two neurons; compared to the unassociated state, it takes a lower threshold of activity in one neuron to stimulate an action potential if the two neurons have become associated by prior heavy activity

**Attachment:** cooperative behavior in which social or intimate engagement with the other person is part of the reward from cooperation

**Attention:** the contents of working memory at any given moment

**Attention-deficit/hyperactivity disorder (ADHD):** a relative deficit in the ability to maintain persistent effort on cognitive tasks, and to inhibit impulsive, stimulus-driven behaviors

**Autism:** a state of social incompetence that results developmentally from asociality

**Autonomic:** relating to the nervous system functions that govern visceral activity and allostatic regulation

**Avoidance:** behavioral bias that overvalues threat and undervalues reward

**Avulsion:** alienation or apparent withdrawal of content from the flow of thought

**Axon:** the part of a neuron that carries the action potential from the nerve cell body to the synapse

**Basal ganglia:** a cluster of subcortical nuclei primarily engaged in the coordination of sequenced action

**Behavior:** actions undertaken for the purpose of satisfying a need or craving or defending against a threat

**Belief:** information acquired without personal experience and held without concrete evidence

**Benzodiazepine:** a GABA-enhancing drug that serves to inhibit neural activity in the brain

**Beta-blockers:** a class of drugs that inhibits certain adrenergic receptors in the autonomic nervous system and peripheral organs

**Bias:** a tendency to favor one emotional consequence over another

**Biopsychosocial:** the prevailing perspective that phenomena at different levels of existence, from molecules to minds to multitudes, are related in a chain of causality

**Bipolar disorder:** a syndrome of mental illness characterized by dramatic changes in emotional and behavioral state into depression and mania

**Borderline (personality):** refers to a persistent pattern of unstable emotions and self-destructive behavior

**Brainstem:** where brain transitions to spinal cord; contains many subcortical nuclei and tracts of neurons

**Bulimia:** food binges followed by compensatory behavior like vomiting, fasting, excessive exercise

**Cannabinoid:** a class of drugs, including marijuana, that induces euphoria by stimulating endocannabinoid receptors

**Catatonia:** a state of mental illness in which the patient is awake but engages in no purposeful behavior

**Catecholamines:** arousing monoaminergic neurotransmitters, namely, dopamine and norepinephrine

**Central sulcus:** the apparent rift in the visible cortex that separates frontal from parietal lobes

**Cerebellum:** a brain structure situated to the rear and below the cerebrum that governs coordination, sequencing, and conditioning

**Character:** a belief one holds about the likely actions of another person

**Cingulate cortex:** a strip of cortex tucked between the two hemispheres that links both to sensory regions of the cortex and to regions involved in memory and emotion

**Circumstantiality:** a manner of speaking in which the speaker digresses frequently but generally returns to the topic at hand

**Classical conditioning:** a specialized form of learning that superimposes new stimulus-driven responses over existing reflexive responses

**Client:** a person who seeks therapeutic intervention but follows advice selectively

**Cognition:** mental function that serves to identify and differentiate objects of perception

**Cognitive impairment:** deficit in the integration of perception, memory, and adaptive behavior

**Communication:** transmission or exchange of experiential knowledge by way of shared symbols

**Compulsion:** a repetitive, irresistible activity that has no adaptive purpose

**Conditioning:** learning that shapes responses, but not necessarily memory

**Conduct disorder:** a pattern of sociopathic behavior in childhood and adolescence

**Consummatory:** behavior aimed to use something immediately at hand to satisfy a drive

**Control:** the capacity to initiate and stop goal-driven action

**Conversion:** (a) an abrupt change in a set of beliefs; (b) behavior that mimics physical signs of illness, usually neurologic illness, usually serving to gain sympathy and attention

**Cooperation:** an agreement to take action predicted to aid another's welfare, in exchange for another's actions that aid one's own welfare

**Corpus callosum:** a band of neurons that connects the right and left sides of the brain

**Cortex:** layers of neuron cell bodies and support cells on the outer surface of the brain

**Cortisol:** a hormone secreted by the outer part of the adrenal gland, stimulated by the brain, which alters body metabolism in order to prepare for protracted adversity, or stress

**Deep brain stimulation (DBS):** a mode of treatment, still under development, in which an electrode passed into a specific area of the brain induces symptomatic improvement

**Dejection:** a miserable, hopeless mood; historically, in medical terminology, has excremental connotations

**Delirium:** a state of disordered brain arousal generally induced by altered physiology or intoxication

**Delusion:** a fixed, false, idiosyncratic belief, usually maintained by an abnormal state of arousal

**Dementia:** a state of impaired cognition in the absence of delirium

**Demoralization:** a state of dysphoric mood, with few if any other symptoms, generally associated with adverse experience

**Dendrite:** part of a nerve cell that receives a signal from another neuron

**Denial:** a belief, often maladaptive, that an adverse event or situation is either not salient or not serious

**Depolarization:** the electrical activity in a neuron that rapidly transmits a signal from one neuron to another

**Depression:** unremitting sadness; the clinical syndrome characterized by malaise, anhedonia, and disruptions in appetitive arousal

**Derailment:** a general term to refer to incomprehensible speech that reflects an apparent disruption in the logical construction of thought; *see also* Flight of ideas; Loosening of associations

**Diagnosis:** a name agreed by clinicians to denote a particular form of illness

**Dimension:** any measurable trait that varies across a population

**Disease:** a complex of symptoms and deficits that follows from an altered state of physiology (that is, a pathophysiologic process)

**Disinhibition:** in this text, specifically refers to the loss of the normal executive function to defer immediate, stimulus-driven behavior in favor of longer-term goals

**Dissociation:** a subjective state in which the perceptions associated with an experience seem to become disconnected from its emotional salience

**Dissolution:** a sense of lost identity (that is, a failure to maintain a stable character); common element of dissociative disorders

**Distractibility/Distraction:** an aspect of inattentiveness denoting the enhanced potential for working memory to be captured by immediate sensory stimuli

**Dopamine:** a monoaminergic neurotransmitter essential in reward and in the arousal of action

**Dopamine inhibitor:** a drug that blocks dopamine from reaching its receptor; *see also* Antipsychotic

**Dorsolateral prefrontal cortex (DLPFC):** a large expanse of frontal cortex in which the sequencing of complex behavior is encoded

**Doubt:** a state of uncertainty when information calls into question the validity of a belief

**Dread:** the stressful fear of some future or potential threat, as opposed to the arousing fear of an immediate threat that induces defensive action

**Drive:** the motive force behind an intention; may reflect an innate appetite or a learned desire

**Dysfluency:** inhibited, diminished, delayed, or telegraphic speech

**Dyskinesia:** any pathological symptom of abnormal movement; includes tics, tremors, choreoform movements, and others

**Dysphoria:** unpleasant, painful, or low mood

**Dysthymia:** a state of chronic low mood and poor hedonic functioning

**Eccentricity:** patterns of behavior that defy social conventions; by definition a hindrance to cooperation

**Egotism:** essentially an impediment to affiliative relationships; when a person unilaterally fails to accept another's cooperative interest as a mutual interest

**Electroconvulsive therapy (ECT):** a treatment for mental illness that involves a series of controlled, electrically induced seizures; the most effective treatment known for severe major depression and catatonia

**Electroencephalogram (EEG):** assessment of brain activity by analysis of magnetic fields generated by populations of active neurons

**Elemental hallucination:** an unformed perception experienced without a stimulus (that is, an unidentifiable sound, image, taste, and so on)

**Elementary (mind):** the basic input (sensory, interoceptive) and motor output functions at the gateways of mental life

**Emotion:** a change in the potential for behavioral activation, minus a specific plan of action; the functional basis of feeling

**Empirical:** evidence-based

**Encephalopathy:** gross alteration in brain function that produces delirium

**Endorphin:** a hormone that diminishes nervous system arousal; the physiological analog of morphine-derived drugs

**Excitatory neurotoxicity:** neuron cell death that may occur due to excessive activation

**Excitement:** in the context of mood, a state of enhanced anticipation of pleasure and drive to pursue it

**Executive:** the cognitive function that weighs the value of competing drives and initiates adaptive action

**Extraversion:** a personality trait measuring one's tendency to be moved by positive experience; in a social context, implies gregariousness

**Extravolition:** the abnormal experience of feeling as if some external force was in control of one's actions; often referred to as a "passivity" delusion

**Fear:** an emotional state of arousal by anticipated threat

**Feeling:** the subjective correlate of emotion; combines interoceptive information with information about context to become a complex source of information in working memory

**Flashbacks:** vivid reconstructions of episodic memory, often of frightening events

**Flight of ideas:** thought-disordered speech in which successive ideas are only tenuously linked together

**Folk psychology:** scientifically and philosophically naïve theories about how the mind works, generated by culture and common experience

**Formed hallucination:** an identifiable perception without sensory stimulus (for example, a voice speaking understandable words, a vision of a specific person, a metallic taste, and so on)

**Formulation:** a structured clinical conclusion about the nature of a patient's problem

**Freedom (of will or choice):** the philosophical concept of mind over matter; that we are free agents who can weigh options and choose a course of action (as opposed to our actions being determined by material or supernatural causes)

**Frontal lobe:** the part of the brain closest to the forehead, integral to executive functioning

**Fugue:** an abnormal mental state in which a person apparently has no recollection for a period of time

**Function:** the contribution of a process to the ends of survival and propagation

**GABA-enhancer:** *see* Benzodiazepine

**Gamma-amino-butyric acid (GABA):** a neurotransmitter that tends to inhibit depolarization

**Gender:** sexual identity; not necessarily congruent with biological determinants of sex

**Genotype:** an individual's genetic pattern; may encompass several or all of a person's alleles

**Glutamate:** an excitatory neurotransmitter integral to information processing and storage

**Grief:** a generally prolonged state of adjustment to the loss of an attachment

**Guilt:** fear of punishment for a transgression, real or imagined

**Gyrus:** outer folds of the brain; the parts of cortex visible on surface inspection

**Habit:** patterns of learned behavior

**Hallucination:** perception without a stimulus

**Hallucinogenics:** a class of drugs that alters perceptions

**Hippocampus:** a subcortical structure integral to sensory integration and memory

**Histrionic:** a personality style that overvalues feeling and undervalues knowledge

**Hostility:** defensive reaction to an inescapable threat

**Hyperfluency:** rapid or pressured speech, difficult to interrupt, often disjointed

**Hypochondriasis:** overvalued idea and anxiety about a disease

**Hypothalamic-pituitary-adrenal (HPA) axis:** self-regulating system that links brain to stress and metabolic hormones

**Hypothalamus:** a cluster of nuclei deep within the brain that directs physiologic signals to adaptive brain-mediated responses

**Hysteria:** a pseudoneurological symptom produced by distress and anxiety

**Identity:** a set of beliefs about one's own values

**Illusion:** a false perception derived from an actual stimulus

**Impulsiveness:** the bias toward action and away from deliberation; the opposite of ambivalence

**Inertia:** a bias toward inaction rooted in a devalued expectation of reward

**Information:** the elemental unit of mental functioning; a complex, neuronally encoded pattern that permits a stimulus to alter behavior, emotion, attention, or memory in a specific way

**Insula:** a region of cortex behind the temporal lobe involved mainly in interoception

**Integral (mind):** functions that transform mental elements into information to store and use to guide adaptive behavior

**Intelligence:** an abstract concept encompassing cognitive fluency and the capacity to discriminate between abstract concepts

**Intention:** a plan of action, aroused and in play; a counterpoint to feeling, in which there is emotional arousal but no plan of action

**Interoception:** source of raw data comprising information about the state of the body

**Intoxication:** a state of delirium brought about by alcohol or drugs

**Introversion:** opposite of extraversion; slowness to warm to the prospects of positive experience, often manifest as social avoidance

**Intrusion:** specifically with respect to thought processes, when a thought seems to have been inserted into consciousness by some external force

**Intrusive memory:** *see* Flashbacks

**Irascibility:** an irritable mood state in which hostile emotions are easily aroused

**Knowledge:** information stored in memory that can be used for mental functioning; also known as semantic memory

**Labile personality:** a set of immature attitudes and chaotic behaviors acquired as a result of having constitutionally unpredictable shifts of emotional state

**Limbic system:** a general (and archaic) term for a set of subcortical structures thought to govern emotion

**Lithium:** in the psychiatric context, a salt that has properties as a mood stabilizer

**Locus coeruleus:** a subcortical structure that transmits norepinephrine throughout the cortex

**Logorrhea:** excessive speech

**Loosening of associations:** thought-disordered speech in which there is no logical connection between ideas

**Maintenance:** in the context of behavioral treatment, the phase after recovery geared toward preventing relapse

**Major depression:** a syndrome characterized by dysphoric mood, anhedonia, anergia, and appetitive dysfunctions

**Maladaptive:** describes behavior that appears to run counter to survival

**Maladjustment:** a state of distress or dysfunction that results from becoming overwhelmed by life challenges

**Malingering:** pretending to be ill in order to acquire some material benefit or advantage

**Mania:** a hyperexcited state in which the mood can range from irritable to euphoric and appetitive behavior breaks free of autoregulation

**Meatware:** a modern colloquial term referring to the biological interface with hardware and software

**Medial septal nucleus:** a subcortical structure that projects cholinergic neurons

**Memory:** the retention of traces from experience within the structure of the brain, so that past experience can inform future actions; can be subdivided into working (*see* Attention), episodic/autobiographical (memory for specific events complete with sensory and narrative context), semantic (*see* Knowledge), and procedural (skill-related learning)

**Mental illness:** used in this book as a blanket term for any brain activity, behavior, propensity, or personal experience that produces dangerous behavior, dysfunctional mental performance, and emotional distress

**Mental retardation:** significantly diminished capacity to perform tasks involving cognitive flexibility and discrimination; to be replaced by "intellectual disability" in the next DSM

**Mind:** the chief organic function of the brain; the capacity to process signals from the environment, from the body, and from past experience into information that guides adaptive behavior

**Misrepresentation:** speaking falsely; makes no assumption about the intention, which is lying if the aim is to spread false information and confabulation if not

**Monoamine oxidase inhibitor (MAO-I):** a pharmaceutical that blocks the metabolism of monoaminergic neurotransmitters, effectively prolonging their availability for stimulation of receptors; used primarily to treat major depression

**Monoaminergic:** referring to a shared chemical aspect of the major neurotransmitters involved in phasic arousal (dopamine, norepinephrine, and serotonin)

**Mood:** a pervasive emotional state that persists without, or despite salient cause for arousal

**Motion:** any kinetic activity of muscles, whether goal-directed or not

**Motivation:** linkage of arousal to an identifiable goal of action

**Motor:** anything related to muscular activity

**Motor strip:** a region of frontal cortex adjacent to the central sulcus (hence bordering on the parietal lobe) that sends out the final signals for muscular contraction

**Myelin:** a pale-colored substance that serves as a sheath to protect neuronal axons and facilitate depolarization

**Narcissism:** a persistent bias toward uneven cooperation that favors one's own interests at the expense of stable affiliation

**Narcolepsy:** a disorder of sleep regulation in which sleepiness frequently arises throughout the day

**Narrative:** a holistic mode of communication in which truth lives in the adequacy, appropriateness, and accuracy of an entire sequence of events rather than in the mechanisms behind events

**Network:** in the context of the brain, a set of neurons associated by frequent use into a functional unit; when one neuron depolarizes, all neurons in the network depolarize

**Neuroleptic:** another term for an antipsychotic drug (that is, a dopamine inhibitor)

**Neuromodulator:** a generic term for drugs that inhibit neurotransmission; specifically includes anticonvulsants

**Neuron:** a cell that specializes in transmitting information

**Neurosis:** a pattern of maladjustment and a tendency to suffer that emerges over time, specifically as a result of emotional vulnerabilities, often manifesting as self-defeating though not self-destructive behavior

**Neuroticism:** specifically, in the five-factor model of personality traits, the tendency to experience suffering under adverse conditions

**Neurotransmitter:** a chemical secreted at the synaptic terminal of a neuron to convey a signal to another neuron

**Noradrenergic:** relating to norepinephrine (that is, noradrenalin) neurotransmission

**Norepinephrine:** a monoaminergic neurotransmitter with the potential to arouse system-wide alterations in body physiology and brain activity to excite heightened vigilance

**Nosology:** a system for classifying medical disorders

**Nucleus:** (a) the central part of any cell, including neurons, in which DNA is stored; (b) a collection of neuronal cell bodies clustered in the brain that generally perform a common function

**Nucleus basalis:** a subcortical structure that projects cholinergic neurons

**Object:** in the context of this book, a mental construct that combines perceptual elements and functional qualities of environmental stimuli into a coherent unit of information

**Objective:** in the context of this book, refers to the program of action associated with obtaining, using, or disposing of an object

**Obsession:** an abnormal mental experience in which an irrational thought or worry recurs repeatedly despite efforts and desire to resist or suppress it

**Occipital lobe:** the part of the cortex onto which visual information first projects

**Oligodendrocyte:** a myelin-containing cell in the brain that serves a supportive role for neurons

**Operant conditioning:** a specialized form of learning in which one is trained to perform an action or series of actions in pursuit of a goal

**Opiate:** a euphoria-inducing drug, analogous to an endorphin, that has both therapeutic properties in pain relief and abuse potential in the form of heroin and other illicit substances

**Oppositional-defiant disorder:** a psychiatric disorder of youth characterized by a persistent refusal to heed authority

**Orbitofronal cortex:** the part of the frontal lobe that sits over the eyes and optic nerves and is involved in emotion and motivation; overlaps with the ventromedial prefrontal cortex

**Orexin/hypocretin:** a polypeptide hormone involved in appetitive regulation

**Organic:** (a) in the context of this book, signifies a bodily function or something done by an organ; (b) in general, a process that can best be explained in biological terms

**Overdependency:** an unstable attachment style in which desire for the other is matched or outweighed by fear of losing the other

**Overvalued idea:** a belief that serves a behavioral function and is held despite its inconsistence with fact and despite maladaptive consequences from holding and acting on it

**Oxytocin:** a polypeptide hormone thought to be involved in the formation of interpersonal attachment, among other things

**Panic:** an acute eruption of fearful emotions and autonomic correlates of defensive arousal (*see* Paroxysm)

**Paranoia:** a set of beliefs that support an intractably fearful outlook; generally experienced as being in the center of constant, impending threat

**Parasuicide:** suicidelike behavior performed without intention of causing death

**Parasympathetic:** aspect of the autonomic nervous system that excites vegetative functions and counters defensive arousal

**Parietal lobe:** expanse of cortex in which sensory input is organized to resolve perception into complex objects

**Paroxysm:** in this book, a sudden surge of fear without apparent stimulus (a panic attack)

**Passive aggressive behavior:** a pattern of feigned cooperative behavior that effectively punishes the other party while acting at the other's bidding

**Pathology:** an abnormality rooted in a dysfunctional brain process

**Patient:** a seeker of medical help who enters into a fully cooperative relationship with the clinician

**Pavlovian conditioning:** *see* Classical conditioning

**Perception:** sensation analyzed and meaningfully represented in the mind

**Personality:** a persistent pattern of biases that drive behavior

**Phasic arousal:** stimulation of brain activity, driven by need

**Phenomena:** events—in this book, primarily of the mental sort

**Phobia:** intense, stimulus-driven fear leading to avoidance of the stimulus

**Plasticity:** the capacity for change in neuronal structure and hence function

**Polypeptide hormones:** a class of hormones comprised of short sequences of amino acids

**Postsynaptic neuron:** the neuron in a network that receives a neurotransmitter from the neuron preceding it in the chain

**Potentiation:** the process by which the strength of a stimulus necessary to depolarize a neuron diminishes after heavy use

**Premotor:** frontal cortex functions that precede output from the motor strip

**Pre-pulse inhibition:** dampening of the responsiveness of a neuron immediately after it has been stimulated

**Pressured speech:** one-sided communication; uninterrupted speech

**Presynaptic neuron:** the neuron in a network that releases a neurotransmitter to stimulate the next neuron in the chain

**Procedure:** a multistep task aimed to find or make something; the end result of operant conditioning

**Projection:** an unfounded assumption that another person's feelings or attitudes reflect one's own perspective

**Pseudoamnesia:** the experience or complaint of forgetting something that was never stored in memory

**Pseudohallucination:** the experience or complaint of false perceptions that do not have the quality of perceptions

**Pseudomemory:** the experience or complaint of recall of events that never happened

**Pseudomotor:** refers to symptoms of paralysis or other loss of control over muscles without neurologic injury

**Pseudosensory:** refers to symptoms of sensory change or loss without neurologic injury

**Psychoanalysis:** psychological theory originating with Sigmund Freud that mental symptoms arise from conflicts in mental life, generally without the person's overt knowledge, and the therapeutic method based on it

**Psychosis:** pathological mental symptom of belief (delusion), perception (hallucination), or action (disorganization)

**Psychosomatic:** physical symptom induced, exacerbated, or perpetuated by emotional distress

**Psychotherapy:** a mode of treatment in which the aim is to lead the patient out of emotional distress and toward adaptive behavior through communication

**Racing thoughts:** the experience of being overwhelmed with ideas

**Raphe nucleus:** serotonin-projecting subcortical structure involved in phasic arousal

**Recovery:** transitional phase in the resolution of an addictive behavior

**Regulation:** with respect to action, the application of information in order to stop or modulate an action (in contrast to control, which also applies to the initiation of action)

**Reward:** brain mechanism to associate an action and object with the satisfaction of a drive

**Ruminations:** worries; fearful thoughts that cannot be alleviated by thinking

**Salience:** the significance of a relationship between two things, or between an object and a drive

**Satiety:** relief of a drive

**Schizoid:** asocial personality

**Schizophrenia:** psychiatric disorder characterized by psychosis, asociality, and poor occupational and executive functioning

**Schizotypal:** eccentric, asocial personality

**Selective serotonin reuptake inhibitor (SSRI):** variety of antidepressant medication that works by preventing the removal of serotonin from the synaptic space

**Sensation:** information about the environment translated into neural signals

**Shame:** painful feeling resulting from the socially enforced loss of cooperation as punishment for a transgression

**Skinnerian conditioning:** *see* Operant conditioning

**Sociopathy:** pattern of anti- or pseudo-cooperative behavior in which one person benefits at the expense of others

**Soma:** the typically bulging part of the neuron in which the cell nucleus is located

**Somatization:** pattern of maladaptive help-seeking behavior for psychosomatic complaints

**Startle:** reflex behavioral reaction to unexpected, strong sensory stimulus

**Stress:** mode of bodily defense against protracted, unpredictable threat that involves cortisol-induced changes in physiological function

**Striatum:** subcortical structures that comprise part of the basal ganglia system

**Subcortical structures:** in the context of this book, refers collectively to all the brain nuclei that contribute to mental functioning

**Substance abuse:** diagnostic term that denotes use of alcohol or drugs that produces adverse consequences

**Substance dependence:** diagnostic term that denotes persistent use of alcohol or drugs, with loss of control over the frequency and intensity of use

**Substantia nigra:** subcortical structure projecting dopamine-secreting neurons, involved in the control of motion

**Suicidality:** attitude and actions that place a positive value on suicide

**Suicide:** an act of self-destruction committed with an intention of ending life

**Sulcus:** recess between gyri, as seen on the surface of the brain

**Sympathetic:** adrenergically mediated aspect of the autonomic nervous system that engages physiology for defensive action

**Symptom:** painful or distressing sensation that provokes medical help-seeking

**Synapse:** end point of a neuron from which neurotransmitters are secreted

**Synaptic cleft:** point connection between neurons; a space into which neurotransmitters are secreted

**Syndrome:** a set of signs and symptoms that cluster and typically follow from a pathological process

**Synthetic (mind):** application of mental capacities to adaptive behavior in the absence of complete or adequate information

**Tangentiality:** mode of speech in which ideas are connected logically, but digress without returning to the point

**Telemission:** the apparent projection or broadcasting of one's thought content to others; the opposite of telepathy, in which one receives the thoughts of others

**Temperament:** trait of emotional responsiveness; component of personality

**Temporal lobe:** brain regions on either lateral aspect of the brain involved in hearing, language, and memory

**Territoriality:** a complex motive combining an attachment to some person, place, thing, or concept with the fear that it is under attack, often resulting in hostile attitude and irritable emotions

**Thalamus:** subcortical structure that serves to organize and synchronize cortical activity

**Theory:** a concept that makes narrative sense of a set of facts

**Thought:** general term for self-conscious mental activity

**Thought broadcasting:** *see* Telemission

**Thought disorder:** general term for incomprehensible communication; *see also* Derailment

**Thought insertion:** *see* Intrusion

**Thought withdrawal:** *see* Avulsion

**Thyroxine:** brain-regulated, metabolism-regulating hormone

**Tonic arousal:** baseline mental activation constituting wakefulness

**Trait:** stable attribute that affects functioning

**Transference:** projection-based feelings a patient develops for a therapist

**Tricyclic antidepressant (TCA):** variety of antidepressant medication

**User:** seeker of medical help who aims primarily for material gain rather than relief of a medical problem

**Value:** anticipated degree of satisfaction from an action

**Ventral tegmental area:** subcortical structure that projects dopamine-secreting neurons to the VMPFC; involved in reward

**Ventromedial prefrontal cortex (VMPFC):** aspect of the frontal cortex involved in the assessment of value between competing choices of action

**Visceral:** refers to functioning of internal organs

**Vulnerability:** propensity to experience distress or dysfunction under stressful circumstances

**Withdrawal:** (a) physiologic response to deprivation from an addictive drug; (b) behavior of social avoidance

**Working memory:** the "theater of consciousness" in which thoughts, feelings, and intentions compete for dominance over behavior

# References

Preface

American Psychiatric Association (1994): *Diagnostic and Statistical Manual of Mental Disorders, Fourth Edition.* Washington, DC: American Psychiatric Association.

Andreasen, NC (2007): DSM and the death of phenomenology in America: an example of unintended consequences. *Schizophr Bull* 33: 108–112.

Bierce, A (1911): *The Devil's Dictionary.* New York: Oxford University Press.

Darwin, C (1859): *The Origin of Species:* New York: Signet Classic (2003 edition).

Freud, S (1949): *An Outline of Psycho-analysis:* Strachey, J, translator. New York: WW Norton & Company.

Galatzer-Levy, IR, Galatzer-Levy, RM (2007): The revolution in psychiatric diagnosis: problems at the foundations. *Perspect Biol Med* 50: 161–180.

Insel, TR, Quirion, R (2005): Psychiatry as a clinical neuroscience discipline. *JAMA* 294: 2221–2224.

Jensen, PS, Hoagwood, K (1997): The book of names: DSM-IV in context. *Dev Psychopathol* 9: 231–249.

Kandel, ER (1998): A new intellectual framework for psychiatry. *Am J Psychiatry* 155: 457–469.

Kendler, KS (2005): Toward a philosophical structure for psychiatry. *Am J Psychiatry* 162: 433–440.

Malmberg, L, Fenton, M (2001): Individual psychodynamic psychotherapy and psychoanalysis for schizophrenia and severe mental illness. *Cochrane Database Syst Rev:* CD001360.

Richards, RJ (1992): The structure of narrative explanation in history and biology. In: Nitecki, MH, Nitecki, DV, eds. *History and Evolution.* Albany: State University of New York Press, pp. 19–53.

Rieff, P (1979): *Freud, the Mind of the Moralist.* Chicago: University of Chicago Press.

Shorter, E (1996): *A History of Psychiatry: From the Era of the Asylum to the Age of Prozac.* New York: John Wiley & Sons.

Thomas, L (1974): *The Lives of a Cell: Notes of a Biology Watcher.* New York: Viking Press.

van Praag, HM (1997): Over the mainstream: diagnostic requirements for biological psychiatric research. *Psychiatry Res* 72: 201–212.

Watson, JD, Crick, FH (1953): Genetical implications of the structure of deoxyribo-nucleic acid. *Nature* 171: 964–967.

Widiger, TA, Clark, LA (2000): Toward DSM-V and the classification of psychopathology. *Psychol Bull* 126: 946–963.

Wittchen, HU (1996): Critical issues in the evaluation of comorbidity of psychiatric disorders. *Br J Psychiatry Suppl* 30: 9–16.

CHAPTER ONE: Organic Mind

Buonomano, DV, Merzenich, MM (1998): Cortical plasticity: from synapses to maps. *Annu Rev Neurosci* 21: 149–186.

Cardinal, RN, Parkinson, JA, Hall, J, Everitt, BJ (2002): Emotion and motivation: the role of the amygdala, ventral striatum, and prefrontal cortex. *Neurosci Biobehav Rev* 26: 321–352.

Castro-Alamancos, MA, Connors, BW (1997): Distinct forms of short-term plasticity at excitatory synapses of hippocampus and neocortex. *Proc Natl Acad Sci USA* 94: 4161–4166.

Charney, DS (2003): Neuroanatomical circuits modulating fear and anxiety behaviors. *Acta Psychiatr Scand Suppl*: 38–50.

Charney, DS, Grillon, C, Bremner, JD (1998): Review: the neurobiological basis of anxiety and fear: circuits, mechanisms, and neurochemical interactions (part I). *The Neuroscientist* 4: 35–44.

Chklovskii, DB, Mel, BW, Svoboda, K (2004): Cortical rewiring and information storage. *Nature* 431: 782–788.

Churchland, PM (1994): *Matter and Consciousness: A Contemporary Introduction to the Philosophy of Mind.* Cambridge: MIT Press.

Critchley, HD (2005): Neural mechanisms of autonomic, affective, and cognitive integration. *J Comp Neurol* 493: 154–166.

Critchley, HD, Wiens, S, Rotshtein, P, Ohman, A, Dolan, RJ (2004): Neural systems supporting interoceptive awareness. *Nat Neurosci* 7: 189–195.

Davidson, RJ, Irwin, W (1999): The functional neuroanatomy of emotion and affective style. *Trends Cogn Sci* 3: 11–21.

Davidson, RJ, Putnam, KM, Larson, CL (2000): Dysfunction in the neural circuitry of emotion regulation—a possible prelude to violence. *Science* 289: 591–594.

Eichenbaum, H (2000): A cortical-hippocampal system for declarative memory. *Nat Rev Neurosci* 1: 41–50.

Fingelkurts, AA, Fingelkurts, AA, Kahkonen, S (2005): Functional connectivity in the brain—is it an elusive concept? *Neurosci Biobehav Rev* 28: 827–836.

Groenewegen, HJ, Uylings, HB (2000): The prefrontal cortex and the integration of sensory, limbic and autonomic information. *Prog Brain Res* 126: 3–28.

Holscher, C (2003): Time, space and hippocampal functions. *Rev Neurosci* 14: 253–284.

Hurley, LM, Devilbiss, DM, Waterhouse, BD (2004): A matter of focus: monoaminergic modulation of stimulus coding in mammalian sensory networks. *Curr Opin Neurobiol* 14: 488–495.

Jackson, F (1986): What Mary didn't know. *The Journal of Philosophy*: 291–295.

Jessop, DS (1999): Stimulatory and inhibitory regulators of the hypothalamo-pituitary-adrenocortical axis. *Baillieres Best Pract Res Clin Endocrinol Metab* 13: 491–501.

Johnson, MH (2001): Functional brain development in humans. *Nat Rev Neurosci* 2: 475–483.

Jones, EG (2001): The thalamic matrix and thalamocortical synchrony. *Trends Neurosci* 24: 595–601.

Kandel, ER (2001): The molecular biology of memory storage: a dialogue between genes and synapses. *Science* 294: 1030–1038.

Mann, JJ (2003): Neurobiology of suicidal behaviour. *Nat Rev Neurosci* 4: 819–828.

McEwen, BS (1998): Stress, adaptation, and disease: allostasis and allostatic load. *Ann NY Acad Sci* 840: 33–44.

McEwen, BS (2003): Mood disorders and allostatic load. *Biol Psychiatry* 54: 200–207.

McHugh, PR, Slavney, PR (1998): *The Perspectives of Psychiatry*. 2nd ed. Baltimore: Johns Hopkins University Press.

Miresco, MJ, Kirmayer, LJ (2006): The persistence of mind-brain dualism in psychiatric reasoning about clinical scenarios. *Am J Psychiatry* 163: 913–918.

Nagel, T (1974): What is it like to be a bat? *The Philosophical Review* 83: 435–450.

Packard, MG, Knowlton, BJ (2002): Learning and memory functions of the basal ganglia. *Annu Rev Neurosci* 25: 563–593.

Pascual-Leone, A, Amedi, A, Fregni, F, Merabet, LB (2005): The plastic human brain cortex. *Annu Rev Neurosci* 28: 377–401.

Paus, T (2001): Primate anterior cingulate cortex: where motor control, drive and cognition interface. *Nat Rev Neurosci* 2: 417–424.

Phelps, EA (2004): Human emotion and memory: interactions of the amygdala and hippocampal complex. *Curr Opin Neurobiol* 14: 198–202.

Price, JL (1999): Prefrontal cortical networks related to visceral function and mood. *Ann NY Acad Sci* 877: 383–396.

Robbins, TW (1997): Arousal systems and attentional processes. *Biol Psychol* 45: 57–71.

Rossi, EL (1996): The psychobiology of mind-body communication: the complex, self-organizing field of information transduction. *Biosystems* 38: 199–206.

Saper, CB (2002): The central autonomic nervous system: conscious visceral perception and autonomic pattern generation. *Annu Rev Neurosci* 25: 433–469.

Sapolsky, RM (1996): Why stress is bad for your brain. *Science* 273: 749–750.

Sarter, M, Bruno, JP (2000): Cortical cholinergic inputs mediating arousal, attentional processing and dreaming: differential afferent regulation of the basal forebrain by telencephalic and brainstem afferents. *Neuroscience* 95: 933–952.

Sawa, A, Snyder, SH (2002): Schizophrenia: diverse approaches to a complex disease. *Science* 296: 692–695.

Schildkraut, JJ (1965): The catecholamine hypothesis of affective disorders: a review of supporting evidence. *Am J Psychiatry* 122: 509–522.

Shortliffe, EH, Buchanan, BG, Feigenbaum, EA (1979): Knowledge engineering for medical decision making: a review of computer-based clinical decision aids. *Proceedings of the IEEE* 67: 1207–1224.

Sprague, RG, Power, MH (1950): Observations on the physiologic effects of cortisone and ACTH in man. *Arch Intern Med (Chic)* 85: 199–258.

Steckler, T, Holsboer, F, Reul, JM (1999): Glucocorticoids and depression. *Baillieres Best Pract Res Clin Endocrinol Metab* 13: 597–614.

Sullivan, GM, Coplan, JD, Kent, JM, Gorman, JM (1999): The noradrenergic system in pathological anxiety: a focus on panic with relevance to generalized anxiety and phobias. *Biol Psychiatry* 46: 1205–1218.

Weiss, JM (1970): Somatic effects of predictable and unpredictable shock. *Psychosom Med* 32: 397–408.

Wise, RA (2008): Dopamine and reward: the anhedonia hypothesis 30 years on. *Neurotox Res* 14: 169–183.

CHAPTER TWO: Elementary Mind

Abed, RT, de Pauw, KW (1998): An evolutionary hypothesis for obsessive compulsive disorder: a psychological immune system? *Behav Neurol* 11: 245–250.

Allen, P, Laroi, F, McGuire, PK, Aleman, A (2008): The hallucinating brain: a review of structural and functional neuroimaging studies of hallucinations. *Neurosci Biobehav Rev* 32: 175–191.

Aston-Jones, G, Cohen, JD (2005): An integrative theory of locus coeruleus-norepinephrine function: adaptive gain and optimal performance. *Annu Rev Neurosci* 28: 403–450.

Aybek, S, Kanaan, RA, David, AS (2008): The neuropsychiatry of conversion disorder. *Curr Opin Psychiatry* 21: 275–280.

Bass, C, Gardner, W (1985): Emotional influences on breathing and breathlessness. *J Psychosom Res* 29: 599–609.

Behrendt, RP (2006): Dysregulation of thalamic sensory "transmission" in schizophrenia: neurochemical vulnerability to hallucinations. *J Psychopharmacol* 20: 356–372.

Berkowitz, L (1989): Frustration-aggression hypothesis: examination and reformulation. Psychological Bulletin 106: 59–73.

Berridge, KC (2004): Motivation concepts in behavioral neuroscience. *Physiol Behav* 81: 179–209.

Bishop, ER, Jr., Holt, AR (1980): Pseudopsychosis: a reexamination of the concept of hysterical psychosis. *Compr Psychiatry* 21: 150–161.

Boksem, MAS, Tops, M (2008): Mental fatigue: costs and benefits. *Brain Research Reviews* 59: 125–139.

Bongers, ME, Tabbers, MM, Benninga, MA (2007): Functional nonretentive fecal incontinence in children. *J Pediatr Gastroenterol Nutr* 44: 5–13.

Botvinick, MM (2008): Hierarchical models of behavior and prefrontal function. *Trends Cogn Sci* 12: 201–208.

Broberger, C (2005): Brain regulation of food intake and appetite: molecules and networks. *J Intern Med* 258: 301–327.

Campbell, N, Boustani, M, Limbil, T, Ott, C, Fox, C, Maidment, I, Schubert, CC, Munger, S, Fick, D, Miller, D, Gulati, R (2009): The cognitive impact of cholinergics: a clinical review. *Clin Interv Aging* 4: 225–233.

Cavedini, P, Gorini, A, Bellodi, L (2006): Understanding obsessive-compulsive disorder: focus on decision making. *Neuropsychol Rev* 16: 3–15.

Chaudhuri, A, Behan, PO (2004): Fatigue in neurological disorders. *The Lancet* 363: 978–988.

Corbetta, M, Shulman, GL (2002): Control of goal-directed and stimulus-driven attention in the brain. *Nat Rev Neurosci* 3: 201–215.

Critchley, HD (2005): Neural mechanisms of autonomic, affective, and cognitive integration. *J Comp Neurol* 493: 154–166.

Eaton, LF, Menolascino, FJ (1982): Psychiatric disorders in the mentally retarded: types, problems, and challenges. *Am J Psychiatry* 139: 1297–1303.

Eilam, D, Zor, R, Szechtman, H, Hermesh, H (2006): Rituals, stereotypy and compulsive behavior in animals and humans. *Neurosci Biobehav Rev* 30: 456–471.

Eriksson, PS, Wallin, L (2004): Functional consequences of stress-related suppression of adult hippocampal neurogenesis—a novel hypothesis on the neurobiology of burnout. *Acta Neurol Scand* 110: 275–280.

Esch, T, Stefano, GB (2004): The neurobiology of pleasure, reward processes, addiction and their health implications. *Neuro Endocrinol Lett* 25: 235–251.

Fagan, PJ (2004): *Sexual Disorders: Perspectives on Diagnosis and Treatment*. Baltimore: Johns Hopkins University Press.

Farah, MJ (1992): Agnosia. *Curr Opin Neurobiol* 2: 162–164.

Gelenberg, AJ (1976): The catatonic syndrome. *Lancet* 1 (7973): 1339–1341.

Glicklich, LB (1951): An historical account of enuresis. *Pediatrics* 8: 859–876.

Gould, SJ (1981): *The Mismeasure of Man*. New York: Norton.

Grafton, ST, Hamilton, AF (2007): Evidence for a distributed hierarchy of action representation in the brain. *Hum Mov Sci* 26: 590–616.

Graybiel, AM (2008): Habits, rituals, and the evaluative brain. *Annu Rev Neurosci* 31: 359–387.

Gross, RG, Grossman, M (2008): Update on apraxia. *Curr Neurol Neurosci Re.* 8: 490–496.

Harvey, SB, Stanton, BR, David, AS (2006): Conversion disorder: towards a neurobiological understanding. *Neuropsychiatr Dis Treat* 2: 13–20.

Hoebel, BG (1997): Neuroscience and appetitive behavior research: 25 years. *Appetite* 29: 119–133.

Hubel, DH (1982): Exploration of the primary visual cortex, 1955–78. *Nature* 299: 515–524.

Johnson, AK, Thunhorst, RL (1997): The neuroendocrinology of thirst and salt appetite: visceral sensory signals and mechanisms of central integration. *Front Neuroendocrinol* 18: 292–353.

Joliot, M, Ribary, U, Llinas, R (1994): Human oscillatory brain activity near 40 Hz coexists with cognitive temporal binding. *Proc Natl Acad Sci USA* 91: 11748–11751.

Jones, BE (2003): Arousal systems. *Front Biosci* 8: s438–s451.

Kakei, S, Hoffman, DS, Strick, PL (1999): Muscle and movement representations in the primary motor cortex. *Science* 285: 2136–2139.

Katz, LC, Crowley, JC (2002): Development of cortical circuits: lessons from ocular dominance columns. *Nat Rev Neurosci* 3: 34–42.

Kertesz, A, Hooper, P (1982): Praxis and language: the extent and variety of apraxia in aphasia. *Neuropsychologia* 20: 275–286.

Kurtz, MM (2006): Symptoms versus neurocognitive skills as correlates of everyday functioning in severe mental illness. *Expert Rev Neurother* 6: 47–56.

Lang, PJ, Davis, M (2006): Emotion, motivation, and the brain: reflex foundations in animal and human research. *Prog Brain Res* 156: 3–29.

Lindenmayer, JP (2000): The pathophysiology of agitation. *J Clin Psychiatry* 61 Suppl 14: 5–10.

Livingstone, M, Hubel, D (1988): Segregation of form, color, movement, and depth: anatomy, physiology, and perception. *Science* 240: 740–749.

Llinas, R, Ribary, U (1993): Coherent 40-Hz oscillation characterizes dream state in humans. *Proc Natl Acad Sci USA* 90: 2078–2081.

Llinas, R, Ribary, U (2001): Consciousness and the brain: the thalamocortical dialogue in health and disease. *Ann NY Acad Sci* 929: 166–175.

Lowe, MR, Butryn, ML (2007): Hedonic hunger: a new dimension of appetite? *Physiology & Behavior* 91: 432–439.

Mataix-Cols, D, Rauch, SL, Baer, L, Eisen, JL, Shera, DM, Goodman, WK, Rasmussen, SA, Jenike, MA (2002): Symptom stability in adult obsessive-compulsive disorder: data from a naturalistic two-year follow-up study. *Am J Psychiatry* 159: 263–268.

Meston, CM, Frohlich, PF (2000): The neurobiology of sexual function. *Arch Gen Psychiatry* 57: 1012–1030.

Mesulam, MM (1998): From sensation to cognition. *Brain* 121 (pt 6): 1013–1052.

Montague, PR, Berns, GS (2002): Neural economics and the biological substrates of valuation. *Neuron* 36: 265–284.

Moscarelli, M (2009): Passive and active schizophrenia: toward a new descriptive micropsychopathology. *Schizophr Bull* 35: 1183–1196.

Moskowitz, AK (2004): "Scared stiff": catatonia as an evolutionary-based fear response. *Psychol Rev* 111: 984–1002.

Neisser, U, Boodoo, G, Bouchard, TJ, Boykin, AW, Brody, N, Ceci, SJ, Halpern, DF, Loehlin, JC, Perloff, R, Sternberg, RJ, Urbina, S (1997): Intelligence: knowns and unknowns. *Annual Progress in Child Psychiatry and Child Development*: 95–133.

Neubauer, AC, Fink, A (2009): Intelligence and neural efficiency. *Neurosci Biobehav Rev* 33: 1004–1023.

Neubauer, DN (2003): *Understanding Sleeplessness: Perspectives on Insomnia*. Baltimore: Johns Hopkins University Press.

Northoff, G (2002): What catatonia can tell us about "top-down modulation": a neuropsychiatric hypothesis. *Behav Brain Sci* 25: 555–577.

Norton, JW, Corbett, JJ. (2000): Visual perceptual abnormalities: hallucinations and illusions. *Semin Neurol* 20: 111–121.

Orford, J (2001): Addiction as excessive appetite. *Addiction* 96: 15–31.

Penfield, W (1975): *The Mystery of the Mind: A Critical Study of Consciousness and the Human Brain*. Princeton, NJ: Princeton University Press.

Pfaff, D, Westberg, L, Kow, LM (2005): Generalized arousal of mammalian central nervous system. *J Comp Neurol* 493: 86–91.

Polk, TA, Simen, P, Lewis, RL, Freedman, E (2002): A computational approach to control in complex cognition. *Brain Res Cogn Brain Res* 15: 71–83.

Rizzolatti, G, Luppino, G (2001): The cortical motor system. *Neuron* 31: 889–901.

Robbins, TW (1997): Arousal systems and attentional processes. *Biol Psychol* 45: 57–71.

Rolls, BJ, Hetherington, M, Burley, VJ (1988): Sensory stimulation and energy density in the development of satiety. *Physiol Behav* 44: 727–733.

Ross, CA (1991): CNS arousal systems: possible role in delirium. *Int Psychogeriatr* 3: 353–371.

Saper, CB, Chou, TC, Elmquist, JK (2002): The need to feed: homeostatic and hedonic control of eating. *Neuron* 36: 199–211.

Saper, CD, Scammell, TE, Lu, J (2005): Hypothalamic regulation of sleep and circadian rhythms. *Nature* 7063: 1257–1263.

Seidman, SN, Rieder, RO (1994): A review of sexual behavior in the United States. *Am J Psychiatry* 151: 330–341.

Siddiqi, N, House, AO, Holmes, JD (2006): Occurrence and outcome of delirium in medical in-patients: a systematic literature review. *Age Ageing* 35: 350–364.

Smith, RP (1981): Boredom: a review. *Human Factors: The Journal of the Human Factors and Ergonomics Society* 23: 329–340.

Stellar, E (1954): The physiology of motivation. *Psychol Rev* 61: 5–22.

Stone, J, Smyth, R, Carson, A, Lewis, S, Prescott, R, Warlow, C, Sharpe, M (2005): Systematic review of misdiagnosis of conversion symptoms and "hysteria." *BMJ* 331: 989.

Strik, W, Dierks, T (2008): Neurophysiological mechanisms of psychotic symptoms. *Eur Arch Psychiatry Clin Neurosci* 258 Suppl 5: 66–70.

Sutcliffe, JG, de Lecea, L (2002): The hypocretins: setting the arousal threshold. *Nat Rev Neurosci* 3: 339–329.

Swanson, LW (2000): Cerebral hemisphere regulation of motivated behavior. *Brain Research* 886: 113–164.

Szasz, TS (1951): Physiologic and psychodynamic mechanisms in constipation and diarrhea. *Psychosom Med* 13: 112–116.

Thompson, WG (1984): The irritable bowel. *Gut* 25: 305–320.

Wheaton, LA, Hallett, M (2007): Ideomotor apraxia: a review. *J Neurol Sci* 260: 1–10.

CHAPTER THREE: Integral Mind

Ainsworth, MD (1962): The effects of maternal deprivation: a review of findings and controversy in the context of research strategy. *Public Health Pap* 14: 97–165.

Alexander, GE, DeLong, MR, Strick, PL (1986): Parallel organization of functionally segregated circuits linking basal ganglia and cortex. *Annu Rev Neurosci* 9: 357–381.

Alvarez, JA, Emory, E (2006): Executive function and the frontal lobes: a meta-analytic review. *Neuropsychol Rev* 16: 17–42.

Anisman, H, Matheson, K (2005): Stress, depression, and anhedonia: caveats concerning animal models. *Neurosci Biobehav Rev* 29: 525–546.

Austin, DW, Richards, JC (2001): The catastrophic misinterpretation model of panic disorder. *Behaviour Research and Therapy* 39: 1277–1291.

Benedetti, F, Mayberg, HS, Wager, TD, Stohler, CS, Zubieta, JK (2005): Neurobiological mechanisms of the placebo effect. *J Neurosci* 25: 10390–10402.

Berridge, KC (2004): Motivation concepts in behavioral neuroscience. *Physiology & Behavior* 81: 179–209.

Berridge, KC, Kringelbach, ML (2008): Affective neuroscience of pleasure: reward in humans and animals. *Psychopharmacology (Berl)* 199: 457–480.

Blanchard, DC, Blanchard, RJ (2003): What can animal aggression research tell us about human aggression? *Horm Behav* 44: 171–177.

Bouton, ME, Mineka, S, Barlow, DH (2001): A modern learning theory perspective on the etiology of panic disorder. *Psychol Rev* 108: 4–32.

Bracha, HS, Bracha, AS, Williams, AE, Ralston, TC, Matsukawa, JM (2005): The human fear-circuitry and fear-induced fainting in healthy individuals—the paleolithic-threat hypothesis. *Clin Auton Res* 15: 238–241.

Bradford, JM (2001): The neurobiology, neuropharmacology, and pharmacological treatment of the paraphilias and compulsive sexual behaviour. *Can J Psychiatry* 46: 26–34.

Braff, DL, Geyer, MA, Swerdlow, NR (2001): Human studies of prepulse inhibition of startle: normal subjects, patient groups, and pharmacological studies. *Psychopharmacology (Berl)* 156: 234–258.

Brewin, CR (2001): A cognitive neuroscience account of posttraumatic stress disorder and its treatment. *Behav Res Ther* 39: 373–393.

Bridger, WH (1961): Sensory habituation and discrimination in the human neonate. *Am J Psychiatry* 117: 991–996.

Cannon, WB (1927): The James-Lange theory of emotions: a critical examination and an alternative theory. By Walter B. Cannon, 1927. *Am J Psychol* 100: 567–586.

Cardinal, RN, Parkinson, JA, Hall, J, Everitt, BJ (2002): Emotion and motivation: the role of the amygdala, ventral striatum, and prefrontal cortex. *Neurosci Biobehav Rev* 26: 321–352.

Castellanos, FX, Tannock, R (2002): Neuroscience of attention-deficit/hyperactivity disorder: the search for endophenotypes. *Nature Reviews Neuroscience* 3: 617–628.

Clarke, DM, Kissane, DW (2002): Demoralization: its phenomenology and importance. *Aust NZ J Psychiatry* 36: 733–742.

Comings, DE, Blum, K (2000): Reward deficiency syndrome: genetic aspects of behavioral disorders. *Prog Brain Res* 126: 325–341.

Cooper, JL, Morrison, TL, Bigman, OL, Abramowitz, SI, Levin, S, Krener, P (1988): Mood changes and affective disorder in the bulimic binge-purge cycle. *International Journal of Eating Disorders* 7: 469–474.

Cota, D, Tschöp, MH, Horvath, TL, Levine, AS (2006): Cannabinoids, opioids and eating behavior: the molecular face of hedonism? *Brain Research Reviews* 51: 85–107.

Cummings, JL (1986): Subcortical dementia. Neuropsychology, neuropsychiatry, and pathophysiology. *Br J Psychiatry* 149: 682–697.

Cummings, JL (1993): Frontal-subcortical circuits and human behavior. *Arch Neurol* 50: 873–880.

Damasio, AR (1999): *The Feeling of What Happens: Body and Emotion in the Making of Consciousness.* New York: Harcourt Brace.

Damasio, H, Grabowski, T, Frank, R, Galaburda, AM, Damasio, AR (1994): The return of Phineas Gage: clues about the brain from the skull of a famous patient. *Science* 264: 1102–1105.

Davis, C, Claridge, G (1998): The eating disorders as addiction: a psychobiological perspective. *Addictive Behaviors* 23: 463–475.

Davis, M (1998): Are different parts of the extended amygdala involved in fear versus anxiety? *Biol Psychiatry* 44: 1239–1247.

Delgado, MR, Olsson, A, Phelps, EA (2006): Extending animal models of fear conditioning to humans. *Biol Psychol* 73: 39–48.

Depue, RA, Iacono, WG (1989): Neurobehavioral aspects of affective disorders. *Annu Rev Psychol* 40: 457–492.

D'Esposito, M (2007). From cognitive to neural models of working memory. *Philos Trans R Soc Lond B Biol Sci* 362:761–772.

Domjan, M (2005): Pavlovian conditioning: a functional perspective. *Annu Rev Psychol* 56: 179–206.

Donahoe, J (1999): Edward L. Thorndike: the selectionist connectionist. *J Exp Anal Behav* 72: 451–454.

Ehlers, A, Hackmann, A, Michael, T (2004): Intrusive re-experiencing in post-traumatic stress disorder: phenomenology, theory, and therapy. *Memory* 12: 403–415.

Escobar, M, Miller, RR (2004): A review of the empirical laws of basic learning in Pavlovian conditioning. *International Journal of Comparative Psychology* 17: 279–303.

Everitt, BJ, Parkinson, JA, Olmstead, MC, Arroyo, M, Robledo, P, Robbins, TW (1999): Associative processes in addiction and reward: the role of amygdala-ventral striatal subsystems. *Ann NY Acad Sci* 877: 412–438.

Fagan, PJ, Wise, TN, Schmidt, CW, Jr., Berlin, FS (2002): Pedophilia. *JAMA* 288: 2458–2465.

Fawcett, J, Busch, KA, Jacobs, D, Kravitz, HM, Fogg, L (1997): Suicide: a four-pathway clinical-biochemical model. *Ann NY Acad Sci* 836: 288–301.

Feldman, CM (1997): Childhood precursors of adult interpartner violence. *Clinical Psychology: Science and Practice* 4: 307–334.

Feldman, MD (1988): The challenge of self-mutilation: a review. *Compr Psychiatry* 29: 252–269.

Fellows, LK (2007): Advances in understanding ventromedial prefrontal function: the accountant joins the executive. *Neurology* 68: 991–995.

Fendt, M, Fanselow, MS (1999): The neuroanatomical and neurochemical basis of conditioned fear. *Neurosci Biobehav Rev* 23: 743–760.

Frank, JD (1974): Psychotherapy: the restoration of morale. *Am J Psychiatry* 131: 271–274.

Freeman, D (2007): Suspicious minds: the psychology of persecutory delusions. *Clinical Psychology Review* 27: 425–457.

Garety, PA, Hemsley, DR, Wessely, S (1991): Reasoning in deluded schizophrenic and paranoid patients: biases in performance on a probabilistic inference task. *J Nerv Ment Dis* 179: 194–201.

Goodman, A (2008): Neurobiology of addiction: an integrative review. *Biochem Pharmacol* 75: 266–322.

Grillon, C (2008): Models and mechanisms of anxiety: evidence from startle studies. *Psychopharmacology (Berl)* 199: 421–437.

Harris, EC, Barraclough, B (1997): Suicide as an outcome for mental disorders. A meta-analysis. *Br J Psychiatry* 170: 205–228.

Haslam, N (2006): Dehumanization: an integrative review. *Personality and Social Psychology Review* 10: 252–264.

Hermans, D, Craske, MG, Mineka, S, Lovibond, PF (2006): Extinction in human fear conditioning. *Biol Psychiatry* 60: 361–368.

Hinson, JM, Jameson, TL, Whitney, P (2003): Impulsive decision making and working memory. *J Exp Psychol Learn Mem Cogn* 29: 298–306.

Holtzworth-Munroe, A, Stuart, GL (1994): Typologies of male batterers: three subtypes and the differences among them. *Psychological Bulletin* 116: 476–497.

Hyman, SE, Malenka, RC, Nestler, EJ (2006): Neural mechanisms of addiction: the role of reward-related learning and memory. *Annu Rev Neurosci* 29: 565–598.

James, W (1884): What is an emotion? *Mind*: 188–205.

John, ER (2001): A field theory of consciousness. *Conscious Cogn* 10: 184–213.

Johnson, SL (2005): Mania and dysregulation in goal pursuit: a review. *Clinical Psychology Review* 25: 241–262.

Joiner, TE, Jr., Brown, JS, Wingate, LR (2005): The psychology and neurobiology of suicidal behavior. *Annu Rev Psychol* 56: 287–314.

Kelley, AE, Berridge, KC (2002): The neuroscience of natural rewards: relevance to addictive drugs. *J Neurosci* 22: 3306–3311.

Kihlstrom, JF (1997): Hypnosis, memory and amnesia. *Philos Trans R Soc Lond B Biol Sci* 352: 1727–1732.

Klonsky, ED (2007): The functions of deliberate self-injury: a review of the evidence. *Clinical Psychology Review* 27: 226–239.

Knudsen, EI (2007): Fundamental components of attention. *Annu Rev Neurosci* 30: 57–78.

Koob, GF, Le Moal, M (2008): Review: Neurobiological mechanisms for opponent motivational processes in addiction. *Philos Trans R Soc Lond B Biol Sci* 363: 3113–3123.

Kopelman, MD (1987): Amnesia: organic and psychogenic. *Br J Psychiatry* 150: 428–442.

Korte, SM (2001): Corticosteroids in relation to fear, anxiety and psychopathology. *Neurosci Biobehav Rev* 25: 117–142.

LaBar, KS, Cabeza, R (2006): Cognitive neuroscience of emotional memory. *Nat Rev Neurosci* 7: 54–64.

Lang, PJ, Davis, M (2006): Emotion, motivation, and the brain: reflex foundations in animal and human research. *Prog Brain Res* 156: 3–29.

Lang, PJ, Davis, M, Ohman, A (2000): Fear and anxiety: animal models and human cognitive psychophysiology. *J Affect Disord* 61: 137–159.

Levy, R, Dubois, B (2006): Apathy and the functional anatomy of the prefrontal cortex-basal ganglia circuits. *Cereb Cortex* 16: 916–928.

Loftus, EF, Davis, D (2006): Recovered memories. *Annu Rev Clin Psychol* 2: 469–498.

Maren, S (2005): Building and burying fear memories in the brain. *Neuroscientist* 11: 89–99.

Marin, RS (1991): Apathy: a neuropsychiatric syndrome. *J Neuropsychiatry Clin Neurosci* 3: 243–254.

Matsumoto, M, Hikosaka, O (2009): Two types of dopamine neuron distinctly convey positive and negative motivational signals. *Nature* 459: 837–841.

McNally, RJ (2005): Debunking myths about trauma and memory. *Can J Psychiatry* 50: 817–822.

Moscicki, EK (1997): Identification of suicide risk factors using epidemiologic studies. *Psychiatric Clinics of North America* 20: 499–517.

Moscovitch, M, Rosenbaum, RS, Gilboa, A, Addis, DR, Westmacott, R, Grady, C, McAndrews, MP, Levine, B, Black, S, Winocur, G, Nadel, L (2005): Functional neuroanatomy of remote episodic, semantic and spatial memory: a unified account based on multiple trace theory. *J Anat* 207: 35–66.

Munroe, RL, Gauvain, M (2001): Why the paraphilias? domesticating strange sex. *Cross-Cultural Research* 35: 44–64.

Naranjo, CA, Tremblay, LK, Busto, UE (2001): The role of the brain reward system in depression. *Prog Neuropsychopharmacol Biol Psychiatry* 25: 781–823.

Ofshe, R, Watters, E (1998): Making monsters. *Society* 35: 364–376.

Parfitt, D.N. (1944): Psychogenic amnesia: the refusal to remember. *Journal of Mental Science* 90:511–531.

Pizzagalli, DA, Jahn, AL, O'Shea, JP (2005): Toward an objective characterization of an anhedonic phenotype: a signal-detection approach. *Biol Psychiatry* 57: 319–327.

Reiss, S (1987): Theoretical perspectives on the fear of anxiety. *Clinical Psychology Review* 7: 585–596.

Rescorla, RA, Solomon, RL (1967): Two-process learning theory: relationships between Pavlovian conditioning and instrumental learning. *Psychol Rev* 74: 151–182.

Rinehart, NJ, McCabe, MP (1997): Hypersexuality: psychopathology or normal variant of sexuality? *Sexual and Relationship Therapy* 12: 45–60.

Robbins, TW (1997): Arousal systems and attentional processes. *Biol Psychol* 45: 57–71.

Sandman, CA, Hetrick, WP (1995): Opiate mechanisms in self-injury. *Mental Retardation and Developmental Disabilities Research Reviews* 1: 130–136.

Schacter, DL (1999): The seven sins of memory: insights from psychology and cognitive neuroscience. *Am Psychol* 54: 182–203.

Schachter, S, Singer, JE (1962): Cognitive, social, and physiological determinants of emotional state. *Psychol Rev* 69: 379–399.

Schultz, W (2006): Behavioral theories and the neurophysiology of reward. *Annu Rev Psychol* 57: 87–115.

Schultz, W, Tremblay, L, Hollerman, JR (1998): Reward prediction in primate basal ganglia and frontal cortex. *Neuropharmacology* 37: 421–429.

Seiden, RH (1978): Where are they now? A follow-up study of suicide attempters from the Golden Gate Bridge. *Suicide Life Threat Behav* 8: 203–216.

Seligman, ME (1972): Learned helplessness. *Annu Rev Med* 23: 407–412.

Seymour, B, O'Doherty, JP, Koltzenburg, M, Wiech, K, Frackowiak, R, Friston, K, Donlan R (2005): Opponent appetitive-aversive neural processes underlie predictive learning of pain relief. *Nat Neurosci* 8: 1234–1240.

Shumake, J, Gonzalez-Lima, F (2003): Brain systems underlying susceptibility to helplessness and depression. *Behav Cogn Neurosci Rev* 2: 198–221.

Simo, LS, Krisky, CM, Sweeney, JA (2005): Functional neuroanatomy of anticipatory behavior: dissociation between sensory-driven and memory-driven systems. *Cereb Cortex* 15: 1982–1991.

Sinha, R (2008): Chronic stress, drug use, and vulnerability to addiction. *Ann NY Acad Sci* 1141: 105–130.

Sodersten, P, Bergh, C, Zandian, M (2006): Understanding eating disorders. *Hormones and Behavior* 50: 572–578.

Southwick, SM, Bremner, JD, Rasmusson, A, Morgan, CA, III, Arnsten, A, Charney, DS (1999): Role of norepinephrine in the pathophysiology and treatment of posttraumatic stress disorder. *Biol Psychiatry* 46: 1192–1204.

Spitzer, RL (1981): The diagnostic status of homosexuality in DSM-III: a reformulation of the issues. *Am J Psychiatry* 138: 210–215.

Squire, LR (1986): Memory functions as affected by electroconvulsive therapy. *Ann NY Acad Sci* 462: 307–314.

Squire, LR, Zola, SM (1996): Structure and function of declarative and nondeclarative memory systems. *Proc Natl Acad Sci USA* 93: 13515–13522.

Squire, LR, Zola-Morgan, S (1991): The medial temporal lobe memory system. *Science* 253: 1380–1386.

Staddon, JE, Cerutti, DT (2003): Operant conditioning. *Annu Rev Psychol* 54: 115–144.

Sullivan, GM, Coplan, JD, Kent, JM, Gorman, JM (1999): The noradrenergic system in pathological anxiety: a focus on panic with relevance to generalized anxiety and phobias. *Biol Psychiatry* 46: 1205–1218.

Tononi, G. (2004). An information integration theory of consciousness. *BMC Neurosci* 5: 42.

Tulving, E (2002): Episodic memory: from mind to brain. *Annu Rev Psychol* 53: 1–25.

Wilson, EO (1970): Competitive and aggressive behavior. *Social Science Information* 9: 123–154.

Winchel, RM, Stanley, M (1991): Self-injurious behavior: a review of the behavior and biology of self-mutilation. *Am J Psychiatry* 148: 306–317.

Wise, RA (2008): Dopamine and reward: the anhedonia hypothesis 30 years on. *Neurotox Res* 14: 169–183.

Yarrow, K, Haggard, P, Heal, R, Brown, P, Rothwell, JC (2001): Illusory perceptions of space and time preserve cross-saccadic perceptual continuity. *Nature* 414: 302–305.

Zalcman, SS, Siegel, A (2006): The neurobiology of aggression and rage: role of cytokines. *Brain Behav Immun* 20: 507–514.

Zola, SM (1998): Memory, amnesia, and the issue of recovered memory: neurobiological aspects. *Clin Psychol Rev* 18: 915–932.

Zola-Morgan, S, Squire, LR, Amaral, DG (1986): Human amnesia and the medial temporal region: enduring memory impairment following a bilateral lesion limited to field CA1 of the hippocampus. *J Neurosci* 6: 2950–2967.

CHAPTER FOUR: Synthetic Mind

Ainslie, G (1975): Specious reward: a behavioral theory of impulsiveness and impulse control. *Psychological Bulletin* 82: 463–496.

Ainsworth, MD (1969): Object relations, dependency, and attachment: a theoretical review of the infant-mother relationship. *Child Dev* 40: 969–1025.

Axelrod, R, Hamilton, WD (1981): The evolution of cooperation. *Science* 211: 1390–1396.

Bandura, AA, Ross, D (1961): Transmission of aggression through imitation of aggressive models. *J Abnorm Soc Psychol* 63: 575–582.

Baron-Cohen, S, Leslie, AM, Frith, U (1985): Does the autistic child have a "theory of mind"? *Cognition* 21: 37–46.

Barsky, AJ, Borus, JF (1999): Functional somatic syndromes. *Ann Intern Med* 130: 910–921.

Bartholomew, K (1990): Avoidance of intimacy: an attachment perspective. *Journal of Social and Personal Relationships* 7: 147–178.

Baumeister, RF, Scher, SJ (1988): Self-defeating behavior patterns among normal individuals: review and analysis of common self-destructive tendencies. *Psychol Bull* 104: 3–22.

Bell, V, Halligan, PW, Ellis, HD (2006): Explaining delusions: a cognitive perspective. *Trends in Cognitive Sciences* 10: 219–226.

Bond, R, Smith, PB (1996): Culture and conformity: a meta-analysis of studies using Asch's line judgment task. *Psychological Bulletin* 119: 111–137.

Bowlby, J (1977): The making and breaking of affectional bonds. I. Aetiology and psychopathology in the light of attachment theory. An expanded version of the Fiftieth Maudsley Lecture, delivered before the Royal College of Psychiatrists, 19 November 1976. *Br J Psychiatry* 130: 201–210.

Bushman, BJ, Baumeister, RF (1998): Threatened egotism, narcissism, self-esteem, and direct and displaced aggression: does self-love or self-hate lead to violence? *J Pers Soc Psychol* 75: 219–229.

Campbell, WK, Foster, JD (2007): The narcissistic self: background, an extended agency model, and ongoing controversies. In: Sedikides, C, Sedikides, S, eds. *Frontiers in Social Psychology: The Self*. Philadelphia: Psychology Press.

Ciaranello, AL, Ciaranello, RD (1995): The neurobiology of infantile autism. *Annu Rev Neurosci* 18: 101–128.

Cloninger, CR, Svrakic, DM, Przybeck, TR (1993): A psychobiological model of temperament and character. *Arch Gen Psychiatry* 50: 975–990.

Clore, GL, Huntsinger, JR (2007): How emotions inform judgment and regulate thought. *Trends Cogn Sci* 11: 393–399.

Constantinidis, C, Procyk, E (2004): The primate working memory networks. *Cogn Affect Behav Neurosci* 4: 444–465.

Costa, PT (1991): Clinical use of the five-factor model: an introduction. *J Pers Assess* 57: 393–398.

Crowe, RR (1974): An adoption study of antisocial personality. *Arch Gen Psychiatry* 31: 785–791.

de Waal, FBM (1988): The communicative repertoire of captive bonobos (Pan paniscus), compared to that of chimpanzees. *Behaviour* 106: 183–251.

Dimberg, U, Thunberg, M, Elmehed, K (2000): Unconscious facial reactions to emotional facial expressions. *Psychol Sci* 11: 86–89.

Eakin, PJ (2004): What are we reading when we read autobiography? *Narrative* 12: 121–132.

Fehr, E, Fischbacher, U (2003): The nature of human altruism. *Nature* 425: 785–791.

Feigl, H, Meehl, PE (1974): The determinism-freedom and body-mind problems. In: *The Philosophy of Karl Popper*. LaSalle, IL: Open Court Publishing Co.

Flaherty, AW (2005): Frontotemporal and dopaminergic control of idea generation and creative drive. *J Comp Neurol* 493: 147–153.

Freud, S (1961): *Civilization and Its Discontents*: Strachey, J, translator. New York: WW Norton & Company.

Ghaemi, SN (2004): The perils of belief: delusions reexamined. *Philosophy, Psychiatry, and Psychology* 11: 49–54.

Gilbert, P (2000): The relationship of shame, social anxiety and depression: the role of the evaluation of social rank. *Clinical Psychology & Psychotherapy* 7: 174–189.

Gu, Q (2002): Neuromodulatory transmitter systems in the cortex and their role in cortical plasticity. *Neuroscience* 111: 815–835.

Gunderson, JG, Ridolfi, ME (2001): Borderline personality disorder: suicidality and self-mutilation. *Ann NY Acad Sci* 932: 61–73.

Harlow, HF, Zimmerman, RR (1959): Affectional responses in the infant monkey; orphaned baby monkeys develop a strong and persistent attachment to inanimate surrogate mothers. *Science* 130: 421–432.

Heinrichs, N, Hofmann, SG (2001): Information processing in social phobia: a critical review. *Clinical Psychology Review* 21: 751–770.

Hinshaw, SP, Stier, A (2008): Stigma as related to mental disorders. *Annu Rev Clin Psychol* 4: 367–393.

Hinson, JM, Jameson, TL, Whitney, P (2003): Impulsive decision making and working memory. *J Exp Psychol Learn Mem Cogn* 29: 298–306.

Howarth, E (1988): Mood differences between the four Galen personality types: choleric, sanguine, phlegmatic, melancholic. *Personality and Individual Differences* 9: 173–175.

Hunter, RC, Lohrenz, JG, Schwartzman, AE (1964): Nosophobia and hypochondriasis in medical students. *J Nerv Ment Dis* 139: 147–152.

Insel, TR, Young, LJ (2001): The neurobiology of attachment. *Nat Rev Neurosci* 2: 129–136.

Kagan, J, Snidman, N (1991): Temperamental factors in human development. *The American Psychologist* 46: 856–862.

Kendler, KS, Gardner, CO, Prescott, CA (2003): Personality and the experience of environmental adversity. *Psychol Med* 33: 1193–1202.

Kiehl, KA (2006): A cognitive neuroscience perspective on psychopathy: evidence for paralimbic system dysfunction. *Psychiatry Res* 142: 107–128.

Kihlstrom, JF (1987): The cognitive unconscious. *Science* 237: 1445–1452.

Kihlstrom, JF (2005): Dissociative disorders. *Annu Rev Clin Psychol* 1: 227–253.

Kunert, HJ, Norra, C, Hoff, P (2007): Theories of delusional disorders: an update and review. *Psychopathology* 40: 191–202.

Lakin, JL, Chartrand, TL, Arkin, RM (2008): I am too just like you: nonconscious mimicry as an automatic behavioral response to social exclusion. *Psychol Sci* 19: 816–822.

Lee, KH, Farrow, TF, Spence, SA, Woodruff, PW (2004): Social cognition, brain networks and schizophrenia. *Psychol Med* 34: 391–400.

Lipowski, ZJ (1988): Somatization: the concept and its clinical application. *Am J Psychiatry* 145: 1358–1368.

Loeber, R (1982): The stability of antisocial and delinquent child behavior: a review. *Child Dev* 53: 1431–1446.

Lothstein, LM (1982): Sex reassignment surgery: historical, bioethical, and theoretical issues. *Am J Psychiatry* 139: 417–426.

Lund, FH (1925): The psychology of belief: a study of its emotional, and volitional determinants. *Journal of Abnormal and Social Psychology* 20: 174–196.

Maciejewski, PK, Zhang, B, Block, SD, Prigerson, HG (2007): An empirical examination of the stage theory of grief. *JAMA* 297: 716–723.

McGinn, C (1989): Can we solve the mind–body problem? *Mind* 98: 349–366.

McKenna, PJ (1984): Disorders with overvalued ideas. *Br J Psychiatry* 145: 579–585.

Meltzoff, AN, Kuhl, PK, Movellan, J, Sejnowski, TJ (2009): Foundations for a new science of learning. *Science* 325: 284–288.

Moll, J, Schulkin, J (2009): Social attachment and aversion in human moral cognition. *Neurosci Biobehav Rev* 33: 456–465.

Murstein, BI, Pryer, RS (1959): The concept of projection: a review. *Psychological Bulletin* 56: 353–374.

Pollak, JM (1979): Obsessive-compulsive personality: a review. *Psychological Bulletin* 86: 225–241.

Potter-Efron, RT, Efron, DE (1993): Three models of shame and their relation to the addictive process. *Alcoholism Treatment Quarterly* 10: 23–48.

Pruitt, DG, Kimmel, MJ (1977): Twenty years of experimental gaming: critique, synthesis, and suggestions for the future. *Annual Review of Psychology* 28: 363–392.

Raine, A (2006): Schizotypal personality: neurodevelopmental and psychosocial trajectories. *Annu Rev Clin Psychol* 2: 291–326.

Reddy, V (2003): On being the object of attention: implications for self-other consciousness. *Trends Cogn Sci* 7: 397–402.

Rhodes, J, Gipps, RGT (2008): Delusions, certainty and the background. *Philosophy, Psychiatry, and Psychology* 15: 295–310.

Roberts, G (1992): The origins of delusion. *Br J Psychiatry* 161: 298–308.

Ruch, W (1992): Pavlov's types of nervous system, Eysenck's typology and the Hippocrates-Galen temperaments: an empirical examination of the asserted correspondence of three temperament typologies. *Personality and Individual Differences* 13: 1259–1271.

Rutter, M (1987): Temperament, personality and personality disorder. *British Journal of Psychiatry* 150: 39–83.

Rutter, M, Kreppner, J, Sonuga-Barke, E (2009): Emanuel Miller Lecture: attachment insecurity, disinhibited attachment, and attachment disorders: where do research findings leave the concepts? *J Child Psychol Psychiatry* 50: 529–543.

Saulsman, LM, Page, AC (2004): The five-factor model and personality disorder empirical literature: a meta-analytic review. *Clinical Psychology Review* 23: 1055–1085.

Schnider, A (2003): Spontaneous confabulation and the adaptation of thought to ongoing reality. *Nat Rev Neurosci* 4: 662–671.

Shapiro, D (1965): *Neurotic Styles*. New York: Basic Books.

Sincoff, JB (1990): The psychological characteristics of ambivalent people. *Clinical Psychology Review* 10: 43–68.

Spanos, NP (1994): Multiple identity enactments and multiple personality disorder: a sociocognitive perspective. *Psychol Bull* 116: 143–165.

Spitzer, M (1997): A cognitive neuroscience view of schizophrenic thought disorder. *Schizophr Bull* 23: 29–50.

Spivak, H, Rodin, G, Sutherland, A (1994): The psychology of factitious disorders: a reconsideration. *Psychosomatics* 35: 25–34.

Svrakic, DM, Lecic-Tosevski, D, Divac-Jovanovic, M (2009): DSM axis II: personality disorders or adaptation disorders? *Curr Opin Psychiatry* 22: 111–117.

Tantam, D (1988): Lifelong eccentricity and social isolation. II: Asperger's syndrome or schizoid personality disorder? *Br J Psychiatry* 153: 783–791.

Vazire, S, Funder, DC (2006): Impulsivity and the self-defeating behavior of narcissists. *Personality and Social Psychology Review* 10: 154–165.

Whittle, S, Allen, NB, Lubman, DI, Yucel, M (2006): The neurobiological basis of temperament: towards a better understanding of psychopathology. *Neurosci Biobehav Rev* 30: 511–525.

Wisniewski, AB, Migeon, CJ (2002): Gender identity / role differentiation in adolescents affected by syndromes of abnormal sex differentiation. *Adolesc Med* 13: 119–128.

Young, LJ, Wang, Z (2004): The neurobiology of pair bonding. *Nat Neurosci* 7: 1048–1054.

Zucker, KJ (2005): Gender identity disorder in children and adolescents. *Annu Rev Clin Psychol* 1: 467–492.

CHAPTER FIVE: Psychiatric Mind

Abraham, PF, Calabrese, JR (2008): Evidenced-based pharmacologic treatment of borderline personality disorder: a shift from SSRIs to anticonvulsants and atypical antipsychotics? *J Affect Disord* 111: 21–30.

Arroll, B, Elley, CR, Fishman, T, Goodyear-Smith, FA, Kenealy, T, Blashki, G, Kerse, N, MacGillivray, S. (2009): Antidepressants versus placebo for depression in primary care. *Cochrane Database Syst Rev*: CD007954.

Bailey, JE, Argyropoulos, SV, Kendrick, AH, Nutt, DJ (2005): Behavioral and cardiovascular effects of 7.5% $CO_2$ in human volunteers. *Depress Anxiety* 21: 18–25.

Bauer, M, Alda, M, Priller, J, Young, LT (2003): Implications of the neuroprotective effects of lithium for the treatment of bipolar and neurodegenerative disorders. *Pharmacopsychiatry* 36 Suppl 3: S250–S254.

Campbell, N, Boustani, M, Limbil, T, Ott, C, Fox, C, Maidment, I, Schubert, CC, Munger, S, Fick, D, Miller, D, Gulati, R (2009): The cognitive impact of anticholinergics: a clinical review. *Clin Interv Aging* 4: 225–233.

Cullen, W (1800): *Nosology: or, a systematic arrangement of diseases, by classes, orders, genera, and species: with the distinguishing characters of each, and outlines of the systems of Sauvages, Linnaeus, Vogel, Sagar, and MacBride*: Printed by C. Stewart and Co. for William Creech.

Faraone, SV, Biederman, J, Spencer, TJ, Aleardi, M (2006): Comparing the efficacy of medications for ADHD using meta-analysis. *Med Gen Med* 8: 4.

Frank, JD, Frank, JB (1991): *Persuasion and Healing: A Comparative Study of Psychotherapy*. 3rd ed. Baltimore: Johns Hopkins University Press.

Friedrich, MJ (1999): Lithium: proving its mettle for 50 years. *JAMA* 281: 2271–2273.

Gao, K, Muzina, D, Gajwani, P, Calabrese, JR (2006): Efficacy of typical and atypical antipsychotics for primary and comorbid anxiety symptoms or disorders: a review. *J Clin Psychiatry* 67: 1327–1340.

Gardner, DM, Baldessarini, RJ, Waraich, P (2005): Modern antipsychotic drugs: a critical overview. *CMAJ* 172: 1703–1711.

Geffken, GR, Ward, HE, Staab, JP, Carmichael, SL, Evans, DL (1998): Psychiatric morbidity in endocrine disorders. *Psychiatr Clin North Am* 21: 473–489.

Hall, RCW, Popkin, MK, Stickney, SK, Gardner, ER (1979): Presentation of the steroid psychoses. *The Journal of Nervous and Mental Disease* 167: 229–236.

Kapur, S, Agid, O, Mizrahi, R, Li, M (2006): How antipsychotics work—from receptors to reality. *NeuroRX* 3: 10–21.

Kiehl, KA (2006): A cognitive neuroscience perspective on psychopathy: evidence for paralimbic system dysfunction. *Psychiatry Res* 142: 107–128.

Kramer, PD (1993): *Listening to Prozac*. New York: Viking.

McElroy, SL, Keck, PE, Jr. (2000): Pharmacologic agents for the treatment of acute bipolar mania. *Biol Psychiatry* 48: 539–557.

McHugh, PR, Slavney, PR (1998): *The Perspectives of Psychiatry*. 2nd ed. Baltimore: Johns Hopkins University Press.

Moos, RH (2008): Active ingredients of substance use-focused self-help groups. *Addiction* 103: 387–396.

Ntais, C, Pakos, E, Kyzas, P, Ioannidis, JP (2005): Benzodiazepines for alcohol withdrawal. *Cochrane Database Syst Rev*: CD005063.

Pagnin, D, de, Q, V, Pini, S, Cassano, GB (2004): Efficacy of ECT in depression: a meta-analytic review. *J ECT* 20: 13–20.

Rassovsky, Y, Kushner, MG, Schwarze, NJ, Wangensteen, OD (2000): Psychological and physiological predictors of response to carbon dioxide challenge in individuals with panic disorder. *J Abnorm Psychol* 109: 616–623.

Rosebush, PI, Mazurek, MF (2010): Catatonia and its treatment. *Schizophr Bull* 26: 239–242.

Shanks, M, Kivipelto, M, Bullock, R, Lane, R (2009): Cholinesterase inhibition: is there evidence for disease-modifying effects? *Curr Med Res Opin* 25: 2439–2446.

Snyder, SH (1973): Amphetamine psychosis: a "model" schizophrenia mediated by catecholamines. *Am J Psychiatry* 130: 61–67.

Soomro, GM, Altman, D, Rajagopal, S, Oakley-Browne, M (2008): Selective serotonin re-uptake inhibitors (SSRIs) versus placebo for obsessive compulsive disorder (OCD). *Cochrane Database Syst Rev*: CD001765.

Thase, ME (2002): What role do atypical antipsychotic drugs have in treatment-resistant depression? *J Clin Psychiatry* 63: 95–103.

APPENDIX A: The Official Version

Akiskal, HS, Pinto, O (1999): The evolving bipolar spectrum. Prototypes I, II, III, and IV. *Psychiatr Clin North Am* 22: 517–534.

Akiskal, HS, Bourgeois, ML, Angst, J, Post, R, Moller, H, Hirschfeld, R (2000): Re-evaluating the prevalence of and diagnostic composition within the broad clinical spectrum of bipolar disorders. *J Affect Disord* 59 Suppl 1: S5–S30.

Battaglia, M, Torgersen, S (1996): Schizotypal disorder: at the crossroads of genetics and nosology. *Acta Psychiatr Scand* 94: 303–310.

Boller, F, Bick, K, Duyckaerts, C (2007): They have shaped Alzheimer disease: the protagonists, well known and less well known. *Cortex* 43: 565–569.

Brandes, M, Bienvenu, OJ (2006): Personality and anxiety disorders. *Curr Psychiatry Rep* 8: 263–269.

Chevaleyre, V, Takahashi, KA, Castillo, PE (2006): Endocannabinoid-mediated synaptic plasticity in the CNS. *Annu Rev Neurosci* 29: 37–76.

Cooper, JL, Morrison, TL, Bigman, OL, Abramowitz, SI, Levin, S, Krener, P (1988): Mood changes and affective disorder in the bulimic binge-purge cycle. *International Journal of Eating Disorders* 7: 469–474.

Fahy, TA (1988): The diagnosis of multiple personality disorder: a critical review. *Br J Psychiatry* 153: 597–606.

Faraone, SV, Biederman, J, Spencer, T, Wilens, T, Seidman, LJ, Mick, E, Doyle, AE (2000): Attention-deficit/hyperactivity disorder in adults: an overview. *Biol Psychiatry* 48: 9–20.

Farmer, A, Elkin, A, McGuffin, P (2007): The genetics of bipolar affective disorder. *Curr Opin Psychiatry* 20: 8–12.

Farre, M, Cami, J (1991): Pharmacokinetic considerations in abuse liability evaluation. *Br J Addict* 86: 1601–1606.

Folstein, MF, Folstein, SE, McHugh, PR (1975): "Mini-mental state": a practical method for grading the cognitive state of patients for the clinician. *J Psychiatr Res* 12: 189–198.

Heim, C, Nemeroff, CB (2009): Neurobiology of posttraumatic stress disorder. *CNS Spectr* 14: 13–24.

Hyman, SE (2007): Can neuroscience be integrated into the DSM-V? *Nat Rev Neurosci* 8: 725–732.

Jureidini, J (2004): Does dissociation offer a useful explanation for psychopathology? *Psychopathology* 37: 259–265.

Kaufman, J, Charney, D (2000): Comorbidity of mood and anxiety disorders. *Depress Anxiety* 12 Suppl 1: 69–76.

Lewis, DA, Lieberman, JA (2000): Catching up on schizophrenia: natural history and neurobiology. *Neuron* 28: 325–334.

Lipowski, ZJ (1988): Somatization: the concept and its clinical application. *Am J Psychiatry* 145: 1358–1368.

Lish, JD, Dime-Meenan, S, Whybrow, PC, Price, RA, Hirschfeld, RM (1994): The National Depressive and Manic-depressive Association (DMDA) survey of bipolar members. *J Affect Disord* 31: 281–294.

Mace, NL, Rabins, PV (2001): *The 36-Hour Day: A Family Guide to Caring for Persons with Alzheimer Disease, Related Dementing Illnesses, and Memory Loss in Later Life.* Warner Books.

MacKinnon, DF, Pies, R (2006): Affective instability as rapid cycling: theoretical and clinical implications for borderline personality and bipolar spectrum disorders. *Bipolar Disord* 8: 1–14.

MacKinnon, DF, Zamoiski, R (2006): Panic comorbidity with bipolar disorder: what is the manic-panic connection? *Bipolar Disord* 8: 648–664.

Mataix-Cols, D, Rosario-Campos, MC, Leckman, JF (2005): A multidimensional model of obsessive-compulsive disorder. *Am J Psychiatry* 162: 228–238.

McHugh, PR, Treisman, G (2007): PTSD: a problematic diagnostic category. *J Anxiety Disord* 21: 211–222.

Mellor, CS (1970): First rank symptoms of schizophrenia. I. The frequency in schizophrenics on admission to hospital. II. Differences between individual first rank symptoms. *Br J Psychiatry* 117: 15–23.

Mones, AG (1998): Oppositional children and their families: an adaptational dance in space and time. *Am J Orthopsychiatry* 68: 147–153.

Nestler, EJ, Barrot, M, DiLeone, RJ, Eisch, AJ, Gold, SJ, Monteggia, LM (2002): Neurobiology of depression. *Neuron* 34: 13–25.

O'Hearn, K, Asato, M, Ordaz, S, Luna, B (2008): Neurodevelopment and executive function in autism. *Dev Psychopathol* 20: 1103–1132.

Rabins, PV, Folstein, MF (1982): Delirium and dementia: diagnostic criteria and fatality rates. *Br J Psychiatry* 140: 149–153.

Raine, A (2002): Biosocial studies of antisocial and violent behavior in children and adults: a review. *J Abnorm Child Psychol* 30: 311–326.

Romano, J, Engel, GL (1944): Delirium: I. Electroencephalographic data. *Arch Neurol Psychiat* 51: 356–377.

Rovner, BW, David, A, Lucas-Blaustein, MJ, Conklin, B, Filipp, L, Tune, L (1988): Self-care capacity and anticholinergic drug levels in nursing home patients. *Am J Psychiatry* 145: 107–109.

Schretlen, DJ, Cascella, NG, Meyer, SM, Kingery, LR, Testa, SM, Munro, CA Pulver, AE, Rivkin, P, Rao, VA, Diaz-Asper, CM, Dickerson, FB, Yolken, RH, Pearlson, GD (2007): Neuropsychological functioning in bipolar disorder and schizophrenia. *Biol Psychiatry* 62: 179–186.

Sciutto, MJ, Eisenberg, M (2007): Evaluating the evidence for and against the overdiagnosis of ADHD. *J Atten Disord* 11: 106–113.

Strakowski, SM, DelBello, MP, Adler, CM (2005): The functional neuroanatomy of bipolar disorder: a review of neuroimaging findings. *Mol Psychiatry* 10: 105–116.

Stuart, S, Noyes, R, Jr. (1999): Attachment and interpersonal communication in somatization. *Psychosomatics* 40: 34–43.

Ustun, TB, Ayuso-Mateos, JL, Chatterji, S, Mathers, C, Murray, CJ (2004): Global burden of depressive disorders in the year 2000. *Br J Psychiatry* 184: 386–392.

Valera, EM, Faraone, SV, Murray, KE, Seidman, LJ (2007): Meta-analysis of structural imaging findings in attention-deficit/hyperactivity disorder. *Biological Psychiatry* 61: 1361–1369.

Weissman, MM, Bland, RC, Canino, GJ, Faravelli, C, Greenwald, S, Hwu, HG, Joyce, PR, Karam, EG, Lee, C-K, Lellouch, J, Lépine, J-P, Newman, SC, Rubio-Stipec, M, Wells, JE, Wickramaratne, PJ, Wittchen, H-U, Yeh, E-K (1996): Cross-national epidemiology of major depression and bipolar disorder. *JAMA* 276: 293–299.

Wells, CE (1979): Pseudodementia. *Am J Psychiatry* 136: 895–900.

Willcutt, EG, Doyle, AE, Nigg, JT, Faraone, SV, Pennington, BF (2005): Validity of the executive function theory of attention-deficit/hyperactivity disorder: a meta-analytic review. *Biol Psychiatry* 57: 1336–1346.

APPENDIX B: The Novice's Guide to Psychiatric Assessment

Beck, JC, White, KA, Gage, B (1991): Emergency psychiatric assessment of violence. *Am J Psychiatry* 148: 1562–1565.

Copello, AG, Templeton, L, Velleman, R (2006): Family interventions for drug and alcohol misuse: is there a best practice? *Curr Opin Psychiatry* 19: 271–276.

Crum, RM, Anthony, JC, Bassett, SS, Folstein, MF (1993): Population-based norms for the Mini-Mental State Examination by age and educational level. *JAMA* 269: 2386–2391.

Follette, W, Cummings, NA (1967): Psychiatric services and medical utilization in a prepaid health plan setting. *Medical Care* 5: 25–35.

Folstein, MF, Folstein, SE, McHugh, PR (1975): "Mini-mental state": a practical method for grading the cognitive state of patients for the clinician. *J Psychiatr Res* 12: 189–198.

Kamphuis, JH, Emmelkamp, PM (2000): Stalking—a contemporary challenge for forensic and clinical psychology. *Br J Psychiatry* 176: 206–209.

Large, MM, Ryan, CJ, Nielssen, OB, Hayes, RA (2008): The danger of dangerousness: why we must remove the dangerousness criterion from our mental health acts. *J Med Ethics* 34: 877–881.

Pompili, M, Innamorati, M, Tatarelli, R (2009): Suicide attempt. *Clinical Neuropsychiatry* 6: 181–187.

Sanderson, K, Andrews, G (2002): Prevalence and severity of mental health-related disability and relationship to diagnosis. *Psychiatr Serv* 53: 80–86.

Simon, RI (2006): Imminent suicide: the illusion of short-term prediction. *Suicide Life Threat Behav* 36: 296–301.

Wei, LA, Fearing, MA, Sternberg, EJ, Inouye, SK (2008): The Confusion Assessment Method: a systematic review of current usage. *J Am Geriatr Soc* 56: 823–830.

Wessely, S, Buchanan, A, Reed, A, Cutting, J, Everitt, B, Garety, P (1993): Acting on delusions. I: Prevalence. *Br J Psychiatry* 163: 69–76.

# Additional Reading

Textbooks on Psychiatry and Psychopathology

Cohen, BJ (2003): *Theory and Practice of Psychiatry.* New York: Oxford University Press.

Fish, FJ (1985): *Fish's Clinical Psychopathology: Signs and Symptoms in Psychiatry.* 2nd ed. Bristol: Wright.

Jaspers, K (1997): *General Psychopathology.* Baltimore: Johns Hopkins University Press.

Kay, J, Tasman, A, Lieberman, JA, eds. (2000): *Psychiatry: Behavioral Science and Clinical Essentials.* Philadelphia: WB Saunders.

Lishman, WA (1998) *Organic Psychiatry: The Psychological Consequences of Cerebral Disorder.* 3rd ed. Wiley-Blackwell.

Sadock, BJ, Sadock, VA (2007): *Kaplan & Sadock's Synopsis of Psychiatry.* 10th ed. Philadelphia: Walter Kluwer / Lippincott Williams & Wilkins.

Sims, AC (1995): *Symptoms in the Mind: An Introduction to Descriptive Psychopathology.* 2nd ed. London: Saunders.

Stoudemire, A, ed. (1998): *Clinical Psychiatry for Medical Students.* 3rd ed. Philadelphia: Lippincott Williams & Wilkins.

General Textbooks on Neurobiology

Kandel, ER, ed. (2000): *Principles of Neural Science.* 4th ed. New York: McGraw-Hill, Health Professions Division.

Shepherd, GM, ed. (2004): *The Synaptic Organization of the Brain.* 5th ed. New York: Oxford University Press.

Squire, LR, ed. (2003): *Fundamental Neuroscience.* 2nd ed. Boston: Academic Press.

Books about Psychiatric Nosology and Pathophysiology

Cooper, JR, Bloom, FE, Roth, RH (2003): *The Biochemical Basis of Neuropharmacology.* 8th ed. New York: Oxford University Press.

Charney, DS, Nestler, EJ, eds. (2005): *Neurobiology of Mental Illness.* 2nd ed. New York: Oxford University Press.

Ghaemi, SN (2007): *The Concepts of Psychiatry: A Pluralistic Approach to the Mind and Mental Illness*. Baltimore: Johns Hopkins University Press.

Hyman, SE, Nestler, EJ (1993): *The Molecular Foundations of Psychiatry*. Washington, DC: American Psychiatric Press.

Pliszka, SR (2004): *Neuroscience for the Mental Health Clinician*. New York: The Guildford Press.

Sadler, JZ, Wiggins, OP, Schwartz, MA (1994): *Philosophical Perspectives on Psychiatric Diagnostic Classification*. Baltimore: Johns Hopkins University Press.

Sadler, JZ, ed. (2002): *Descriptions and Prescriptions: Values, Mental Disorders, and the DSMs*. Baltimore: Johns Hopkins University Press.

## Books on the Nature of Mind

Block, N, Flanagan, O, Guzeldere, G, eds. (1996): *The Nature of Consciousness: Philosophical Debates*. Cambridge: MIT Press.

Chalmers, DJ (1996): *The Conscious Mind: In Search of a Fundamental Theory*. New York: Oxford University Press.

Damasio, AR (1999): *The Feeling of What Happens: Body and Emotion in the Making of Consciousness*. New York: Harcourt Brace.

Dennett, DC (1991): *Consciousness Explained*. Boston: Little, Brown and Co.

Glynn, I (1999): *An Anatomy of Thought: The Origins and Machinery of the Mind*. London: Weidenfeld & Nicolson.

Hundert, EM (1989): *Philosophy, Psychiatry, and Neuroscience: Three Approaches to the Mind*. New York: Oxford University Press.

LeDoux, JE (1996): *The Emotional Brain: The Mysterious Underpinnings of Emotional Life*. New York: Simon & Schuster.

Linden, DJ (2007): *The Accidental Mind*. Cambridge: Belknap Press of Harvard University Press.

Llinas, R (2001): *I of the Vortex: From Neurons to Self*. Cambridge: MIT Press.

Lyons, W, ed. (1995): *Modern Philosophy of Mind*. London: Orion Publishing Group, Ltd.

Searle, JR (1992): *The Rediscovery of the Mind*. Cambridge: MIT Press.

# Index

## About the Author

Dean F. MacKinnon, M.D., is an associate professor of psychiatry at the Johns Hopkins School of Medicine. He studied intellectual history as an undergraduate at the University of Pennsylvania before attending medical school at the University of California, San Diego. After a psychiatric residency at Johns Hopkins and a fellowship in affective disorders and psychiatric genetics, he joined the faculty. In addition to clinical work focused on affective disorders, he has been involved in research on the causes of affective and anxiety disorders and runs the first-year medical student course on brain, mind, and behavior.

# About the Cover

From left to right, top to bottom: (1) Rorschach card no. 1. (2) Diagram of the brain by René Descartes, 1664. (3) Dissection of the brain by Johann Christian Reil, 1812. (4) Nodes of intercortical connectedness across the brain, from Hagmann, P et al., 2008. Mapping the structural core of human cerebral cortex. *PLoS Biology* 6(7): e159. (5) Diagram depicting social transmission of life satisfaction in a large cohort, from Fowler, JH and Christakis, NA, 2008. Dynamic spread of happiness in a large social network. *BMJ* 337: a2338. Used and adapted with permission of the authors. (6) Map of human cortex based on local variation in the structure and arrangement of cortical cells, by Korbinian Brodmann, 1909. (7) Positron Emission Tomography (PET) scan of a person with Alzheimer disease. (8) Neuronal pathways in the cortex, from Gigandet, X et al., 2008. Estimating the confidence level of white matter connections obtained with MRI tractography. *PLoS ONE* 3(12): e4006. (9) Rorschach card no. 8.

## DATE DUE